Tourette's Syndrome
and Tic Disorders

WILEY SERIES IN CHILD AND ADOLESCENT MENTAL HEALTH

Joseph D. Noshpitz, Editor

FATHERLESS CHILDREN

by Paul L. Adams, Judith R. Milner, and Nancy A. Schrepf

DIAGNOSIS AND PSYCHOPHARMACOLOGY OF CHILDHOOD AND ADOLESCENT DISORDERS

by Jerry M. Wiener

INFANT AND CHILDHOOD DEPRESSION: DEVELOPMENTAL FACTORS

by Paul V. Trad

TOURETTE'S SYNDROME AND TIC DISORDERS: CLINICAL UNDERSTANDING AND TREATMENT

by Donald J. Cohen, Ruth D. Bruun, and James F. Leckman

Tourette's Syndrome and Tic Disorders: Clinical Understanding and Treatment

Edited by
Donald J. Cohen
Child Study Center
Yale University School of Medicine

Ruth D. Bruun
Cornell University Medical College

James F. Leckman
Child Study Center
Yale University School of Medicine

WILEY

A Wiley-Interscience Publication
JOHN WILEY & SONS
New York   Chichester   Brisbane   Toronto   Singapore

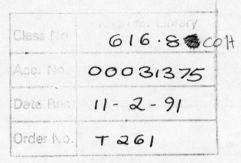
Library of Congress Cataloging-in-Publication Data:

Tourette's syndrome and tic disorders : clinical understanding and
    treatment / edited by Donald J. Cohen, Ruth D. Bruun, James F.
    Leckman.

    p.   cm. — (Wiley series in child and adolescent mental
health)
    "A Wiley-Interscience publication."
    Includes bibliographies and indexes.
    ISBN 0-471-62924-3
    1. Gilles de la Tourette's syndrome. 2. Tic. I. Cohen, Donald
J. II. Bruun, Ruth Dowling. III. Leckman, James F. IV. Series.
    [DNLM: 1. Gilles de la Tourette's Disease. WM 197 T727]

RC375.T68 1988
616.8′3—dc19
DNLM/DLC
for Library of Congress   87-29449
                                                          CIP

Printed in the United States of America

10 9 8 7 6 5 4 3 2 1

Contributors

Nathan H. Azrin, Ph.D., Professor of Psychology, Nova University School of Psychology, Ft. Lauderdale, Florida

Joel D. Bregman, M.D., Instructor, Child Study Center, Yale University School of Medicine, New Haven, Connecticut

Ruth Dowling Bruun, M.D., Clinical Associate Professor of Psychiatry, Cornell University Medical College, New York, New York

Mariann M. Clubb, B.A., Assistant in Research, Child Study Center, Yale University School of Medicine, New Haven, Connecticut

Donald J. Cohen, M.D., Director, Child Study Center, Irving B. Harris Professor of Child Psychiatry, Pediatrics and Psychology, Yale University School of Medicine, New Haven, Connecticut

Brenda G. Comings, M.S.W., L.C.S.W., private practice, Duarte, California

David E. Comings, M.D., Director, Department of Medical Genetics, City of Hope Medical Center, Duarte, California

Gerald Erenberg, M.D., Section of Child Neurology, Director, Learning Disabilities Clinic, Cleveland Clinic Foundation, Cleveland, Ohio

Stanley Fahn, M.D., H. Houston Merritt Professor of Neurology, Director, Movement Disorder Group, Columbia University College of Physicians & Surgeons, and Neurological Institute of New York, New York, New York

Karen Gammon, M.S., R.N., Clinical Research Nurse, Department of Neurology, Johns Hopkins Hospital, The Johns Hopkins University School of Medicine, Baltimore, Maryland

Gerald S. Golden, M.D., Shainberg Professor of Pediatrics, Professor and Acting Chairman of Neurology, Director, Child Development Center, University of Tennessee, Memphis, Tennessee

Rosa A. Hagin, Ph.D., Professor, Division of Psychological and Educational Services, Fordham University, and Director, School Consultation Center, Fordham University, New York, New York

Maureen T. Hardin, M.S.N., Associate Research Scientist, Child Study Center, and Lecturer, School of Nursing, Yale University School of Medicine, New Haven, Connecticut

John E. Kugler, M.S., Graduate Assistant, Doctoral Program in School Psychology, Fordham University, New York, New York

James F. Leckman, M.D., Neisen Harris Associate Professor of Child Psychiatry and Pediatrics, Child Study Center, Yale University School of Medicine, New Haven, Connecticut

Abbey S. Meyers, Executive Director, National Organization for Rare Disorders, Commissioner, National Commission on Orphan Diseases, New Fairfield, Connecticut

Harvey Moldofsky, M.D., Professor of Psychiatry and Medicine, University of Toronto, and Psychiatrist-in-Chief, Toronto Western Hospital, Toronto, Ontario, Canada

Sharon I. Ort, R.N., M.P.H., Associate Research Scientist, Child Study Center, Yale University School of Medicine, New Haven, Connecticut

David L. Pauls, Ph.D., Assistant Professor, Human Genetics, Child Study Center and Human Genetics, Yale University School of Medicine, New Haven, Connecticut

Alan L. Peterson, M.S., Ph.D., Candidate in Clinical Psychology, Nova University School of Psychology, Ft. Lauderdale, Florida

Mark A. Riddle, M.D., Assistant Professor of Psychiatry and Pediatrics, Child Study Center, Yale University School of Medicine, and Associate Medical Director, Child Psychiatry Inpatient Service, Yale-New Haven Hospital, New Haven, Connecticut

Paul Sandor, M.D., Assistant Professor of Psychiatry, University of Toronto, and Head, Psychobiological Medicine Unit, Toronto Western Hospital, Toronto, Ontario, Canada

Arthur K. Shapiro, M.D., Director of the Tourette and Tic Laboratory and Clinic, New York, New York

Elaine Shapiro, Ph.D., Co-Director of the Tourette and Tic Laboratory and Clinic, New York, New York

Archie A. Silver, M.D., Professor of Psychiatry, Director, Child and Adolescent Psychiatry, University of South Florida Medical School, Tampa, Florida

Harvey S. Singer, M.D., Associate Professor, Departments of Neurology and Pediatrics, The Johns Hopkins University School of Medicine, Baltimore, Maryland

Kenneth E. Towbin, M.D., Assistant Clinical Professor of Pediatrics and Psychiatry, Child Study Center, Yale University School of Medicine, New Haven, Connecticut, Medical Director, Riverview Hospital, Middletown, Connecticut

Richard Trifiletti, M.D., Visiting Clinical Fellow in Pediatrics, Columbia Presbyterian Hospital, New York, New York

Fred R. Volkmar, M.D., Harris Assistant Professor of Psychiatry, Pediatrics, and Psychology, Child Study Center, Yale University School of Medicine, New Haven, Connecticut

John T. Walkup, M.D., Postdoctoral Fellow in Child Psychiatry, Child Study Center, Yale University School of Medicine, New Haven, Connecticut

Emanuel C. Wolff, M.D., Associate Clinical Professor of Psychiatry, Child Study Center, Yale University School of Medicine, New Haven, Connecticut

Gwendolyn E.P. Zahner, Ph.D., Associate Research Scientist, Child Study Center, Yale University School of Medicine, New Haven, Connecticut

Series Preface

This series is intended to serve a number of functions. It includes works on child development; it presents material on child advocacy; it publishes contributions to child psychiatry; and it gives expression to cogent views on child rearing and child management. The mental health of parents and their interaction with their children is a major theme of the series, and emphasis is placed on the child as individual, as family member, and as a part of the larger social surround.

Child development is regarded as the basic science of child mental health, and within that framework research works are included in this series. The many ethical and legal dimensions of the way society relates to its children is the central theme of the child advocacy publications, as well as a primarily demographic approach that highlights the role and status of children within society. The child psychiatry publications span studies that concern the diagnosis, description, therapeutics, rehabilitation, and prevention of the emotional disorders of childhood. And the views of thoughtful and creative contributors to the handling of children under many different circumstances (retardation, acute and chronic illness, hospitalization, handicap, disturbed social conditions, etc.) find expression within the framework of child rearing and child management.

Family studies with a central child mental health perspective are included in the series, and explorations into the nature of parenthood and the parenting process are emphasized. This includes books about divorce, the single parent, the absent parent, parents with physical and emotional illnesses, and other conditions that significantly affect the parent-child relationship.

Finally, the series examines the impact of larger social forces, such as war, famine, migration, and economic failure, on the adaptation of children and families. In the largest sense, the series is devoted to books that illuminate the special needs, status, and history of children and their families within all perspectives that bear on their collective mental health.

Joseph D. Noshpitz

Children's Hospital Medical Center, and
The George Washington University
Washington, D.C.

Preface

The centennial of Georges Gilles de la Tourette's classic paper describing the syndrome of multiple motor and phonic tics associated with strange behavioral symptoms was celebrated in 1985. This paper stemmed from work done at Charcot's clinical laboratory at the Salpetriere Hospital, one of the most fertile settings for work in neurology and psychiatry in the history of medicine. Few original descriptions have so well weathered the decades.

The clinical picture of a school-age boy blinking, making faces, sticking out his tongue, thrusting his arms, jerking his legs, coughing, hawking, spitting, shouting various phrases, and moving without stopping has now been seen wherever physicians have looked for it, in every culture and social class. While other disorders have come and gone, including the grand hysterias with which it was originally contrasted, Tourette's Syndrome (TS) has retained its stability as a clinical condition with clearly definable characteristics. The major clinical manifestations continue to be the multiform and polymorphous symptomatology, affecting all muscle groups and many forms of speech, with one symptom dropping off and another taking its place; waxing and waning over hours, weeks, and months; the capacity for the patient to suppress symptoms for shorter or longer periods of time; and the not-infrequent remission or marked improvement during adolescence.

Some observations from the first years of the study of TS have only recently reemerged as accurate, such as the familial clustering and probable genetic transmission of the condition, as well as its etiological relationship to some forms of obsessive-compulsive disorder. Other thoughts about the disorder that attracted attention over the years are now known to be incorrect, such as the theory that TS might lead to dementia or that its roots could be found in psychodynamics of aggression or etiologically explained within the context of psychoanalytic theory of neurosis or character.

During the century of its treatment and study, virtually every form of environmental and biological approach has been used, and success has been claimed for many. Complications in the assessment of the efficacy of the different drugs and procedures have arisen from various sources, including the patient's desire to be well; the family's wish to minimize or exaggerate symptoms; the waxing and waning course; the responsivity of symptoms to environmental context; and, at times, specific and nonspecific benefits of treatments. The therapeutic situation was dramatically altered in the 1960s with the advent of neuroleptic medications, which have profound and prolonged impact on the symptoms of TS. The broad acceptance of haloperidol quickly led clinicians to define appropriate dosage levels, areas of symptomatic improvement, and the nature of side effects. While increased experience has shown that haloperidol is not the "magic bullet" that is hoped for and that its use can be associated with serious unwanted physical effects, its value in suppressing the symptoms of TS is universally recognized. However, recent reports of treatment-emergent dyskinesias following long-term treatment with haloperidol and other neuroleptics in TS patients compellingly underline the need for safer agents to be developed.

With the introduction of effective pharmacological treatment a new phase of clinical understanding and research concerning TS was initiated. This phase has been characterized by the utilization of various methods of biomedical research to study possible alterations in central nervous system metabolism, particularly dopaminergic functioning, and clinical trials with various agents that affect brain function. The agents that have been used derive almost exclusively from the broader field of psychiatry and medicine, rather than from original research relating to TS, but the results have led to an expanded clinical armamentarium.

During the last decade, there has been a marked increase in the recognition of the prevalence of TS. It was once thought to be a rare disorder, one a clinician might see once in a lifetime of practice and talk about for years afterward; we now know that TS may affect up to 1 person in every 2500 in its full-blown form and perhaps a single person in several hundred in its milder variants. Newer research has helped elucidate the spectrum of conditions related to TS—such as chronic multiple tics and obsessive–compulsive disorder—and has expanded the number of individuals who might benefit from clinical care and research concerning TS. The increased recognition of patients with TS is a result of several factors. One major force has been the availability of effective treatment, which, of course, has encouraged physicians and others to make the diagnosis. Another factor, which is in a sense almost uniquely American, has been the extraordinary achievements of the national Tourette Syndrome Association (TSA). The TSA started as a parent self-help group and has developed into the leading advocate for research, public and professional education, and services for individuals with TS. One example of the achievements of TSA was the organization of a clinical symposium on TS, which was an important stimulus for this volume.

A third factor that has increased the recognition of TS and has done a good deal to "demystify" it and remove it from the "exotic disorders" found at the end of textbook chapters has been the serious commitment of clinical researchers to understanding TS and associated conditions. This research commitment stems from concern about the care and management of patients with TS, on one hand, and the belief that TS is a model neuropsychiatric condition that can help reveal information of broad applicability to other conditions. Thus clinical research on TS has moved ahead the frontier of understanding of the mode of genetic transmission of a complex disorder, modes of studying CNS metabolism, and new approaches to drug treatment and evaluation.

The emphasis on biological factors in the pathogenesis of TS may have obscured, at some points, the awareness that individuals with TS are whole people who must deal with the serious and persistent problems of their disorder and its treatment. Also, the search for the biological base and cure of TS may have led clinicians away from thinking about phenomena that were of great interest at other phases of the history of TS: that TS affects individuals at the core of their experience of themselves as being in control of their own movements, statements, and thoughts. Since living a life is in very large part attempting to try to understand what one is doing, it is easy to see the enormity of the developmental tasks of children and adults with TS. At this point in the history of our knowledge about TS, one of the responsibilities of clinicians is to balance the expanding knowledge about neurobiological and genetic factors with an appreciation of all the other factors that help a

patient move along as normally as possible with psychological development and social adjustment. Indeed, some evidence suggests that just
such factors may mediate the expression and severity of the disorder.

In providing clinical care to TS patients, many areas of a patient's life
need to be considered: the functioning of the family, and how parents
and siblings are responding to the disorder and trying, or finding it
impossible, to be supportive; the provisions of the school, especially for
children with learning and attentional problems and symptoms that are
disruptive; the acceptance into a peer group; the choice of a career
and the acceptance into the world of work; the pleasures of intimacy,
formation of a marital bond, and concerns about family planning; and
barriers experienced by all individuals with a medical problem or handicap that requires legal action and advocacy. Among these areas are the
individual's most intimate, personal experience, his or her inner world
and mode of personal adaptation.

During the last several years, clinicians have become familiar with
many hundreds of TS patients, and have been able to follow them over
the course of decades and in relation to various treatments. It is now
clear that the majority of TS patients suffer from mild difficulties for
which no specific treatment, or perhaps only reassurance and guidance,
are needed. The most severely afflicted patients are a minority. Even
for these, entry into the mainstream of life is almost always possible.
We know very little about what makes the difference between a milder
expression of TS and a serious, fully disabling form of the disorder.
What we do know, however, suggests that there is a great deal of importance in early diagnosis and careful, considerate (and, we might say,
rather conservative) medical and therapeutic management. Parents
need a physician who understands the disorder and can help them
through periods of exacerbation and crisis. Medication must be used
judiciously and with serious concern about side effects, and only when
symptoms interfere with development. Educational and social planning
may be central. What is critical to later adaptation is the child's sense
of himself or herself as competent and loved. This mandates the avoidance by family and physicians of any interventions that may make a
person with tics feel that he or she is a "chronic problem patient." This
is not always an easy prescription to follow.

This volume provides an orientation to the care of individuals with
TS. Early chapters describe the classification, natural history, and major
clinical characteristics of the disorder. Parts 3 and 4 provide a detailed
discussion of different approaches to intervention and different areas
of functioning that require consideration. The individuality of the TS
patient—that is, what sort of a person he or she is, and not simply the
fact of the TS symptoms—is emphasized as important to planning any

treatment. This biopsychological approach to the management of the individual with TS is summarized in the final chapter.

This volume also offers material about areas that require further investigation and remain controversial. One such example is the relation between the use of stimulant medication and the precipitation or worsening of tic disorders. Where there are differences of opinion, we have tried to reflect these in the chapters; at points, chapters appear to overlap because of our desire to provide as much balance as possible where there are differences among clinical investigators with deep and serious engagement with TS.

We have learned a great deal during the past years that has been translated into treatment and guidance of individual patients. It is to be anticipated, at this point, that the pace of knowledge will increase during the next several years. We now expect that there will be fundamental new knowledge about etiology, perhaps including the identification of the gene and the pathogenetic line leading from DNA to its expression as a clinical syndrome. Along with this, we should have a better understanding of the nongenetic environmental and psychological factors that mediate the expression of the genetic vulnerability. This knowledge should lead to more specific medications and clinical interventions, some of which may be preventative in nature.

The prospects for individuals with TS thus seem brighter now than at any time during the past century. We can be hopeful that within several years a discussion of the clinical care of individuals with TS will be much shorter and, at the same time, will more profoundly demonstrate the intrinsic links between biology, clinical disorder, and the care of patients.

In conclusion, we would like to acknowledge the contributions of Ms. Sue Lynn Levi and the other leaders and members of the Tourette Syndrome Association, as well as the many years of support for clinical and basic research on TS provided by Mr. H. B. Pearl and the Gateposts Foundation.

Donald J. Cohen
Ruth D. Bruun
James F. Leckman

New Haven, Connecticut
New York, New York
New Haven, Connecticut
March 1988

Contents

Part I

Diagnosis, Natural History, Assessment and Etiology

CHAPTER ONE

Descriptive and Diagnostic Classification of Tic Disorders

James F. Leckman
Donald J. Cohen

OVERVIEW

Public awareness of and scientific interest in tic disorders have increased dramatically over the past decade. Once considered rare disorders of passing medical interest, tic disorders now are the focus of intense research efforts that show promise of identifying specific genetic and nongenetic factors that are involved in their transmission and expression (Leckman Riddle, & Cohen, Chapter 7, this volume). As our knowledge has grown, so has the awareness that the general class of tic disorders encompasses a much broader range of phenotypic expression. Although the cardinal features of these disorders remain the repetitive motor and/or phonic tics, other behavioral symptoms and mental states frequently co-occur with tics and may be etiologically related. These associated symptoms include premonitory sensory urges, stimulus-bound behaviors, obsessive thoughts, compulsive behaviors, mood lability, irritability, and behavioral disinhibition. Attentional problems, impulsivity, motoric hyperactivity, and specific learning problems also frequently are associated with tic disorders, particularly among children referred for clinical evaluation.

Although the etiologic role of genetic and nongenetic factors in the expression of tic disorders is an area of active investigation (Pauls & Leckman, Chapter 6, this volume), no specific pathogenic factors have yet been identified, and no sensitive and specific diagnostic tests are available. Consequently, the diagnostic classification of tic disorders in the *Diagnostic and Statistical Manual of Mental Disorders* (APA, 1980, 1986) is conventional and based solely on observable signs and symptoms and duration.

DEFINITION

Tics *per se* are sudden, repetitive, stereotyped motor movements or phonic productions. They can be characterized by their anatomical location, number, frequency, duration, intensity, and complexity (Leckman, Towbin, Ort & Cohen, Chapter 4, this volume). They are often more easily recognized than precisely defined. The tics usually are perceived as involuntary but may be accompanied by premonitory sensory "urges." In such instances, patients may experience a tic as a partially "voluntary" act performed to relieve an urge. Tics typically can be suppressed actively for brief periods of time (seconds to minutes). Tics typically occur in bouts and their intensity often is quite variable within a 24-hour period. They tend to be more pronounced during periods of stress or fatigue and are less severe when an individual is asleep, absorbed in an activity, or placed in a novel or highly structured situation.

Tics may also be triggered by environmental stimuli, such as watching television or hearing someone cough. Over longer intervals of time, tics wax and wane in severity. Specific tics presenting in a particular anatomical location at a particular time may alter in intensity and complexity or totally disappear so that over weeks to months a changing and bewildering array of tics can be seen in an individual patient.

Motor Tics

Motor tics usually begin with brief bouts of transient tics involving the face or head. A typical report involves bouts of eye blinking of variable intensity beginning in kindergarten or in the early school years. These symptoms often disappear after a few weeks only to reappear at a later point in time (see Fig. 1.1). Some authors report a rostral–caudal progression of motor tics, with tics of the face, head, and shoulders appearing earlier and in a higher proportion of patients than motor tics involving the extremities or the torso (Jagger et al., 1982). The observed range of motor tics is extraordinary, so that virtually any voluntary motor movement can emerge as a motor tic. Exhibit 1.1 presents a brief compendium of some of the more common motor tics.

Motor tics may be described as simple or complex. *Simple motor tics* are sudden, brief (usually less than 1 second in duration), meaningless movements. Common examples include eye blinking, facial grimacing, mouth movements, head jerks, shoulder shrugs, and arm and leg jerks. Younger patients often are totally unaware of the simple motor tics.

Exhibit 1.1.   *MOTOR TICS*

Simple Motor Tics: Sudden, Brief,
Meaningless Movements

Examples: eye blinking, eye movements, grimacing, nose twitching, mouth movements, lip pouting, head jerks, shoulder shrugs, arm jerks, abdominal tensing, kicks, finger movements, jaw snaps, tooth clicking, rapid jerking of any part of the body

Complex Motor Tics: Slower, Longer,
More "Purposeful" Movements

Examples: sustained "looks," facial gestures, biting, touching objects or self, throwing, banging, thrusting arms, gestures with hands, gyrating and bending, dystonic postures, copropraxia (obscene gestures)

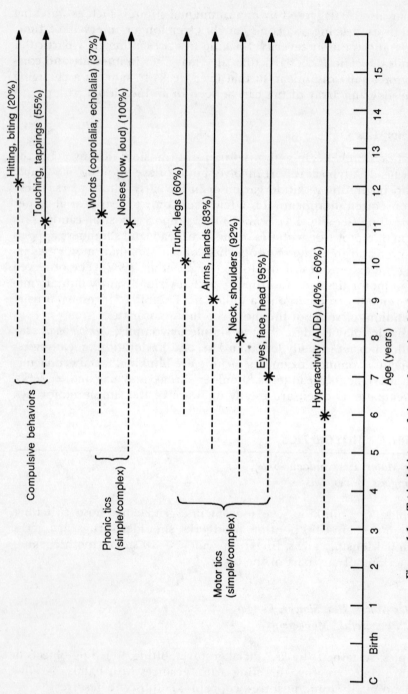

Figure 1.1. *Typical history of tics and associated behaviors progressing at different ages from transient episodes (broken lines) to sustained periods (solid lines). (Adapted from Jagger et al., 1982.)*

Over time, many patients develop *complex motor tics,* which are sudden, more purposive appearing, stereotyped movements of longer duration. Examples are myriad and include facial gestures and movements such as brushing hair back, possibly in combination with head jerk, and body shrugs. Gyrating, bending, and more dystonic appearing movements of the torso are also seen. These complex motor tics rarely are seen in the absence of simple motor tics. Paroxysms, or continuous orchestrated displays of simple and complex motor tics, can occur in more severe cases. Lewd and obscene gestures with hands or tongue (copropraxia) and self-abusive acts (hitting the face, biting a hand or wrist) are observed in a small number of patients. At times, it may be difficult to distinguish complex tics from compulsions. It is also important to differentiate simple and complex tics from motor dyskinesias and hyperkinetic movement disorders (Fahn & Erenberg, Chapter 3, this volume).

The degree of impairment and disruption associated with particular motor tics is variable and a salient clinical feature. Partly dependent on frequency, intensity, complexity, and duration of specific tics, estimates of impairment also need to include the impact on the individual's self-esteem, family life, social acceptance, school or job functioning, and physical well-being. For example, a very frequent simple motor wrist tic may be less impairing than an infrequently occurring, forceful copropraxic gesture. Patients are often aware of their complex motor tics and their impact on other people, setting the stage for detrimental intrapsychic consequences. The mental elaborations associated with the behaviors may also have a detrimental effect on self-esteem and limit socialization. Physical injuries, including blindness from retinal detachment, also can occur in a small minority of adolescent and adult cases secondary to severe self-abusive tics.

The natural history of tics is variable, but these tics usually diminish in frequency and intensity in adulthood (Bruun, Chapter 2, this volume). Noticeable but not impairing tics often persist into adulthood. In some adult patients, the tic repertoire becomes more stable with fewer tics being present and the fluctuations in frequency and intensity less marked (Bruun, Chapter 2, this volume).

Phonic Tics

Phonic or vocal tics usually appear after the onset of motor tics (8 to 15 years of age). Less than 5 percent of patients have isolated phonic tics in the absence of motor symptoms. Phonic tics often show a similar progression from transient episodes to more sustained periods of phonic symptoms (see Fig. 1.1). Again, the range of possible phonic or vocal symptoms is extraordinary with any noise or sound having the potential to be enlisted as a tic (see Exhibit 1.2). As with motor tics,

Exhibit 1.2. PHONIC TICS

Simple Phonic Symptoms: Sudden, Meaningless
Sounds or Noises

Examples: throat clearing, coughing, sniffling, spitting, screeching, barking, grunting, gurgling, clacking, hissing, sucking, and innumerable other sounds

Complex Phonic Symptoms: Sudden,
More "Meaningful" Utterances

Examples: syllables, words, phrases, statements such as "shut up," "stop that," "oh, okay," "I've got to," "okay honey," "what makes me do this?," "how about it," or "now you've seen it," speech atypicalities (unusual rhythms, tone, accents, intensity of speech); echo phenomenon (immediate repetition of one's own or another's words or phrases); and coprolalia (obscene, inappropriate, and aggressive words and statements)

---

phonic symptoms are characterized by their number, frequency, duration, intensity (volume), and complexity (noises vs. syllables or words). Associated sensory "urges" (sometimes localized to the throat) similar to the premonitory sensory phenomena associated with motor tics are commonplace, as are reports of the tics being triggered by specific and/or nonspecific environmental stimuli.

Simple phonic tics are fast, meaningless sounds or noises that can be characterized by their frequency, duration, volume intensity, and potential for disrupting speech. Sniffing, throat clearing, grunting, barks, and high-pitched squeaks are common simple phonic symptoms. *Complex phonic tics* are quite diverse and can include syllables, words or phrases, as well as odd patterns of speech in which there are sudden changes in the rate, volume, and/or rhythm. Immediate echo phenomena such as repeating words and phrases are common in some patients (echolalia and palilalia). In a minority of patients coprolalia is present in which obscene or socially inappropriate syllables, words, or phrases are expressed, at times in a loud explosive manner. Complex phonic tics are rarely if ever present in the absence of simple phonic tics and motor tics of one sort or another. Provocative and insulting phonic symptoms have a high potential for stigmatizing the patient and his or her family and can indirectly lead to physical injury.

The natural history of phonic symptoms is variable, with most patients showing a clear decrease in the frequency and intensity of the symptoms in adulthood (Bruun, Chapter 2, this volume). However, stable patterns of vocal tics may continue, and in a few unfortunate adult patients, disabling, explosive coprolalia can be persistent.

Tic-Related Mental States

Many patients with tic disorders report a variety of mental states associated with their tics. Eloquent descriptions of these phenomena have appeared in first-person and biographical accounts of celebrated ticquers (Lees, 1985). These phenomena are more frequently reported by adults and include premonitory sensory urges that are reported to prompt the tics, complex states of inner conflict over if and when to yield to these urges, and a sensation of relief that frequently accompanies the performance of a tic. Those patients with stimulus-bound tics may also report the distress and frustration over the unwitting acts of others that may provoke their tic symptoms; for example a person's cough or gesture may set off a bout of tics in response. Complex permutations of these mental events are also frequently encountered. They include needing to perform the tic a certain number of times or in a particular way to satisfy the internal urge. Other patients report the emergence of urges to perform more complex acts that are dangerous, forbidden, or simply senseless and bizarre such as touching a hot iron or putting the car in reverse gear while driving down a highway or touching the breast of an unknown woman in an adjacent seat or shouting out in a quiet church service. This lowering of the stimulus barrier has led Cohen (1980) to view severe tic disorder as a model neuropsychiatric disorder that exists at the interface of mind and body. One severely affected individual recently described this by saying, "My mind and body are constantly going at it. Both are incredibly strong, like two bulls with locked horns, and if one side gets the upper hand, I tic. If the other side gets the upper hand, I go crazy with these thoughts and urges."

Associated Behavioral Traits

Motor and phonic tics often do not appear in isolation from other behavioral problems. In some instances these behavioral problems may overshadow the tic disorder altogether. Exhibit 1.3 presents a list of some of the behavioral syndromes frequently seen in tic disorder patients. As noted earlier and elsewhere in this volume, the relationships between tic disorders and these behavioral traits are controversial. While some may be etiologically related, such as obsessive–compulsive

Exhibit 1.3. **ASSOCIATED BEHAVIORAL TRAITS**

Developmentally inappropriate inattention and impulsivity, disinhibition of thoughts and actions

Motoric hyperactivity and restlessness

Learning disabilities

Emotional lability, increased irritability, maniclike behavior

Obsessive–compulsive behaviors

Heightened anxiety, phobias, separation anxiety

Depressive reactions

disorder, others may be comorbid conditions that interact with the pathobiology of the tic syndrome to complicate its course and presentation.

Viewed from the perspective of the natural history of tic disorders, developmentally inappropriate levels of motoric hyperactivity, impulsivity, and inattention frequently precede the onset of motor and phonic tics. In clinic populations, nearly 50 percent of all patients with tic disorders have symptoms of *attention deficit disorder* (ADD). Some authors view the ADD as component of tic disorders (Comings & Comings, Chapter 8, this volume). Others, relying on epidemiologic and family interview data, have come to view the ADD as a comorbid condition that complicates the course and management of the tic disorder (Pauls, Hurst et al., 1986). Such problems may be significantly more prevalent in clinic populations. Other behavioral problems that may appear early in the course of a tic disorder include *specific developmental disorders* (learning disabilities) that can cover the entire gamut of math, language, and reading problems. These difficulties, with the possible exception of math problems, are likely to be comorbid conditions, etiologically unrelated to tic disorders but capable of influencing the course of illness (Hagin, Chapter 15, this volume).

Mood lability and periods of behavior disinhibition are reported to occur more frequently in patients with a tic disorder (Riddle, Hardin, Ort, Leckman, & Cohen, Chapter 10, this volume). Rarely, manic like symptoms have been observed in adolescent and adult patients.

Later in the natural history of tic disorders, 10 to 40 percent of patients report *obsessional thoughts* and exhibit *compulsive behaviors* and rituals (Towbin, Chapter 9, this volume). In a few cases, the tic symptoms appear to be replaced largely by the obsessive–compulsive behaviors that can be extremely severe and disabling. Clinical attention has focused on the degree of senselessness and ego dystonia associated with these symptoms. Many tic disorder patients report an internal need to perform complex acts in a stereotyped manner (tying shoes, symmetrical touching, etc.) but deny that the act is troublesome to them. They also frequently are unaware of any internal resistance to the performance of the ritual acts. Arthur Shapiro and others have proposed the term *impulsions* to distinguish these acts from true compulsions. On the other hand, a sizable proportion of tic disorder patients have classical obsessive-compulsive disorder (OCD) as reviewed by Towbin (Chapter 9, this volume). Recent family interview data support the remarkable hypothesis that tic disorders and some forms of OCD are linked etiologically (Pauls & Leckman, 1986).

Other behavioral traits seen in association with severe tic disorders include anxiety states and depressive reactions that may be secondary to the tic symptoms. Still other traits seen in combination with tic disorders may constitute chance associations in unfortunate individuals, such as autism or mental retardation. The hypothesis that etiological factors underlying such pervasive developmental disorders may contribute to the vulnerability to express a tic disorder, however, cannot be discounted.

ETIOLOGY

Ideally, the classification of tic disorders will eventually be based on precise knowledge of the pathobiology of these disorders (Leckman, Riddle, Cohen, Chapter 7, this volume). Although the results of recent family genetic studies are suggestive that a single major autosomal gene is involved in the transmission of some tic disorders (Pauls & Leckman, 1986), no biological markers of this vulnerability have been conclusively identified. Should this promise be fulfilled and the putative gene located on a chromosome, closely flanking genetic markers could be employed in at-risk families to identify vulnerable individuals.

In the absence of precise knowledge of etiology, well-documented pathophysiological mechanisms potentially could serve as a rational basis for diagnostic classification and treatment intervention. Although a number of central neurochemical systems have been implicated in tic disorders, including cholinergic, serotonergic, noradrenergic, GABAergic, endogenous opioid, and gender-specific neuroendocrine systems, the strongest evidence supports the role of midbrain dopaminergic systems acting in concert with compensatory and modulating neurotransmitter systems (Leckman & Riddle, Cohen, Chapter 7, this volume). Despite the disappointing results of early studies, neuroimaging techniques also show promise of providing relevant and neuroanatomically precise information that may clarify the role of these systems in the pathophysiology of tic disorders and establish accurate techniques to monitor the course of these disorders.

CLINICAL EVALUATION

Exhibit 1.4 presents a schematic outline of clinically relevant areas that should be explored in patients presenting with a tic disorder. The anatomical location, number, frequency, intensity, complexity, and degree of disruption associated with the motor and phonic tics should be documented. Other characteristics, including the onset and course of the tic disorder, should also be recorded. In particular, it is worthwhile to explore with the patient associated mental phenomena that, at times, may precede or co-occur with the tics. It is also important to assess the role of external stimuli in triggering tic symptoms. Taken together, these data provide the basis for determining the degree of impairment associated with the motor and phonic tic phenomena. Other pertinent information includes the long-term effect of the tic disorder on the individual's self-esteem and the impact on his or her family life and social contacts. It also is important to assess the direct impact of the tics on the patient's current educational or work placement. Finally, one must assess the potential risk of physical injury secondary to the tics.

Instruments that enable across-patient comparison of tic behaviors are reviewed in detail in a subsequent chapter (Leckman, Towbin, Ort, & Cohen, Chapter 4, this volume). These include the Tourette Syndrome Symptom List (Cohen Shaywitz, Leckman, 1984), which is a parent- or self-rated instrument, and the Tourette Syndrome Global Scale (Harcherick, Leckman, Detlor, & Cohen, 1984), which is completed by experienced clinicians. Another clinical instrument is the Shapiro Tic Severity Scale developed by Shapiro and Shapiro (unpublished data), for use in a clinical drug trial. Although videotape ratings can be very precise, the waxing and waning of the symptoms and their variation, even over the course of a day, require that the period of assessment span an interval of at least a week.

In order to assess an individual adequately, it also is important to understand the context in which the tics are occurring. This involves a careful look at the current living circumstances of the individuals, their circumstances in school or work placement, and their relationships with peers. It is imperative to have some idea of how the patients views their symptoms and to assess the intrapsychic sequelae of the symptoms. The "choice" of some complex tics may have psychodynamic meaning that is clinically important to understand. In the case of young children, it is essential to have a good sense of their cognitive level of functioning

Exhibit 1.4.   CLINICAL EVALUATION OF TIC DISORDERS

Tics: Anatomic location, number, frequency, intensity, complexity, degree of interference

Onset: Age, character (sudden, gradual, associated with stress)

Course: Waxing and waning, suppressibility, duration, factors associated with worsening or improvement

Associated Mental Phenomena: Sensory urges, mental tics

Impairment: Impact on self-esteem, social adaptation, educational or job performance, risk of physical injury

Obsessive–Compulsive Symptoms and Behaviors: Obsessive worries and thoughts, simple rituals ("evening-up," ordering behaviors), full-fledged obsessive–compulsive disorder

Other Behavioral or Emotional Problems: Attentional problems, mood lability and increased irritability, major depression, and anxiety disorders

Relationship with Family and Peers: Premorbid history, period from onset to diagnosis, current social adjustment, marital status

Life Events: Relationship of life events to onset and exacerbations of tics, stability of family life, coping skills and social supports

Behavioral History of Extended Family: Tics, attentional problems, hyperactivity, learning problems, obsessive–compulsive behaviors

Past Medical and Developmental History: Prenatal events, birth history, developmental delays, medication exposures, injuries, asthma, migraine, other disorders of arousal, and allergies

Physical and Neurological Examination: "Soft," nonlocalizing neurological signs, minor EEG abnormalities, CAT scan usually negative

Medication Status: Response to medications, adequacy of trials

School Status: Cognitive level, specific learning problems, adequacy of placement

Employment Status: Job difficulties associated with tic behaviors or related phenomena. Adequacy of placement given patient's native abilities and whether or not there are any other problems that may impair their performance in school. This could include attention deficit disorder or specific learning problems. In assessing children's school placement, it also is important to establish how well tic disorders are understood by the teachers and administrative personnel of the school.

Maintaining close involvement with teachers and other school personnel in evaluating and treating a child with a tic disorder can be critically important. If these individuals can be helped to understand that the tics are a result of a neurologic condition and are performed involuntarily, often significant shifts in attitude can be observed and can have a markedly beneficial effect on the child's attitude and adjustment.

The presence and extent of obsessive–compulsive symptoms also needs to be assessed in patients presenting with a tic disorder. Although only a minority of patients present with full-fledged and impairing obsessive–compulsive disorder, a large number of tic disorder patients have obsessive worries and compulsive behaviors. Towbin's Chapter in this volume (Chapter 9) explores this area in more detail and reviews relevant epidemiologic data concerning the association of obsessive–compulsive symptoms and tic disorders.

Some clinicians have found an increased frequency of irritability and mood lability in patients with a tic disorder (Riddle, Hardin, Ort, Leckman, & Cohen, Chapter 10, this volume). Anxiety disorders other than obsessive–compulsive disorder also may occur more frequently in tic disorder patients. Other emotional difficulties frequently encountered in this population include major depression that may occur in a reaction to the inability to control the body, as well as other adverse physical and psychological consequences that sometimes attend a severe tic disorder.

As with other neuropsychiatric disorders, it is important to document the past medical and developmental history. One should pay particular attention to potential neurological insults such as adverse perinatal events, serious head injuries, and exposure to CNS medications.

A thorough physical and neurological examination should be performed on all patients presenting with a tic disorder. Nonlocalizing neurologic signs have been reported in a significant minority of tic disorder patients, as have minor EEG abnormalities, such as increased slow wave and posterior spikes (Shapiro, Shapiro, Bruun, & Sweet, 1978; Volkmar et al., 1984). Although the EEG has continued to remain a part of the baseline evaluation of tic disorder patients, we and others have found that the CAT scan usually has not revealed significant information in the absence of any specific neurologic signs. The usefulness of other imaging techniques has not been fully evaluated.

The final chapter of this volume (Towbin, Leckman, Riddle, Bruun, & Cohen) offers additional information on the clinical assessment of individuals with tic disorders.

DIAGNOSTIC CLASSIFICATION

Ideally, diagnostic classifications are based on a thoroughgoing knowledge of specific etiological or pathophysiologic mechanisms. In the absence of such knowledge, conventional and to some extent arbitrary diagnostic categories of the tic disorders have developed. Both DSM-III and DSM-IIIR focus exclusively on the presence or absence of motor and phonic tics, the age of onset of the tic behaviors, and their duration (APA, 1980, 1987). Whether these clinically observable traits are the most salient vis-à-vis the range of symptoms associated with the underlying etiological factors is unclear and the object of ongoing empirical research.

Tourette's Syndrome

The most severe form of tic disorder is a persistent motor and phonic tic disorder best known by the eponym Gilles de la Tourette's syndrome (TS). The DSM-IIIR criteria are presented in Exhibit 1.5 and are contrasted schematically with criteria DSM-III in Table 1.1.

TS is an uncommon disorder that can be chronic and disabling. Many of the most dramatic tic symptoms, such as coprolalia and copropraxia and the paroxysms of self-abusive and injurious tics described earlier, are seen almost exclusively in TS patients. Similarly, the complex array

Table 1.1. Comparison of DSM-III and DSM-IIIR Diagnostic Categories

	Tics			
	Motor	Phonic	Onset	Duration
DSM-III				
Tourette's Syndrome	X and	X	2 to 15 years	> 1 year
Chronic motor tic disorder	X	—	?	≥ 1 year
Transient tic disorder	X	—	"childhood"	≥ 1 month,< 1 year
Atypical tic disorder	?	?	?	?
DSM-IIIR				
Tourette's Syndrome	X and	X	< 21 years	> 1 year
Chronic motor or vocal tic disorder	X or	X	< 21 years	> 1 year
Transient tic disorder	X or	X	< 21 years	≥ 2 weeks, < 1 year
Tic disorder not otherwise specified	?	?	?	?

X = Symptom required for diagnosis

Exhibit 1.5.   DSM-IIIR: TIC DISORDERS

___

Diagnostic Criteria for Tourette's Disorder (307.23)

1. Both multiple motor and one or more vocal tics have been present at some time during the illness, although not necessarily concurrently.
2. The tics occur many times a day (usually in bouts), nearly every day or intermittently throughout a period of more than a year.
3. The anatomic location, number, frequency, complexity, and severity of the tics change over time.
4. Onset before age 21.
5. Occurrence not exclusively during psychoactive substance intoxication or known central nervous system disease, such as Huntington's chorea and post–viral encephalitis.

Diagnostic Criteria for Chronic Motor or Vocal Tic Disorder (307.22)

1. Either motor or vocal tics, but not both, have been present at some time during the illness.
2. The tics occur many times a day, nearly every day, or intermittently throughout a period of more than a year.
3. Onset before age 21.
4. Occurrence not exclusively during psychoactive substance intoxication or known central nervous system disease, such as Huntington's chorea and post–viral encephalitis.

Diagnostic Criteria for Transient Tic Disorder (307.21)

1. Single or multiple motor and/or vocal tics.
2. The tics occur many times a day, nearly every day for at least 2 weeks, but for no longer than 12 consecutive months.
3. No history of Tourette's or chronic motor or vocal tic disorder.
4. Onset before age 21.

Diagnostic Criteria for Tic Disorder Not Otherwise Specified (307.20)

Tics that do not meet the criteria for a specific tic disorder. An example is a tic disorder with onset in adulthood.

___

of tic-related mental states is most commonly encountered in TS patients. On the other hand, the current diagnostic criteria are such that patients could satisfy the criteria without being seriously impaired by their motor and phonic tics. Such cases are commonplace in family-genetic studies and may occur in epidemiologic studies, as well (Zahner, Clubb, Leckman, & Pauls, Chapter 5, this volume). In clinical settings, patients at times will present with mild TS but with an otherwise complicated behavioral history, such as severe ADD and specific developmental disorders. In such cases, it is important not to overdiagnose TS and attribute all of the child's behavioral problems to TS, *per se.* Issues of impairment obviously are critical in assessing the need for clinical intervention. The rating instruments that have been developed for this purpose are discussed in a subsequent chapter (Leckman, Towbin, Ort, & Cohen, Chapter 4, this volume).

Chronic Motor or Vocal Tic Disorder

This category replaces the DSM-III category of chronic motor tic disorder (see Exhibit 1.5 and Table 1.1). It simply broadens the nosologic domain to include the rare individuals with chronic vocal tics. Although adequate epidemiologic studies of chronic tics have not been performed, this disorder presumably is more common than TS. Family studies suggest that, among at-risk family members, chronic tics are at least two to three times more prevalent than TS. Family-genetic studies strongly support an etiologic relationship between chronic motor tic disorder and TS. The empirical basis for including individuals with a chronic vocal tic disorder in the same diagnostic category comes from recent studies of large kindreds in which a small number of relatives of TS probands reported only chronic vocal tics. In each instance, the chronic vocal tics were simple in character, and, although they caused some difficulty, they did not significantly impair the individual.

Longitudinal studies of patients with chronic tic disorders have not been performed. Anecdotal clinical information suggests that the natural history is variable and resembles in form that of TS patients, with most patients showing a decrease in tic frequency and intensity of tics in adulthood.

Transient Tic Disorder

Almost invariably a disorder of childhood, transient tic disorder usually is characterized by one or more simple motor tics that wax and wane in severity over weeks to months. Much less commonly, transient, simple vocal tics may occur. By definition (Exhibit 1.5), a transient tic disorder has a duration of less than a year. However, the tic symptoms may come and go intermittently over a period of several years. Frequently, their emergence is associated with periods of increased stress.

This disorder is relatively common, particularly among school-age boys. Although the symptoms can be a source of considerable distress to the patients and their families, the tic symptoms usually are mild and do not interfere with school performance or peer relationships.

Tic Disorder Not Otherwise Specified

This category is reserved for those tic disorders that cannot readily be placed into one of the categories already mentioned because of their age of onset, duration, or unusual character.

CONCLUSION

The past decade has seen considerable progress in our understanding of tic disorders (Cohen & Leckman, 1984). Although the nosology of tic disorders is still based solely on features of the clinical presentation and course, advances in the areas of molecular genetics and neuroimaging may radically alter this over the next few years. It may be possible to classify individuals on the basis of their genetic vulnerability and monitor their progress using neuroanatomically precise methods and improved neurochemical and neuroendocrine techniques.

REFERENCES

American Psychiatric Association. (1980). *Diagnostic and statistical manual of mental disorders* (3rd ed.). Washington, DC: Author.

American Psychiatric Association. (1987). *Diagnostic and statistical manual of mental disorders* (3rd ed. revised). Washington, DC: Author.

Bliss, J. Sensory experiences of Gilles de la Tourette Syndrome. *Archives of General Psychiatry, 37,* 1343–1347.

Cohen, D.J. (1980). The pathology of the self in primary childhood autism and Gilles de la Tourette's syndrome. In B.J. Binder, (Ed.), *The Psychiatric Clinics of North America, 3,* 383–402.

Cohen, D.J., & Leckman, J.F. (1984). Current developments in Tourette's syndrome: Advances in treatment and research, an introduction. *Journal of the American Academy of Child Psychiatry, 23,* 123–125.

Cohen, D.J., Leckman, J.F., & Shaywitz B.A. (1984) Tourette's Syndrome and other tics. In D. Shaffer, A.A. Ehrhardt, & L. Greenhill (Eds.) *Diagnosis and Treatment in Pediatric Psychiatry.* New York: MacMillan Free Press. pp. 3–28.

Harcherik, D.F., Leckman, J.F., Detlor, J., & Cohen, D.J. (1984). A new instrument for clinical studies of Tourette's syndrome: A preliminary report. *Journal of the American Academy of Child Psychiatry, 23,* 153–160.

Jagger, J., Prusoff, B.A., Cohen, D.J., Kidd, K.K., Carbonari, C.M., & John, K. (1982). The epidemiology of Tourette's syndrome: A pilot study. *Schizophrenia Bulletin, 8,* 267–278.

Leckman, J.F., Walkup, J.T., Riddle, M.A., Towbin, K.E., & Cohen, D.J. (1987). Tic disorders. In H.Y. Meltzer, W. Bunney, J. Coyle, J. Davis, I. Kopin, C. Schuster, R. Shader, & G. Simpson, (Eds.) *Psychopharmacology. The Third Generation of Progress.* New York: Raven. pp 1239–1246.

Lecs, A.J. (1985) *Tics and Related Disorders.* Edinburgh: Churchill Livingstone.

Pauls, D.L., Hurst, C., Kruger, S.D., Leckman, J.F., Kidd, K.K., & Cohen, D.J. (1986). Evidence against a genetic relationship between Tourette's syndrome and attention deficit disorder. *Archives of General Psychiatry, 43,*(12), 1177–1179.

Pauls, D.L., & Leckman, J.F. (1986). The inheritance of Gilles de la Tourette syndrome and associated behaviors: Evidence for an autosomal dominant transmission. *New England Journal of Medicine, 315,* 993–997.

CHAPTER TWO

The Natural History of Tourette's Syndrome

Ruth Dowling Bruun

OVERVIEW

During the past two decades a great deal of information has accumulated concerning the onset and early years of patients with Tourette's syndrome (TS) but there is much less known about long-term prognosis. Interestingly, the first TS patient to be well documented in medical literature, the Marquise de Dampierre, is also one of the oldest whose symptoms have been described in any detail (Gilles de la Tourette, 1885; Itard, 1825). This unfortunate woman was seen by the most prominent neurologists of her time, including Charcot. Her symptomatology remained florid, causing her to be a recluse until her death at the age of 86 years. Although the Marquise de Dampierre has been considered a prototype for the disorder, contemporary research has suggested that the prognosis for the average TS patient is considerably better. Recent literature has been primarily concerned with childhood, adolescent, or young adult cases. This chapter traces the natural history of Tourette's syndrome throughout life, based on studies in the literature and data from 350 patients in my own clinical experience (both from private practice and from clinics at two hospitals in New York City). Most of the previously published data on early symptomatology have come from 11 studies, chosen either because they included large numbers of patients or for their geographic and cultural distribution. In summarizing these data and including my own patients, there are 2463 patients (although there may be a small number of duplications). Between a quarter and a third of these patients are from outside North America (141 from Asia and 567 from Europe). The largest number of patients (650) in any single study are those reported by Shapiro and Shapiro (1982). Earlier data from these same investigators include 76 patients from other studies and 145 from their own (Shapiro, Shapiro, Bruun, & Sweet, 1976). The later report on 650 patients presumably includes the original 145, a few of whom are also included in my data. Other large studies are by Abuzzahab and Anderson (1976, 485 patients); Comings and Comings (1985; 250 patients); and Stefl (1984, 431 patients). Smaller, well-documented studies were chosen for cross-cultural comparisons. These include Lees, Robertson, Trimble, and Murray (1984, 53 patients from Great Britain); Pakkenberg, Regeur, Fog, and Pakkenberg (1982, 18 patients from Denmark); Asam (1982, 16 patients from Germany); Nomura and Segawa (1982; 100 patients from Japan); Lieh Mak, Chung, Lee and Chen (1982; 15 patients from Hong Kong); and Chen and Lu Fei (1983, 19 patients from the People's Republic of China).

ONSET OF TS SYMPTOMS

The mean age of onset in 10 studies (1382 patients) was 7.2 years (see Table 2.1). The range of onset age is defined in DSM-III as 2 to 15, and most investigators have thus excluded cases that began outside of this age spread. However, Abuzzahab and Anderson mention 15 patients whose symptoms began after the age of 20, and there have been 3 patients in my practice (not in the 350) whose symptoms began at age 19 and who otherwise fit all the criteria for a diagnosis of TS.

One hundred eighty-six of my patients (53 percent) recalled an eye tic as their first symptom, either as a single symptom or with others. Most commonly, this consisted of eye blinking, but rolling the eyes and opening them wide were also frequent. Forty-six patients (13 percent) reported other facial tics such as grimacing, nose twitching, or licking or biting of the lips as a first symptom. Vocalizations were the presenting symptom in 46 patients (13 percent). Most commonly these consisted of sniffing, throat clearing, coughing, or grunting. Spitting was considered a vocalization and also was common.

Coprolalia was the initial symptom in only 5 patients (1.4 percent). Other initial symptoms were movements of the head or neck (14 percent), upper extremities (6 percent), lower extremities (1 percent), and trunk (0.6 percent).

Table 2.1. Age of Onset of TS Symptoms

Study	Number of Patients	Male/Female Ratio	Age of Onset
Abuzzahab & Anderson, 1976	485	2–1	7.5
Shapiro et al., 1976	76[a]	3–1	7.3
Shapiro & Shapiro, 1982	650	3–1	—
Nomura & Segawa, 1982	100	5.6–1	6.1
Assam, 1982	16	7–1	8.0
Lieh Mak et al., 1982	15	—	9.4
Pakkenberg et al., 1982	18	3.5–1	6.3
Chen & Lu Fei, 1983	19	3.8–1	8.0
Lees et al., 1984	53	3–1	7.0
Stefl, 1984	431	3.5–1	—
Comings & Comings, 1985	250	4–1	6.8
Bruun, 1986	350	3.4–1	5.8
Average or total	2463	3–1	7.2

[a]A study of 221 patients, of which 145 are included in the 650 patients in 1982 study.

Other investigators had similar experiences with presenting symptomatology. Of those who reported the symptoms by percentage, eye
tics were found to be first in 20 to 53 percent of patients. Total facial
tics as presenting symptoms ranged from 45 to 73 percent, vocalizations
from 13 to 47 percent and coprolalia from 0 to 9 percent (see Table
2.2).

Onset of TS as a simple tic has been reported to occur in 50 to 70
percent of cases (Nomura & Segawa, 1982; Shapiro & Shapiro, 1976).
Since all of these data depend on the memory of patients and their
families and an initial symptom often may not be recognized as such,
the accuracy of these figures is only approximate. However, all investigators agree that eye and other facial tics are most common and that
coprolalia is rare as a presenting symptom.

PROGRESSION OF SYMPTOMS

After the initial tic or tics, others will appear over a period of weeks to
months, either to replace the original ones or to be added to them. Early
in the course of this disorder there are likely to be periods of complete
or almost complete remission. However, the general trend in those who
go on to develop the full syndrome will be toward more obvious and
more bothersome symptoms. The Shapiros write of such a change occurring over a 3-month period after onset of the initial symptom(s)
(1976). However, other investigators have not found any definite time
period between onset of tics and their progression. Symptoms may be
static for long periods of time or may appear and remit in a matter of
days. Occasionally a patient will experience an acute onset of multiple
symptoms with no prior history of tic.

Cephalocaudal progression of the development of motor tics has

Table 2.2. *Initial Symptoms (in percentages)*

	Eye	All Facial	Vocal	Coprolalia	Other
Shapiro et al., 1976	42	54	33	9	29
Shapiro & Shapiro, 1982	35	45	—	1	—
Nomura & Segawa, 1982	35	>50	>25	0	~50
Lieh Mak et al., 1982	20	73	13	0	7
Pakkenberg et al., 1982	50	56	39	0	50
Chen & Lu Fei, 1983	—	68	47	—	32
Comings & Comings, 1985	48	66	32	3	—
Bruun, 1986	53	66	13	1	22

been suggested by some investigators (Jagger et al., 1982; Nomura & Segawa, 1982). Although it is true that less common tics (those of legs and trunk) tend to have a later mean age of onset, an orderly cephalo-caudal progression of symptoms only rarely occurs. This sort of progression has not been found to be characteristic of the disorder by the Shapiros, who have carefully documented the early course of TS in the largest number of patients (1982). It has been present in less than 10 percent of my patients.

Vocal tics are found by most investigators to have a later mean age of onset than motor tics. This is particularly true for coprolalia, which has been found to begin at a mean age ranging from 3.8 to 7.5 years after the onset of motor tics (Comings & Comings, 1985; Nomura & Segawa, 1982).

Following is a history that would be familiar to all those who treat TS.

Tim, age 9, began to have persistent eye blinking at age 6–½, followed a few months later by sniffing. His pediatrician was unconcerned but referred him to an opthalmologist and later to an allergist. No diagnosis was made, but the sniffing stopped and the eye blinking almost disappeared for several months. At the age of 8 Tim began shaking his head, as if tossing his hair out of the way of his eyes. Blinking increased at the same time. A haircut did not effect an improvement. A year and a half later he started to make grunting noises and grimaces. He was finally referred to a neurologist on the suggestion of the school nurse and the diagnosis of TS was made.

RANGE OF SYMPTOMS

The range of symptoms as reviewed by Leckman and Cohen (Chapter 1, this volume) and described in the literature is enormous. As more than one of my older patients has said to me, "You name it and I've done it." The frequency of the occurrence of various simple symptoms in different patient samples is summarized in Table 2.3.

Abuzzahab and Anderson noted certain cross-cultural differences in the frequency of symptoms of their patient sample (e.g., more eye tics in Italy). However, the sample consisted of case reports assembled from different reporting physicians and may well represent cross-cultural differences in the physicians rather than the patients. No other significant differences have been noted in the foreign studies, nor have cross-cultural differences been noted in the large American studies.

Complicated movements such as dancelike foot movements, jumping, touching of objects or body parts, smelling hands, and so on were re-

Table 2.3. *Cumulative Symptoms (in percentages)*

	Face	Head and Neck	Upper Extremities	Lower Extremities	Trunk	Coprolalia
Abuzzahab & Anderson, 1976	92	53	78	54	—	58
Shapiro et al., 1976	97	79	81	55	54	60
Shapiro & Shapiro, 1982	—	71	46	28	26	33
Nomura & Segawa, 1982	>90	~75	>60	<50	50–60	23[a]
Asam, 1982	—	—	—	—	—	38
Lieh Mak et al., 1982	—	—	—	—	—	60
Pakkenberg et al., 1982	>94	94	—	—	>56	22
Chen & Lu Fei, 1983	84	58	84	58	53	21
Lees et al., 1984	94	89	51	40	41	20
Comings & Comings, 1985	82	63	—	—	—	33
Bruun, 1986	98	74	64	29	28	33
Average of all	>90	70–80	60–70	40–50	40–50	30–40

[a]4% = *true*; 19% = *quasi.*

ported by 238 (68 percent) of my patients. These types of movements are reported to occur in 73 percent of the Shapiros' first sample (1976). Lees and colleagues (1984) also find them to be quite common, particularly compulsive touching of objects, such as hot things, sharp knives, door handles, erotic textures, as well as breasts and other body parts of other people. Nomura and Segawa reported less frequently seen complicated movements and Comings and Comings define these movements somewhat differently ("a tic in one part of the body ... reproducibly followed by a secondary tic"), and find an incidence of 21 to 24 percent. Such stereotyped movement sequences also occur fairly frequently in my patients, although I have no exact data on them.

The incidence of copropraxia (e.g., "giving the finger" or grabbing genitals—one's own or others') varies greatly from one patient sample to another (2 to 21 percent) (Lees et al., 1984; Shapiro & Shapiro, 1976). This is undoubtedly due to variant symptom characterization by different physicians. Thus the same gestures Lees and colleagues describe as copropraxia are called grade 1 exhibitionism by Comings and Comings.

Self-abusive tics such as hitting oneself or lipbiting are reported by most investigators, but again, categorized or defined differently. In my patient group only 7 percent of patients had self-abusive symptoms se-

vere enough to inflict significant damage upon themselves as, for example, a young boy who snapped his shoulder joint until it became markedly swollen or another who bit his lip so severely that he had to wear
a mouthpiece. Comings and Comings report a 13 percent incidence of
self-abusive behavior, while the Shapiros and Lees and colleagues mention it without reporting an incidence figure. Pakkenberg and colleagues (1982) noted it in one of their 18 patients while Nee, Caine,
Polinski, Eldridge, and Ebert (1980) found the highest incidence (40
percent) in one of their patient groups but do not state the parameters
used to define it.

Echolalia and echopraxia are described in most patient samples, the
incidence varying from 23 to 43 percent for echolalia and from 10 to
21 percent for echopraxia (Abuzzahab & Anderson, 1976; Lees et al.,
1984; Shapiro & Shapiro, 1976). Palilalia and other speech irregularities
such as blocking, stuttering, and irregular word accentuation as well as
mental coprolalia and mental palilalia have been noted by many investigators including myself. Nomura and Segawa divided coprolalia into
the categories *true* (only 4 percent) and *quasi* (19 percent). Although a
precise definition of these terms is unclear, the term *coprolalia* is usually
interpreted quite broadly, most investigators including any socially inappropriate words or phrases.

The Shapiros have recently called special attention to another sort of
tic, which they term *sensory*. This refers to a disturbing internal sensation
that is premonitory to, or actually causes, a motor tic. The patient will
execute a movement in order to relieve the sensation or sensory tic.
These have previously been described by other authors and are recognized by most physicians involved in the treatment of TS (Bullen &
Hemsley, 1983; Jagger et al., 1982; Shapiro, 1985a).

ASSOCIATED SYMPTOMS

Organic stigmata such as minor, nonspecific abnormalities on neurological examination and/or on EEG and significant disparity between
verbal and performance IQ scores have been documented by most investigators to occur more frequently in TS patients than in control populations. Attention deficit disorder, hyperactivity, learning disabilities,
sleep disorders, and enuresis have also been reported to be associated
with TS to a significant degree. Other associated symptoms include obsessive–compulsive behavior, sexually inappropriate and antisocial behavior (Abuzzahab & Anderson, 1976; Comings & Comings, 1985; Glaze,
Jankovic, & Frost, 1983; Hagin, Beecher, Papano, & Kreeger 1982; Lees
et al., 1984; Nee et al., 1979; Shapiro & Shapiro, 1976, 1982; Stefl, 1984).

Obsessive–compulsive symptomatology, learning disabilities, attention deficit disorder, and behavioral complications of TS are discussed elsewhere in this volume (Towbin, Chapter 9). Obsessive-compulsive symptomatology was described by 147 (42 percent) of my TS patients. In most cases these symptoms are minor, but 58 patients (16 percent) found them severe enough to overshadow tics and vocalizations at times. Obsessive–compulsive symptoms varied from the common, such as the patient who had to switch a light on and off three times, to the bizarre, such as the patient who filed her teeth with a nail file in order to even them up. It was frequently noted by parents that a TS child insisted on having a word or a phrase repeated over and over until it sounded "right." Other compulsions included dangerous behavior such as flicking a cigarette lighter in one's own face, never near enough to do damage, or running across the street just in front of oncoming cars. In my review simple touching tics were not counted as true compulsive behaviors.

Antisocial and inappropriate sexual behavior is considered to be frequently associated with TS by Comings and Comings (1985), who find that 44 percent of their patients have discipline problems, 42 percent have problems with anger and violence, and 14 percent manifest some form of exhibitionism. However, grade 1 exhibitionism is defined as sexual touching of selves or others, and only grade 3 (6 percent) involves public exhibitionism. Here, again, classification becomes a problem since touching can be considered a tic, a compulsion, copropraxia, or inappropriate sexual behavior. Another study mentioning inappropriate sexual activity, done by Nee, Caine, Polinsky et al. (1980) found a 32 percent incidence. The sort of inappropriate behavior was not described. My patient sample included 7 patients over the age of 16 (5 percent) who had been exhibitionistic in public or semipublic places. Two of these had been charged with sexual offenses.

Anger and violent behavior was a serious problem (according to families or, in one case, the employer) for 33 patients (9 percent) of my sample, but led to trouble with the law in only 3. Antisocial behavior, including alcohol and drug abuse, stealing, and minor infractions of the law, was known to be a problem in 32 patients (9 percent). Two have been charged and are awaiting trial, and 3 were placed in treatment centers or imprisoned. Lieh Mak and colleagues (1982) had 2 out of 15 patients who had been in trouble with the law. However, both of these were also afflicted with ADD. This was not necessarily characteristic of the lawbreakers in my sample. The Japanese patients in Nomura and Segawa's study (1982) were noted to have a high percentage of psycho-behavioral problems (66 percent in males, 47 percent in females). These were described as being spoiled, hyperactive, and inattentive rather than as the more severe problems mentioned earlier.

The Shapiros, in contrast to other investigators, state:

Other clinical reports in the literature that most patients with TS are characterized by excessive aggressivity, impulsivity, sexuality, self-destructiveness, obsessive–compulsiveness, enuresis, sleep disorders and antisocial behavior, and other psychopathology are not supported by our controlled and clinical observations. (1982, p. 384).

They suggest, rather, that these behaviors are associated with ADD (which 33 percent of their patients are said to have).

VARIATIONS IN DEGREE AND QUALITY OF SYMPTOMS

All investigators agree that tics and vocalizations have periods of waxing and waning. There is, however, no consensus as to a periodicity in this variation. It is my experience that a few patients can anticipate times when their tics will worsen or abate (e.g., worsening in spring, concurrent with pollen allergy). This predictability, however, is rare. More often, a patient will suddenly develop a symptom after months of relative stability. The symptom may last a day or may persist for months. It may disappear suddenly or gradually fade away. Most patients will have one or two long-standing, familiar tics while others will come and go. Patients often report that periods of severe emotional stress will cause their symptoms to increase in severity and/or frequency. However, this is not necessarily the case, and patients will sometimes express surprise that their condition did not worsen during a stressful time. A few women patients have reported that their symptoms increase premenstrually, but this has never been satisfactorily documented.

The daily variations of tic severity are usually somewhat more predictable. Excitement, anxiety, and impatient anticipation will cause an increase, while concentration on an absorbing activity such as playing a musical instrument or making love will produce a decrease. Thus an athletically inclined young patient may report that he manifests the whole gamut of his symptoms while waiting for action in a game but that the tics virtually disappear when he is running with the ball. Similarly, an actress with moderately severe TS never has to worry about her symptoms while onstage.

Symptoms are generally pronounced when patients relax their self-vigilance. This may be when they are alone in a bathroom or bedroom. It may also be when they come home after a day of work or school and sit down to relax with their families. Watching television is frequently mentioned as a time when symptoms increase, perhaps because it induces relaxation without involvement. Most patients cite either the early evening hours or bedtime as the worst time of the day for tics. It is often hard for patients to get to sleep since a conscious effort to relax without any outside stimulus seems to produce more tics. Thus although it is unusual for a patient not to have some control over the symptoms of TS, the very act of concentrating on not doing a tic may tend to bring that tic on. During the course of a day at work or school the control may be easier to exert. Some patients seem to gain mastery over their tics almost unconsciously, while others can attain control only with great inner effort.

ADOLESCENCE

What happens to the "typical" TS patient as he or she becomes an adolescent? Early adolescence is often the time that coprolalia is first manifested. Although it has been suggested that this may relate to an increased awareness of sexuality, it is reasonable also to understand coprolalia simply as a symptom that tends to appear later in the course of the disorder (Lees et al., 1984; Mahler, 1949; Shapiro & Shapiro, 1976). Adolescence is a difficult time of life for almost everyone. It is a time when social pressures are of great importance, when acceptance outside of the family is a paramount issue, and the need to conform to the standards of one's peers is strongest. To suffer from a disease that causes one to appear strange, even bizarre, is perhaps most difficult to bear at this time of life. It may be because of this that clinicians often find themselves spending a disproportionate amount of time with adolescent TS patients and their families. Symptoms seem to occur somewhat more unpredictably during the teenage years, and when they do they may cause greater concern than they would at another age. A symptom that may not be bothersome at the age of 8 may be acutely embarrassing at 15 when dating or getting a summer job becomes important. It is my impression that symptoms during early adolescence are not necessarily worse but change in nature more rapidly and, being more unpredictable, become harder to live with. This may be related to the physical changes that are occurring at this time or may be based on emotional factors or, more likely, both.

When investigating adolescents specifically, one finds little information in the TS literature. Lucas (1970) reported a gradual amelioration of symptoms in late adolescence or early adulthood. Erenberg, Cruse, Rothner & Rothner (1987) sent a questionnaire to 58 patients between the ages of 15 and 25. Seventy-three percent of the patients reported their tics to be either diminished or mostly gone as they reached late adolescence or early adulthood. Although medication was a factor in this study, there were twice as many patients under 18 on medication as over 18, strongly suggesting a spontaneous trend toward amelioration of symptoms during later teenage years.

ADULT YEARS

Nee and colleagues (1982), using a retrospective rating system, found that 40 percent of 30 adult patients considered their symptoms to be at their worst during the first decade after onset. Sixty-seven percent of these patients experienced symptomatic relief during the second decade. Since the average age of onset was 8, this would put the turning point at 18. In this study improvement continued gradually throughout life except for a slight period of worsening during the fourth decade. Medication did not appear to account for the trend toward improvement in this study.

Asam (1979) followed up 29 patients with multiple tics. Of the 16 Tourette's patients, 3 had no symptoms as adults while 9 of the remaining 13 ticquers had remissions as adults. Lieh Mak and colleagues (1982) reported 1 spontaneous remission in their 15 patients.

Remissions were reported in 5 out of 33 patients followed up by Moldofsky (1985). Two of these were originally rated as mild, but 3 had once been severe. Singer (1985) reviewed the course of 120 patients and also found a trend toward improvement. At the last evaluation mild symptoms were found in all previously mild patients, in 71 percent of those originally rated as moderate, 44 percent of those initially rated as moderately severe, and 18 percent of those who were once severe. These patients were both on and off medication.

The Shapiros (1985) report a 16 percent rate of spontaneous remission in their 650 patients but do not state the length of these remissions. A. Shapiro has noted (1985b) that 25 percent of their adolescent patients improve markedly and then continue to be only mildly affected throughout later life while many of the others improve later in adulthood. He also notes an increase in symptoms experienced by some patients during their twenties or thirties (at least a decade earlier than the increase noted by Nee et al., 1982).

Many other investigators have reported remissions ranging from 6 months to 3 years. The remission rate in the larger studies ranges from 3 to 18 percent of patients for periods of less than a year and from 1 to 4 percent for periods of a year or greater (Abuzzahab and Anderson, 1976; Bruun et al., 1976; Lees et al., 1984).

In order to study the later course of TS, data from my patient group were examined in three ways: an evaluation of all patients at different ages; a retrospective study of patients who are 30 or older; and a longitudinal study of patients who have been followed continuously for 5 to 15 years.

EVALUATION OF PATIENTS AT DIFFERENT AGES

Of the 350 patients, 162 were age 20 or younger, 67 were in their twenties, 77 in their thirties, 23 in their forties, 9 in their fifties, and 12 over the age of 60 (the oldest being 81 years of age). All except 3 patients were symptomatic at the time of follow-up, although several had had long remissions in the past. All patients were rated for severity (mild, moderate, marked, severe) by criteria used since 1970 (Bruun et al., 1976). As may be seen (Fig. 2.1), none of the patients over the age of 50 were rated as marked or severe, and 90 percent were in the mild category. Although there is not a clear-cut pattern of tic diminution with increasing age, there does appear to be a trend in this direction. Each decade after age 20 contains a higher percentage of mild cases with the exception of the age span from 40 to 50 (this corresponds with the findings of Nee et al. previously mentioned). Although medication may play a role in this trend toward amelioration, it is clearly not the causative factor. Only 10 out of 21 patients over 50 were on medication, and all were on smaller doses than they had once required. In the 20–30 and 30–40 age groups 63 patients (44 percent) had discontinued medication while 110 (68 percent) of the younger patients were on medication.

It is particularly striking in this group that almost half of the patients were children. One would expect the percentage to be much lower if the severity of most cases was constant throughout life.

RETROSPECTIVE STUDY OF PATIENTS OVER 30

Of the 121 patients, 63 stated that they had spontaneously improved (not attributable to medication) and had remained improved. Forty-three (36 percent) had first experienced the improvement in their late teens and had continued to improve gradually thereafter or had improved to a certain level where they had stabilized, although continuing to have minor fluctuations. Eleven of those who improved (9 percent of the total) did not do so until their early twenties, and 6 more (another 5 percent) not until their late twenties or early thirties. Three elderly patients (2 women and 1 man) noted a definite improvement in their fifties.

Nineteen patients (16 percent) stated that they had grown gradually worse or had rather suddenly worsened, 3 in their twenties and 3 in their early thirties. One patient attributed this worsening to a head in-

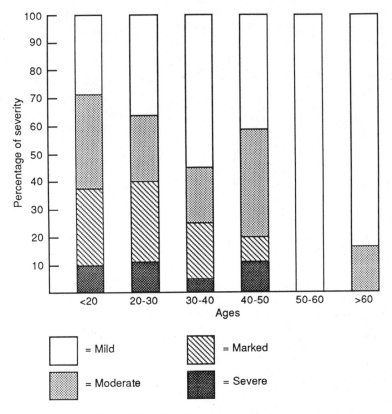

Figure 2.1. Severity of symptoms by age.

jury. The others could give no reason. Twenty-eight patients felt that they had not changed after the first decade beyond the normal waxings and wanings of the syndrome. The 11 remaining patients, though most had improved, could not estimate how they would be without medication or could not recall any coherent pattern to the severity of their symptoms prior to treatment.

Thus of the adult patients who continued to be symptomatic enough to seek medical attention, 57 percent said that they had improved spontaneously after adolescence.

LONGITUDINAL STUDY

One hundred thirty-six patients had been followed for 5 to 15 years. Six of these patients had never been treated and had been followed either because they were related to another TS patient or because they had been diagnosed and had agreed to periodic follow-up although refusing medication. Of the 130 patients who had been medicated, 128 had been on haloperidol at one time. Only 43 remained on this medication, 10 of these being on a combination of haloperidol and clonidine. Twenty-four patients were on clonidine, 12 of these on clonidine alone. Twelve patients were on pimozide (1 on pimozide plus clonidine), and 14 were on various other medications (thiothixene, fluphenazine, trifluperazine, trazodone, doxepin, lithium, clonazepam, diazepam, alprazolam, guanabenz, and high doses of lecithin) alone or in combination. Thirty-seven patients were on no medication. Three of these felt that dietary changes were responsible for their improvement.

Of these 136 patients, 18 were originally rated as severe, 39 as marked, 41 as moderate, and 38 as mild. At last evaluation 5 were severe, 6 were marked, 33 were moderate, 85 were mild, and 7 were in remission. Of the 37 patients off medication, all but 2 were over the age of 18. Three of these were rated as moderate or marked while the rest were either mild or in remission.

Of this whole patient group, 4 were retarded, 13 disabled due to emotional disorders, 18 had been treated for depression at some time during their lives, and 23 were known to be or to have been drug or alcohol abusers.

LIFE ADJUSTMENT

The data presented thus far have their obvious limitations. There may be a bias toward including more severe cases, as less severe cases might be less likely to remain in treatment or to seek a second or third opinion. In addition, the evaluations done by me and by the patients were subjective and had no internal checking system. Furthermore, when an evaluation was completed only core symptoms of TS, tics and vocalizations, were recorded. The patients tended to take a more holistic view when they did retrospective evaluations. Thus there may be one symptom that, while technically no worse than another, still becomes a source of particular concern and causes a patient to feel that he or she is worse. A common example of this is coprolalia, which, while just another symptom, is far more distressing to the average patient than a head tic. It is also true that obsessive–compulsive symptoms, unless in the form of tics, are likely to cause a patient discomfort while not even entering into consideration in the rating system.

Perhaps it would be better to look at the overall adjustment or coping facility of these patients than to look at their symptoms alone. Although this too has its obvious pitfalls, it seems a worthwhile endeavor.

There has been only one large study that has explored the life adjustments of TS patients in any depth. This is the Ohio study done in 1983 through a questionnaire to which 431 patients (or parents) from the membership of the Ohio chapter of the Tourette Syndrome Association responded. Only 36 percent of the adults in this study were employed full-time. Fifteen percent were employed part-time, 18 percent were looking for work, 17 percent were unemployed but not looking for work, and 8 percent never worked. Other employment data may be seen in Table 2.4. Of these over the age of 19, 46 percent were married, 46 percent had never married, and 9 percent were divorced or separated. While the employment figures are strikingly worse than those of the general population in the Ohio area, the matrimonial figures are approximately the same.

Another striking finding of the Ohio study was the high rate of behavioral problems that patients reported, extreme temper, aggressive behavior, extreme anxiety, and mood swings being reported to be frequent problems by one-quarter to one-third of the respondents (Stefl, 1984). More than half of the members of this study had sought some sort of

Table 2.4. Life Adjustment (in percentages)

	Stefl Ohio Study	Bruun
Never married	46	35
Married	46	54
Divorced or separated	9	9
Widowed	—	2
Employed full time	36	56
Employed part time	15	5
Not employed	34	25
Retired	2	2
Housekeepers	4	6
Never worked	8	—
Other	2	1
Receiving SS benefits	4	9
Employed:		
1. Professional, technical, managerial, executive	28	35
2. Clerical sales, etc.	30	33
3. Laborer, operative, service, domestic	25	18
4. Craftsmen	10	—
5. Artists	—	13
6. Students	4	8
7. Army	—	1
Self-employed	—	5

counseling, and many had sought several types. Respondents were asked to indicate how well they felt they had adjusted to TS. Sixteen percent indicated no coping problems, 46 percent said they had adjusted well in most respects, while the remaining 38 percent admitted to some or significant coping problems. Coping ability was unrelated to sex or income level but correlated well to the severity of symptoms. There seemed to be a gradually decreasing ability to cope with increasing age.

Other studies have glimpsed the difficulties faced by TS patients. Jagger and colleagues (1982) questioned patients about their social adjustment. They found that 67 percent of 75 patients (members of the Connecticut chapter of the Tourette Syndrome Association) had sought mental health counseling of some sort. Fifty percent felt that their relationship with their family was adversely affected by TS, 38 percent that social contact outside of the home was affected severely or substantially, and 81 percent that their job performance was either severely or substantially affected.

Asam (1982) comments that all of her 16 patients were subject to immense psychic stress and that they were socially isolated. Ten of her 16 patients drifted downward to a lower social class than that of their parents.

Lieh Mak and colleagues (1982), in their follow-up of 15 patients in Hong Kong, reported that the patients with low intelligence and EEG abnormalities had a downward drift in social class. Social adjustment was considered good in 7, fair in 3, and poor in 5.

In my patient group there were 179 patients over the age of 21. Of these, 44 (25 percent) were unemployed. Seventeen patients were receiving unemployment benefits either for TS or for other conditions. Eleven patients were housekeepers, 15 were students, either in college or graduate school, 4 were retired, 2 were in correctional facilities, and 9 were employed part-time (4 of these were also attending college or graduate school).

Of the remaining 100 patients, 35 percent held jobs as professionals. Three of these were medical doctors, 2 were lawyers, 18 were teachers, social workers, or other health care professionals, 3 were ministers, and the remainder were in executive positions in business. Thirty-three percent held clerical or sales jobs. Eighteen percent were laborers, waiters, or cooks or worked as drivers (trucks, cabs, etc.). Thirteen percent were in the arts, mostly in acting or music. One patient was in the army (having concealed his condition). Of those employed in various categories 13 patients were self-employed. Two patients who were otherwise unemployable worked in the family business.

Thirty-five percent had never been married, 54 percent were married, 9 percent were divorced or separated, and 2 percent widowed. These figures are rather striking for the New York area. TS patients seem to get married and stay married.

Overall, my patient group seemed to be doing somewhat better than the Ohio group. This may be attributed to different recruitment methods. Patients who join the Tourette Syndrome Association tend to be those for whom TS has had a fairly profound effect. Others may shy away from such an organization.

CONCLUSION

It appears from the data collected and presented here that at least half of TS patients can expect some improvement as they reach maturity and that a sizable group will continue to improve throughout their lives. Many patients no longer need treatment as they grow older. Many others require less medication than they once did. It is interesting that all the lengthy remissions in my patient group occurred before the age of 30. Do many patients go into remission and stay that way? Unfortunately, we are still lacking enough data to know what percentage of cases will improve or remit. Almost all studies in the literature have disproportionately large numbers of children compared to adults. In my group of 350 there were only 179 patients over the age of 21. What happens to the adults? Why don't they come for diagnosis if they are still afflicted with the symptoms of TS? Have many of them improved sufficiently that the symptoms are no longer a concern to them? Or have they simply resigned themselves to living with the disorder, perhaps managing to conceal the tics from most people around them or thinking that they do so? I have occasionally spoken with concerned family members who are convinced that a relative has TS but will not even discuss the possibility. Whatever the answers to these questions, an effort should be made to identify more adult TS patients or former patients. One approach to this endeavor would be to contact the families of known TS patients. Another would be more public education.

Another area to be investigated is that of distinguishing aspects of the cases that improve spontaneously or respond well to medication from aspects of those that don't. It has been suggested that obsessive–compulsive symptoms carry a poorer prognosis with them (Asam, 1982; Corbett, Matthews, Connell, & Shapiro, 1969; Moldofsky, 1985) or that hyperactivity or age of onset may have a negative implication for prognosis (Comings & Comings, 1985; Lieh Mak, 1982). Available data do not confirm or disprove these possibilities, yet the presence of comorbid or associated problems increases the burden on a patient's development.

As today's TS children receive treatment that controls their symptoms and enables them to lead more normal lives, will they have a better future? Will they adapt and cope more effectively because of early diagnosis, treatment, and the understanding of their parents and teachers? There is no evidence that treatment will change the natural course of the disease, but it may have a significant effect on life adjustment.

REFERENCES

Abbuzahab, F.S., Sr., & Anderson, F.O. (1976). Gilles de la Tourette's syndrome. *International Registry,* (Vol. 1). St. Paul, MN: Mason.

American Psychiatric Association (1980). *Diagnostic and Statistical manual of mental disorders* (3rd ed.). Washington, DC: Author.

Asam, U. (1979). Katamnestische Untersuchung von über jugendliche Patienten mit multiplen Tics unter spezieller Berusksichtigung des Gilles de la Tourette-Syndroms. *Acta Paedopschiatrica, 45,* 51–63.

Asam, U. (1982). A follow-up study of Tourette syndrome In A.J. Friedhoff, & T.N. Chase (Eds.), *Gilles de la Tourette Syndrome.* New York: Raven.

Bruun, R.D., Shapiro, A.K., Shapiro, E., Sweet, R., Wayne, H., & Solomon, G.E. (1976). A follow-up of 78 patients with Gilles de la Tourette's syndrome. *American Journal of Psychiatry, 133,* 944–947.

Bullen, J.G., & Hemsley, D.R. (1983). Sensory experience as a trigger in Gilles de la Tourette's syndrome. *Journal of Behavioral Therapy & Experimental Psychiatry, 14,* 197–201.

Chen, H.B., & Lu Fei, H.W. (1983). Tourette's syndrome: Report of 19 cases. *Chinese Medical Journal, 96,* 45–50.

Comings, D.E., & Comings, B.G. (1985). Tourette's syndrome: Clinical and psychological aspects of 250 cases. *American Journal of Human Genetics, 37,* 435–450.

Corbet, J.A., Matthews, A.M., Connell, P.H., & Shapiro, D.A. (1969). Tics and Gilles de la Tourette's syndrome: A follow-up study and critical reviews. *British Journal of Psychiatry, 115,* 1229–1241.

Erenberg, G., Cruse, R.P., Rothner, D.O. and Rothner, A.D. (1987). The Natural History of Tourette Syndrome: A Follow-Up Study. *Annals of Neurology, 22,* 383–385.

Gilles de la Tourette, G. (1885). Étude sur une affection nerveuse, caractérisée par de l'incoordination motrice accompagnée d'echolalie et de corprolalie. *Archives de Neurologie, 9,* 19–42, 158–200.

Glaze, D.G., Jankovic, J., & Frost, J.D. (1983). Sleep in Gilles de la Tourette's syndrome: Disorder of arousal. *Neurology, 33,* 586–592.

Hagin, R.A., Beecher, R., Papano, G., & Kreeger, H. (1982). Effects of Tourette syndrome on learning. In A.J. Friedoff, & T.N. Chase (Eds.), *Gilles de la Tourette Syndrome.* New York: Raven.

Itard, J.M.G. (1825). Mémoire sur quelques fonctions involontaires des appareils de la locomotion de la préhension et de la voix. *Archives of General Medicine, 8,* 385–407.

Jagger, J., Prusoff, B., Cohen, D.J., Kidd, K., Carbonari, C., & John, K. (1982). The epidemiology of Tourette syndrome: A pilot study. *Schizophrenia Bulletin, 2,* 267–278.

Lees, A.J., Robertson, M., Trimble, M.R., & Murray, N.M.F. (1984). A clinical study of Gilles de la Tourette's syndrome in the United Kingdom. *Journal of Neurology, Neurosurgery & Psychiatry, 47,* 1–8.

Lieh Mak, F., Chung, S.Y., Lee, P., & Chen, S. (1982). Tourette syndrome in the Chinese: A follow-up of 15 cases. In A.J. Friedhoff, & T.N. Chase (Eds.), *Advances in neurology* (Vol. 35). New York: Raven.

Lucas, A.R. (1970). Gilles de la Tourette's syndrome: An overview. *New York State Journal of Medicine, 70,* 2197–2200.

Mahler, M.A. (1949). Psychoanalytic evaluation of tics: A sign and symptom of psychopathology. *Psychoanalytic Study of the Child, 3–4,* 279.

Moldofsky, H. (1985, June). *Natural history of Gilles de la Tourette's syndrome.* Presented at Tourette Syndrome Association Conference, June 1985, New York City.

Nee, L.E., Caine, E.D., Polinsky, R.J., Eldridge, R., & Ebert, M.H. (1980). Gilles de la Tourette's syndrome: Clinical and family study of 50 cases. *Annals of Neurology, 7,* 41–49.

Nee, L.E., Polinsky, R.J., & Ebert, M.H. (1982). Tourette syndrome: Clinical and family studies. In A.J. Friedhoff, & T.N. Chase (Eds.), *Gilles de la Tourette Syndrome.* New York: Raven.

Nomura, Y., & Segawa, M. (1982). Tourette syndrome in Oriental children: Clinical and pathophysiological considerations. In A.J. Friedhoff, & T.N. Chase (Eds.), *Gilles de la Tourette Syndrome.* New York: Raven.

Pakkenberg, B., Regeur, L., Fog, R., & Pakkenberg, H. (1982). Gilles de la Tourette's syndrom. *Ugeskrift for Laeger, 144,* 3078–3081.

Shapiro, A.K. (1985a, April). Presentation at meeting for DSM-III revision, New York City.

Shapiro, A.K. (1985b, October). Presentation at First National Clinical Symposium on Tourette Syndrome. New York City.

Shapiro, A.K., & Shapiro, E. (1982). An update on Tourette syndrome. *American Journal of Psychotherapy, 36,* 379–390.

Shapiro, A.K., Shapiro, E., Bruun, R.D., & Sweet, R.D. (1976). *Gilles de la Tourette's syndrome.* New York: Raven.

Singer, H. S. (1985, June). Natural History of Tourette syndrome. Presentation at Tourette Syndrome Association Conference June 1985, New York City.

Stefl, M.E. (1983). *The Ohio Study.* Initial report of data prepared for Tourette Syndrome Association.

Stefl, M.E. (1984). Mental health needs associated with Tourette syndrome. *American Journal of Public Health, 74,* 1310–1313.

CHAPTER THREE

Differential Diagnosis of Tic Phenomena: A Neurologic Perspective

Stanley Fahn
Gerald Erenberg

INTRODUCTION

Tics are divided into those that consist of involuntary movements (motor tics) and those that consist of involuntary sounds (phonic tics). When the latter are present, the designation of Tourette's syndrome has been applied. Whether pure motor tics or tics that are transient and not chronic are distinct disorders and separate from Tourette's syndrome is debatable. At present it seems prudent to consider all tic syndromes under the same "umbrella" with different severities and clinical course denoting differences within the spectrum (Leckman & Cohen, Chapter 1, this volume).

Both motor and phonic tics are classified as abnormal involuntary movements, also referred to as hyperkinesias or dyskinesias. The characteristic phenomenology of tics must therefore be contrasted to that of other types of dyskinesias. First, the phenomenologic definition of tics needs to be clearly stated; then other dyskinesias can be compared to these definitions. Both motor and phonic tics can be divided into complex and simple. Motor tics can be further subdivided into clonic and tonic forms.

MOTOR TICS

Definitions and Phenomenology

Simple Motor Tics.   Simple motor tics are basically abrupt, sudden, single, isolated movements without coordinated sequential patterns. Examples include a shoulder shrug, head jerk, dart of the eyes, and twitch of the nose. Most of the time such simple tics can be repetitive, such as a run of eye blinking or a run of a few simple tics in a row. In this manner, the tics change from simple to complex. It is reasonable to view simple tics as *formes frustes* of complex tics. Their existence, however, increases the complexity of the differential diagnosis, since rapid, simple tics by themselves have similarities to myoclonic and choreic jerks.

Complex Motor Tics.   Complex motor tics can be defined as a coordinated pattern of sequential movements making a complex involuntary sudden and abrupt movement (Fahn, 1982). Examples of complex tics include such acts as touching the nose, touching other people, shaking the head with shrugging of shoulders, kicking the legs, and jumping. Obscene gesturing (copropraxia) is another example of complex motor tics. Mannerisms, whether complex or simple, are considered physiologic rather than pathologic (Fahn, 1982). On the other hand, the resemblance between mannerisms and tics is close, and when physiologic mannerisms become pathologic tics depends more upon when the movements become disturbing to the individual or society. Thus mannerisms can blend into tics. There are few dyskinesias that resemble complex motor tics. The major ones are akathitic movements and stereotypies. Akathitic movements, that is, movements that occur as a result of an inner feeling of restlessness, can resemble quite closely the movements of complex tics. Akathitic movements include caressing the scalp, crossing and uncrossing the legs, arising from a chair and pacing about. Stereotypies, or repetitively identical movements occurring over and over again in the same pattern, can be complex, such as chewing movements seen in tardive dyskinesia.

Clonic and Tonic Tics. The terms *clonic* and *tonic* refer to the duration of the abnormal movement, representing brief and sustained contractions, respectively. Most often, tics are brief and therefore of the clonic variety. Myoclonus and chorea, when these are mild and intermittent movements, closely resemble simple, clonic tics. Tonic tics, by their sustained contraction, must be differentiated from dystonic movements.

Ocular Tics. Involuntary ocular movements are an important differentiation point. Tics can be manifested as ocular movements, whether a brief jerk or more sustained eye deviation. Very few other dyskinesias involve ocular movements. The exceptions are (1) opsoclonus (dancing eyes), which is a form of myoclonus; (2) ocular myoclonus (rhythmic vertical oscillations at a rate of 2 Hz), which often accompanies palatal myoclonus, and (3) oculogyric spasms (a sustained deviation of the eyes) associated with neuroleptics or as a consequence of encephalitis lethargica.

Abruptness. Unless they are very severe, the movements of tics are not continual. Rather they are intermittent, abrupt bursts of motor movements, occurring on a background of normal, quiescent behavior. This pattern most easily separates tics from other dyskinesias because most other types of dyskinesias are continual. The major group of dyskinesias noted by not being continuous are those referred to as paroxysmal dyskinesias, which are usually choreic or dystonic (Lance, 1977), and the excessive startle syndromes, also known as hyperekplexia (Andermann & Andermann, 1986). Hyperekplexias are induced by a stimulus, usually a specific stimulus for that affected individual. Thus this presents no problem in differentiation from tics. Akathitic movements and myoclonic jerks are not infrequently intermittent so can resemble the abrupt nature of tics. Mild chorea (usually in the early stages of Huntington's disease) can also be abrupt, transient, brief jerks, but as chorea worsens, it is typically continual and flowing from one muscle to another. When tics are very severe, they are more frequent, and can resemble a continual string of abnormal movements. In such a situation, they can more closely resemble chorea and dystonia.

Suppressibility. Another important feature of tics, especially if mild or moderate in severity, is that they can be suppressed voluntarily for various periods of time. It is not uncommon for patients complaining of tics to be free of abnormal movements in the doctor's office during the interview and examination because of this suppressibility. This feature is helpful in the differential diagnosis. Although many dyskinesias, including chorea, tremor, and stereotypic and akathitic movements, can be suppressed volitionally, these suppressions are mild and very brief at best. Usually myoclonus, dystonia, and athetosis are not suppressible. More of a problem is when the tics are severe; they are then usually not suppressible and can be continual, more closely resembling dystonia.

Abnormal Sensations. Many patients with tics, when questioned, report an urge to make the tic movement. This urge immediately precedes the movement. In other words, patients experience an uncomfortable feeling or sensation that is relieved by carrying out the movement (the tic). When tics are suppressed, this sensation continues, and the urge to move increases in intensity. The subsequent movement provides relief, and there may even be an increase of tic movements to obtain this relief if the tics have been suppressed for a considerable period of time. There are two other dyskinesias in which the patient experiences such sensations with an urge to carry out a movement. These are akathisia (a feeling of restlessness that is relieved by moving) and the restless legs syndrome (a feeling of crawling sensations in the skin of the legs that is also relieved by moving). It is of interest that both akathisia (Walters, Hening, Chokroverty, & Fahn, 1985) and the restless legs syndrome (Walters, Hening, Cote, & Fahn, 1986) can be improved with opioids. Perhaps tics have a similar pharmacologic response.

Stress and Relaxation. As is the case for other dyskinesias, emotional stress can increase the severity and frequency of tics. Likewise, relaxation can decrease the abnormal movements of the dyskinesias, including tics. There is one exception, however. Many patients with tics who have spent much of the day suppressing them in public will have an outpouring of tics in the privacy of their home. This tends to coincide with a period of relaxation, including the watching of television.

Concentrating on a mental task usually suppresses the tics. Perhaps such mental activity interferes with the expression of the unpleasant sensation that precedes the tics.

    Presence During Sleep. Sleep studies have revealed that tics occur during REM and NREM sleep (Glaze, Frost, & Jankovic, 1983). This contrasts with most other dyskinesias with a few exceptions. One of these is the restless legs syndrome. One part of its spectrum is periodic movements in sleep, formerly and erroneously called nocturnal myoclonus (Lugaresi, Cirignotta, & Montagna, 1986; Walters et al., 1986). Myoclonus, particularly rhythmical segmental myoclonus, and the painful legs–moving toes syndrome both occur when the patient is awake or asleep, but these are continuous dyskinesias and are not abrupt on a background of normal motor behavior.

    Table 3.1 summarizes the phenomenology of motor tics and lists the other dyskinesias that must be differentiated from tics.

Table 3.1. Phenomenology of Motor Tics and the Dyskinesias Resembling Them

Phenomenology of Tics	Other Dyskinesias
Simple clonic tics	Myoclonic jerks
	Choreic twitches
Complex clonic tics	Akathitic movements
	Mannerisms
Complex and simple tonic tics	Dystonic movements
Ocular movements	Opsoclonus
	Ocular myoclonus
	Oculogyric spasms
Abruptness	Paroxysmal dyskinesias
	Mild chorea
	Arrhythmic myoclonus
	Hyperekplexia
Suppressibility	Akathitic movements
	Stereotypic movements
	Choreic movements
Sensation relieved by tic	Akathitic movements
	Restless legs syndrome
Increase with stress	Most dyskinesias
Lessens with relaxation	Most dyskinesias
Increases with relaxation	None
Present during sleep	Periodic movements in sleep
	Painful legs, moving toes
	Rhythmical segmental myoclonus

Differentiation from Other Motor Dyskinesias

Table 3.2 lists the various types of hyperkinetic disorders. Only some of them need be considered because others, such as tremor, show no resemblance to tics. A more full description is available elsewhere (Fahn, in press).

Brief definitions and descriptions of the motor phenomenology of the dyskinesias listed in Table 3.1 are presented in alphabetical order to allow the reader to differentiate between these and motor tics. Identification of the dyskinesia is based on clinical observations, with little help coming from laboratory tests. Once the appropriate identification of the dyskinesia is made, then a clinical determination of the etiology of the movement disorder is attempted.

1. *Akathitic movements.* Akathisia (from the Greek, meaning unable to sit still) refers to a feeling of inner restlessness, which is relieved by moving about. The movements carried out by the patient with akathisia are fairly typical. When sitting, the patient may stroke the scalp, cross and uncross the legs, rock the trunk, squirm in the chair, and often get out of the chair and pace back and forth. Occasionally, the patient may make repeated moaning sounds. If akathisia affects a specific body part, that part may give a sensation of burning or pain, again relieved by moving that body part. Akathisia most commonly occurs as a side effect of neuroleptic

---

Table 3.2.   Hyperkinetic Movement Disorders

1. Akathitic movements
2. Athetosis
3. Ballism
4. Chorea
5. Dysmetria
6. Dyssynergia
7. Dystonia
8. Hyperekplexia
9. Myoclonus
10. Nocturnal dyskinesias
11. Painful legs–moving toes
12. Paroxysmal dyskinesias
13. Periodic movements in sleep
14. Restless legs
15. Stereotypy
16. Stiff-man syndrome
17. Tics
18. Tremor

medication. As such, it presents in two forms; acute akathisia and tardive akathisia. Acute akathisia occurs in the early phases of neuroleptic therapy and worsens as the dosage of medication is increased; it is relieved by discontinuing the neuroleptic. Tardive akathisia commonly accompanies tardive dyskinesia and, like tardive dyskinesia, is aggravated by discontinuing the neuroleptic; it is usually relieved by increasing the dose of the offending drug that masks it.

2. *Ballism.* Ballistic movements are very-large-amplitude choreic movements. Because of the speed of choreic movements, these large-amplitude excursions are expressed by flinging and flailing movements when they involve proximal musculature. Ballism is most frequently unilateral and due to a lesion of the contralateral subthalamic nucleus or multiple small infarcts (lacunes) in the contralateral striatum.

3. *Chorea.* Choreic movements are involuntary, irregular, purposeless, nonrhythmic, abrupt, rapid, flowing, unsustained movements. Such movements can be partially suppressed, and the patient with chorea can "hide" some of the movements by incorporating them into semipurposeful movements, known as parakinesia. Chorea is usually accompanied by motor impersistence, the inability to maintain a sustained contraction. Motor impersistence is detected by inability to keep the tongue protruded and by "milkmaid" grips due to inability to keep the fist in a sustained tight grip.

4. *Dystonia.* Dystonic movements are twisting movements that tend to be sustained at the peak of the movement, are frequently repetitive, and often progress to prolonged abnormal postures. The speed of the movement varies widely from slow (athetotic dystonia) to shocklike (myoclonic dystonia). Symptomatic dystonia often begins as fixed postures (tonic form), but idiopathic dystonia usually begins as the kinetic (clonic) form. Idiopathic dystonic movements typically occur when the affected body part is carrying out a voluntary action (action dystonia) and are not present when that body part is at rest. With progression of the disorder, dystonic movements can appear when other parts of the body are voluntarily moving (overflow), and with further progression the dystonic movements can be present when the affected body part is "at rest."

5. *Hyperekplexia.* The term *hyperekplexia* refers to excessive startle reaction to a sudden, unexpected stimulus in which the motor reaction can be a short or prolonged complex motor act.

6. *Myoclonus.* Myoclonic jerks are sudden, brief, shocklike involun-

tary movements caused by muscular contractions (positive my-oclonus) or inhibitions (negative myoclonus). The most common form of negative myoclonus is asterixis. Myoclonus can appear as irregular (arrhythmic) jerks, rhythmical jerks that persist even during sleep, such as in palatal myoclonus, and oscillatory jerks that occur in a burst and then fade. Rhythmic myoclonus is typi-cally due to a structural lesion of the brain stem or spinal cord (segmental myoclonus). Myoclonic jerks occurring in different body parts are often synchronized, a feature that may be specific for myoclonus. Another typical feature of myoclonus is that the jerks can be triggered by sudden stimuli, such as sound, light, visual threat, or movement. Myoclonus has a relationship to epi-lepsy in that both seem to be the result of hyperexcitable neurons.

7. *Painful legs–moving toes.* This is a syndrome in which the toes of one foot are in continual flexion–extension motion, associated with a deep pain in the ipsilateral leg. In some patients with this disorder but not in others, there is evidence for a lesion of one of the lumbar roots.

8. *Paroxysmal dyskinesias.* The paroxysmal dyskinesias are composed of various types of dyskinetic movements, particularly chore-oathetosis and dystonia, that occur "out of the blue" and then disappear after minutes to hours. The patient can remain normal for months between attacks, or there can be several attacks per day. Paroxysmal kinesigenic choreoathetosis is the best described; it is stimulated by a sudden movement, lasts seconds to a few min-utes, can be hereditary or symptomatic, and usually can be treated with anticonvulsants. In addition to being choreic, these movements can be dystonic. Paroxysmal (nonkinesigenic) dys-tonia is often familial, is triggered by stress, fatigue, caffeine, or alcohol, and can last minutes to hours. It is more difficult to treat than the kinesigenic variety, but often responds to clonazepam and sometimes to acetazolamide.

9. *Periodic movements in sleep and restless legs syndrome.* Periodic move-ments in sleep are part of the spectrum of the restless legs syn-drome; one or more parts of the spectrum may be present in any individual. The most common is the presence of unpleasant dysesthesias in the legs occurring in the evening and at night, typically described as crawling sensations beneath the skin, and relieved by walking about. Periodic movements in sleep are another part of the clinical spectrum, in which dorsiflexion of the foot and flexion of the knee and thigh occur simultaneously at intervals around 20 seconds, and which can awaken the patient from sleep. This type of dyskinesia had previously been known

(incorrectly) as nocturnal myoclonus. Other dyskinesias, such as brief myoclonic jerks or more sustained dystonic movements, may occur while the patient is awake in the late evening.

10. *Stereotypy.* Stereotypic movements are simple or complex movements that repeat themselves continuously. These can be as rapid as choreic movements, but their repetition, in contrast to the flowing, nonrepetitive movements of chorea, separates these two disorders. Classical tardive dyskinesia presents as stereotypy, and most commonly affects the oral–buccal–lingual region, although the extremities and trunk can also be involved.

PHONIC TICS

Definitions and Phenomenology

When tics involve the vocal apparatus to cause the production of sounds, the resulting noises are called phonic or vocal tics. Sniffing can also be a phonic tic, involving nasal passages and not the vocal apparatus. In order to combine all sounds due to tics, the term *phonic tics* seems more appropriate than the term *vocal tics*. Phonic tics can range from single throat clearing sounds and grunts to verbalizations and the utterance of obscenities (coprolalia). Thus like motor tics, phonic tics can be divided into simple and complex tics. Throat clearing and sniffing represent simple phonic tics, whereas barking and verbalizations would be considered complex phonic tics. Coprolalia can be a form of complex phonic tics. If vocalizations are present, the term *Tourette's syndrome* is usually applied to the patient. This syndrome lies within the spectrum of tics.

Differentiation of Phonic Tics

Involuntary phonations occur in only a few other neurologic disorders beside tics. These include the moaning seen with akathisia and parkinsonism, and L-dopa toxicity; the brief sounds seen in oromandibular dystonia and Huntington's disease; and the sniffing and spitting occasionally encountered in Huntington's disease.

ETIOLOGIC DIFFERENTIATION OF TICS

In addition to discussing the differential diagnosis of motor and phonic phenomena that resemble tics, we need to discuss the etiologic differentiation of tics, that is, tics with other than idiopathic or hereditary causes. Acquired causes of tics include drugs, carbon monoxide intoxication, degenerative diseases, head trauma, and encephalitis (Fahn, 1982). In the last few years neurologists have realized that tics are one part of the spectrum of the neuroacanthocytosis syndrome (Spitz, Jankovic, & Killian, 1985).

Some children and adults have tics with other forms of neurologic disorders. It is not known, however, whether the occurrence of tics in these other disorders represents the coincidental occurrence of independent events or exceeds that expected by random coincidence. There have been single case reports of Tourette's syndrome with Duchenne muscular dystrophy (Lewis & Bertorini, 1982), tuberous sclerosis (Matthews, 1981), and anorexia nervosa (Annibali, Kales, & Tan, 1986; Larocca, 1984). Although a possible relationship to epilepsy has been suggested (Marra, Reynolds, & Dahl, 1980), a review of 200 Tourette's syndrome patients found no more than the expected number of patients who had a coexisting seizure disorder (Erenberg, Cruse, & Rothner, 1986).

The largest number of reports have described the occurrence of Tourette's syndrome in patients with various combinations of mental retardation, abnormal behavior, and sensory deprivation. Some of these patients have had chromosomal abnormalities identified as the cause of their developmental abnormalities. These include cases in patients with XYY karyotype (Merskey, 1974), triple X and 9p mosaicism (Singh, Howe, Jordan, & Hara, 1982), fragile X syndrome (Kerbeshian, 1984), and trisomy 21 (Barabas, Wardell, Sapiro, & Matthews, 1986; Karlinsky, Sandor, Berg, Moldofsky, & Crawford, 1986; Lederman, Erenberg, & Wassman, 1985). Tourette's syndrome and mental retardation have been described in patients with visual impairment (Burd & Kerbeshian, 1985; Kerbeshian & Burd, 1986; Parraga & Butterfield, 1983) as well as hearing impairment (Golden & Greenhill, 1981). These sensory impaired patients all had autisticlike behavior, and others have also described Tourette's syndrome in patients with autism (Barabas & Matthews, 1983; Realmuto & Main, 1982). Psychotic behavior was found in most cases of Tourette's syndrome reported in mentally retarded persons (Golden & Greenhill, 1981; Reid, 1984).

The diagnosis of Tourette's syndrome in patients with various developmental disorders may be difficult since peculiar motor movements and language distortions are not unusual in retarded, autistic, or psychotic persons (Volkmar & Bregman, Chapter 11, this volume). Such persons may have complex stereotyped movements, compulsive behavior, odd vocalizations, echolalia, echopraxia, or coprolalia. A further confounding factor is introduced when patients are treated with neuroleptic drugs, since both persistent and transient Tourette's syndrome have been reported following withdrawal of chronic neuroleptics (Klawans, Falk, Nausieda, & Weiner, 1978; Singer, 1981). Careful attention to the history of ever-changing motor and vocal tics, however, usually allows a distinction to be made between Tourette's syndrome and the manneristic behavior otherwise present in developmentally handicapped persons.

Both the tics of Tourette's syndrome and the manneristic behavior of developmental disorders may represent a common clinical expression of underlying central nervous system dysfunction. The incidence of reported abnormal historical events and abnormal findings on physical examination is considerably higher in such patients than in those with only Tourette's syndrome. Possible neurochemical abnormalities may link together the movement disorders seen in developmental abnormalities, Tourette's syndrome, and the reactions to withdrawal of neuroleptics (Cohen & Young, 1977).

There are practical implications as to whether the movements and mannerisms seen in patients with various neurodevelopmental disorders are due to Tourette's syndrome or not. Although a variety of neuroleptic agents have been used, the best anti-tic response in Tourette's syndrome has been seen with haloperidol, fluphenazine, and pimozide (See Part 4 of this volume). A trial of one of these agents is warranted if the motor and vocal tics are causing management problems or a decline in the individual's usual level of function. Proper treatment can benefit the patient by eliminating socially disruptive behavior. The response to medication in multiply handicapped persons is no different than that in persons with only Tourette's syndrome. Drug effect must be monitored closely to avoid the possible side effects of depression, cognitive blunting, lethargy, and excessive weight gain. The possibility of an increased risk of dyskinetic reactions has been raised (Golden & Greenhill, 1981), and drug dosages should be increased slowly.

Other medications that can be used in the treatment of patients with Tourette's syndrome and other neurologic disorders include clonidine and clonazepam. On the other hand, medications commonly used for hyperactivity and attentional deficits must be used with caution. Golden (1974) was the first to report the development of Tourette's syndrome after the administration of methylphenidate. Since then, this occurrence has been reported following the use of dextroamphetamine and pemoline. The use of psychostimulants is not always associated with development or increase in tic activity (Erenberg, Curse, & Rothner, 1985), but it is possible that persons with central nervous system dysfunction may be more sensitive to this reaction, which is thought to be secondary to increased dopaminergic activity.

It is hoped that further advances in our understanding of the basic mechanisms in Tourette's syndrome and in developmental disorders will clarify the relationship between involuntary movements and manneristic behavior seen in both conditions. The diagnosis of Tourette's syndrome in a person previously diagnosed as mentally retarded, autistic, or psychotic does not mean that the developmental disorder was caused by Tourette's syndrome. It should represent not an additional burden to the patient, but rather a possible clue to a medication program that may alleviate some of his or her medical problems.

REFERENCES

Andermann, F., & Andermann, E. (1986). Excessive startle syndromes: Startle disease, jumping, and startle epilepsy. *Advances in Neurology, 43,* 321–338.

Annibali, J.A., Kales, J.D. & Tan, T. L. (1986). Anorexia nervosa in a young man with Tourette's syndrome. *Journal of Clinical Psychiatry, 47,* 324–326.

Barabas, G., & Matthews, W.S. (1983). Coincident infantile autism and Tourette syndrome: A case report. *Dev Behav Pediatr, 4,* 280–281.

Barabas, G., Wardell, B., Sapiro, M., & Matthews, W.S. (1986). Coincident Down's and Tourette's syndrome: Three case reports. *Journal of Child Neurology, 1,* 358–360.

Burd, L., & Kerbeshian, J. (1985). Tourette syndrome, atypical pervasive developmental disorder and Ganser syndrome in a 15-year-old, visually impaired, mentally retarded boy. *Canadian Journal of Psychiatry 30,* 74–76.

Cohen, D.J, & Young, G.J. (1977). Neurochemistry and child psychiatry. *Journal of the American Academy of Child Psychiatry, 16,* 353–411.

Erenberg, G., Cruse, R.P., & Rothner, A.D. (1985). Gilles de la Tourette's syndrome: Effects of stimulant drugs. *Neurology, 35,* 1346–1348.

Erenberg, G., Cruse, R.P. & Rothner, A.D. (1986). Tourette syndrome: An analysis of 200 pediatric and adolescent cases. *Cleveland Clinic Quarterly, 53,* 127–131.

Fahn, S. (1982). The clinical spectrum of motor tics. *Advances in Neurology, 35,* 341–344.

Fahn, S. (in press). What are the basal ganglia diseases? In L. Findley & M. Gresty (Eds.), *Disorders of the basal ganglia.* New York: Macmillan.

Glaze, D.G., Frost, J.D., & Jankovic, J. (1983). Gilles de la Tourette's syndrome. Disorder of arousal. *Neurology, 33,* 586–592.

Golden, G.S. (1974). Gilles de la Tourette's syndrome following methylphenidate administration. *Developmental Medicine and Child Neurology, 16,* 76–78.

Golden, G.S., & Greenhill, L. (1981). Tourette syndrome in mentally retarded children. *Mental Retardation, 19,* 17–19.

Karlinsky, H., Sandor, P., Berg, J.M., Moldofsky, H., & Crawford, E. (1986). Gilles de la Tourette's syndrome in Down's syndrome—A case report. *British Journal of Psychiatry, 148,* 601–604.

Kerbeshian, J., & Burd, L. (1986). A second visually impaired, mentally retarded male with pervasive developmental disorder, Tourette disorder and Ganser's syndrome: A diagnostic classification and treatment. *International Journal of Psychiatry in Medicine, 16,* 67–75.

Kerbeshian, J., Burd, L., & Martsolf, J.D. (1984). Fragile X syndrome associated with Tourette symptomatology in a male with moderate mental retardation and autism. *Dev Behav Pediatr, 5,* 201–203.

Klawans, H.L., Falk, D.K., Nausieda, P.A., & Weiner, W.J. (1978). Gilles de la Tourette syndrome after long-term chlorpromazine therapy. *Neurology, 28,* 1064–1068.

Lance, J.W. (1977). Familial paroxysmal dystonic choreoathetosis and its differentiation from related syndromes. *Annals of Neurology, 2,* 285–293.

Larocca, F.E.F. (1984). Gilles de la Tourette's (the movement disorder). The association with a case of anorexia nervosa in a boy. *International Journal of Eating Disorders, 3,* 89–93.

Lederman, R.J., Erenberg, G., & Wassman, E.R. (1985). Tourette's syndrome in patients with mongolism. *Neurology, 35,*(Suppl. 1), 223.

Lewis, J.A., & Bertorini, T.E. (1982). Duchenne muscular dystrophy and Tourette syndrome. *Neurology, 32,* 329.

Lugaresi, E., Cirignotta, F., Coccagna, G., & Montagna, P. (1986). Nocturnal myoclonus and restless legs syndrome. *Advances in Neurology, 43,* 295–307.

Marra, T.R., Reynolds, N.C., & Dahl, D.S. (1980). Tourette syndrome, an acquired encephalopathy? A report of two cases with epileptiform dysrhythmia. *Clinical Electroencephalography, 11,* 118–123.

Matthews, K.L. (1981). Familial Gilles de la Tourette's syndrome associated with tuberous sclerosis. *Texas Medicine 77,* 46–49.

Merskey, H. (1974). A case of multiple tics with vocalization (partial syndrome of Gilles de la Tourette) and XYY karyotype. *British Journal of Psychiatry, 125,* 593–594.

Parraga, H.C., & Butterfield, P.T. (1983). Tourette's syndrome and anophthalmia in a girl: Complex differential diagnosis. *Canadian Journal of Psychiatry, 28,* 206–209.

Realmuto, G.M., & Main, B. (1982). Coincidence of Tourette's disorder and infantile autism. *Journal of Autism and Developmental Disorders, 12,* 367–372.

Reid, A.H. (1984). Gilles de la Tourette syndrome in mental handicap. *Journal of Mental Deficiency Research, 28,* 81–83.

Singer, W.D. (1981). Transient Gilles de la Tourette syndrome after chronic neuroleptic withdrawal. *Developmental Medicine and Child Neurology, 23,* 518–521.

Singh, D.N., Howe, G.L., Jordan, H.W., & Hara, S. (1982). Tourette's syndrome in a black woman with associated triple X and 9p mosaicism. *Journal of the National Medical Association, 74,* 675–682.

Spitz, M.C., Jankovic, J., & Killian, J.M. (1985). Familial tic disorder, parkinsonism, motor neuron disease, and acanthocytosis: A new syndrome. *Neurology, 35,* 366–370.

Walters, A., Hening, W., Chokroverty, S., & Fahn, S. (1985). Opioid responsiveness of neuroleptic-induced akathisia. *Annals of Neurology, 18,* 137.

Walters, A., Hening, W., Cote, L., & Fahn, S. (1986). Dominantly inherited rest-less legs with myoclonus and periodic movements of sleep: A syndrome re-lated to the endogenous opiates? In S. Fahn, C.D. Marsden, & M.H. Van Woert (Eds.) *Myoclonus.* Advances in Neurology. (Vol 43). New York: Raven, 309–319.

CHAPTER FOUR

Clinical Assessment of Tic Disorder Severity

James F. Leckman
Kenneth E. Towbin
Sharon I. Ort
Donald J. Cohen

OVERVIEW

The extensive research over the past 25 years into the development of assessment measures for tic disorders speaks to the demand in both clinical practice and research for specific, valid, and reliable instruments. In the clinical setting, instruments are useful to document the course of illness and to monitor the waxing and waning of symptoms during treatment. These needs arise similarly in drug research trials and metabolic studies (Leckman, Walkup, Riddle, Towbin, & Cohen, 1987; Shapiro & Shapiro, 1984). Other research strategies may require special methods of assessment such as self-report survey instruments for epidemiologic studies (Stefl, 1983), or measures of tic number, frequency, intensity, duration, complexity, and anatomical distribution for phenomenological or natural history studies. Family-genetic and twin studies, a new and promising area of investigation, also have particular requirements in order to permit decisions on whether family members have ever had TS during their lifetime.

As clinical knowledge and theoretical advances accrue, new instruments are often needed to study in more detail aspects of tic disorders. These investigations, using refined assessment techniques, can lead to further advances in the field. For example, clinical observation suggested that obsessive–compulsive symptoms (OCS) are frequently associated with Tourette's syndrome (TS) (Gilles de la Tourette, 1885; Meige & Feindel, 1907). This led to more detailed and exact questions about the occurrence of OCS in family-genetic and epidemiologic studies (Pauls, Kruger, Leckman, Cohen, & Kidd, 1984). The preliminary results of such a study using this advanced methodology suggest that some forms of obsessive-compulsive disorder (OCD) may be etiologically related to TS and other tic disorders. If confirmed, these provocative results may lead to revisions of nosology, assessment instruments, and methodology in treatment studies in both TS and OCD research.

DIFFICULTIES IN ASSESSMENT

Although the symptoms associated with TS range from barely discernible to dramatic, most are observable, overt clinical phenomena. Such a range of severity and form makes objective quantification difficult. The complexities of behavioral manifestations (Leckman & Cohen, Chapter 1, this volume) often defy specification and direct subject-to-subject comparison. For example, how are we to understand a patient's sequence of twisting the wrist, bringing his hand to his mouth, and then alternatively kissing and biting his wrist? Should this be one tic or many? How is it possible to compare this patient's symptoms to those of another who has only nonstop guttural noises?

A second formidable problem is the variability of symptom expression over time. The waxing and waning of symptoms over weeks to months, progressing from one set of motor and phonic tics to another, poses similar difficulties in comparison and specification. Are the eye blinking and facial grimace observed today "equal" in some sense to last month's shoulder jerk? Even during brief intervals of minutes to hours the environmental influences and the capacity to suppress symptoms voluntarily pose substantive obstacles to efforts to assess the symptoms objectively. A common example is provided by the patient who, for instance, arrives in the consulting room displaying an occasional tic, while his distraught parents report that he was "tic"-ing nonstop in the car minutes earlier.

A third problem stems from the need for reliable historical information from multiple informants, most of whom have a limited knowledge of TS and have no experience in making valid severity estimates across patients. For the mother whose son just started making low clicking noises in school, his symptoms may be "extreme," or the "worst ever," when she compares them to his earlier eye blinking and transient throat-clearing tics.

AVAILABLE METHODS

The model for clinical and research assessments is derived from the traditional global impression formed in the consulting room after direct patient observation and review of the available historical information from multiple sources (patient, family members, teachers).

Parental and Self-Reports

Structured parental and/or self-reports have been devised for use in epidemiologic studies, family-genetic studies, and longitudinal studies. Examples include the Tourette Syndrome Questionnaire (TSQ) (Jagger, Prusoff, Cohen, Kidd, Carbonari, & John, 1982), originally developed for an epidemiologic survey. The TSQ's best application appears to be systematically obtaining relevant historical information such as demographic data, developmental history, the course of tic behaviors, and the impact of TS on the individual's life. A quick review of this instrument prior to a clinical consultation can promote a more focused, productive interview. Another parent and/or self-report was created for the landmark needs assessment survey conducted for the TSA of Ohio by Stefl and coworkers (1983).

The Tourette Syndrome Symptom List (Appendix 4.1), a clinical instrument, was developed at Yale to assist parents in making daily or weekly ratings of tic behaviors (Cohen, Leckman, & Shaywitz, 1984). The form asks the respondent to identify and estimate the frequency and disruption of current tics (simple and complex motor and phonic) and behavioral symptoms. This instrument has been successfully applied in monitoring the longitudinal course of TS patients and documenting changes during drug trials.

None of the instruments comprehensively address the associated "behavioral" symptoms of inattention, impulsivity, motoric hyperactivity, irritability, and mood liability. Currently, ancillary scales, such as the Conners Parent Questionnaire, are necessary to evaluate the symptoms of attention deficit disorder (ADD) (Goyette, Connors & Ulrich, 1978). Coverage of obsessive–compulsive symptoms has proved especially difficult. Part of the difficulty may arise from the need to appreciate the patient's subjective experience of symptoms in a self-rating, and the unreliability of the presence of symptoms alone as a measure of obsessive–compulsive severity. Although several scales, unpublished and not validated, have been used for research in drug trials for obsessive–compulsive disorder, they have not been routinely employed in studies of symptoms in TS patients. As we learn more about the phenomenology of obsessions and compulsions in TS, more appropriate self-rated measures may become available. One scale that may be a promising source of self-report information applicable in both adult and child populations is the Leyton Obsessional Inventory-Child Version (Berg, Rapoport, & Flament, 1986) developed at NIMH for diagnostic assessment of childhood OCD.

While self- or parental reports can be useful adjuncts, the information is often of variable quality. Instruction about their proper use is needed to ensure the validity of the ratings. Reviewing what is required for accurate rating is crucial. One caveat to be kept in mind is that under some circumstances the use of self- or parental reports can be detrimental. Clinical experience suggests that, using these instruments, families who anxiously keep children under constant "tic surveillance" may create an environment of undue pressure that can increase family tension and tic symptoms.

Clinician–Observer Ratings

Efforts to develop valid and reliable clinician ratings have led in two directions. One is to base ratings on a microanalysis of tic behaviors recorded during videotaped protocols. Currently, the most highly developed of these methods were devised by Shapiro and Shapiro (1984) and Tanner, Goetz, and Klawans (1982). Both call for counting tics under several different conditions (alone and with examiner in room; quietly sitting and then reading or performing some other task). Despite the minute-to-minute variations in the frequency of tics observed in response to novel or highly structured settings, high levels of reliability can be achieved using these techniques. Meaningful changes in clinical state can be successfully documented (Shapiro & Shapiro, 1984). Countering these advantages, these methods are cumbersome, require technical support, and are labor-intensive. Nevertheless, they can provide a valuable clinical record and may provide a direct insight into the pathophysiology of the disorder.

A second approach is to make clinical judgments about the frequency and disruption of tic behaviors after examining the patient and reviewing details of the patient's progress over a time interval. The Tourette Syndrome Severity Scale (TSSS) developed by Shapiro and Shapiro (1984) and the Tourette Syndrome Global Scale (TSGS) developed at Yale (Harcherick, Leckman, Detlor, & Cohen, 1984) are the most widely used of these scales (Appendixes 4.2 and 4.3).

The TSSS is a scale developed for use in a clinical trial of pimozide. There are five questions which the clinician must answer: How many tics are there? Are the tics noticeable to others? Do the tics elicit comments? Is the patient considered odd or bizarre? And, do the tics interfere with functioning? (Shapiro, Shapiro, & Eisenkraft, 1983).

The TSGS is a multidimensional scale of TS symptoms and social functioning comprising eight individually rated dimensions. These are subsequently summed into an overall global score. The scale ranges from 0 (no symptoms) to 100 (severe nonstop incapacitating TS symptoms). The TSGS has two domains, tics and social functioning, which contribute equally to the global score and can be used separately. The *tic domain* consists of four dimensions: simple motor tics, complex motor tics, simple phonic tics, and complex phonic tics. Each dimension is rated according to frequency and degree of disruption. The *social function domain* contains three dimensions: behavioral problems, motor restlessness, and level of school or occupational functioning. These social dimensions are each rated on a continuous scale of 0 (no impairment) to 25 (severe impairment).

Preparing for a randomized clinical trial, we have recently assessed the interrater agreement for these scales and examined their concurrent validity. Six raters (four child psychiatrists and two clinical nurse specialists) participated in the study. Each independently rated nine videotaped interviews in which TS patients (9 to 27 years old) and their families were systematically questioned about tic symptoms over the previous week. Other ratings were also performed, including global adjustment on the 100-point Global Adjustment Scale, (GAS) for children (Shaffer et al., 1983) or adults (Endicott, Spitzer, & Fleiss, 1976). The interclass correlations across raters were above .80, indicating a high level of agreement (See Table 4.1). The TSGS tic domain score was not

Table 4.1.   Agreement Between Six Raters on TS Symptomatology

	Intraclass Correlation (r_{cc})
Tourette Syndrome Global Scale (TSGS)	
Overall tics	.89
Overall social functioning	.93
Global score	.94

significantly correlated with the overall level of social adjustment as rated on the GAS (See Table 4.2), suggesting that some degree of discriminant validity exists for these scales. These results are consistent with previous reliability and validity reports on these instruments. (Harcherick, Leckman, Detlor, & Cohen, 1984).

The TSGS permits separate estimates of frequency and disruption across four types of tic behaviors. This scheme has allowed us to examine the relationship between overall severity of motor and phonic tics in 63 TS patients. The results indicate that the four types of tics, simple motor, complex motor, simple phonic, and complex phonic, are partially independent. Frequency and disruption for each tic domain were also highly intercorrelated (see Table 4.3 and Table 4.4).

Both scales require additional development. For the TSGS, for example, the final score has some undesirable psychometric properties in which the multiplication of frequency by disruption scores exaggerates small differences in tic severity and potentially exaggerates the weight

Table 4.2.   Concurrent Validity of the Domain Scores of the Tourette Syndrome Global Scale (TSGS) with the Tourette Syndrome Severity Scale (TSSS) and the Global Adjustment Scale (GAS)

	TSGS		GAS
	Social	Global	
TS Global Scale (TSGS)			
Total tics	.83*	.94***	−.65
Social functioning		.97***	−.92***
Global score			−.85**

* $p < .05$
** $p < .01$
*** $p < .001$

Table 4.3. *Agreement Between Motor and Phonic Tic Severity on the TSGS* *(N = 63)*

TSGS Variable	Pearson Correlation (r)
Total motor vs. total phonic tics	.60
Simple vs. complex motor tics	.59
Simple vs. complex phonic tics	.35

of the social and behavioral scales out of proportion to the tic symptom scales (Harcherick et al., 1984).

Clinician-rated instruments are also available for the assessment of OC symptoms. To date, clinical studies of TS have not included such measures in assessing outcome. The Comprehensive Psychopathology Rating Scale—Obsessive–Compulsive Disorder Subscale (CPRS-OC) (Asberg, Montgomery, and Perris, 1977; Thoren, Asberg, Cronholm & Bertilisson, 1980) and the NIMH obsessive–compulsive rating instrument (Insel, Murphy, Cohen, Alterman, Kilts & Linnoila, 1983) are two measures used for assessment of OC symptoms in drug trials of OCD patients. Although a full discussion of their strengths and weaknesses is beyond the scope of this report, neither is wholly adequate. The recently developed Yale-Brown Obsessive Compulsive Scale shows considerable promise and is the most comprehensive of the available OCD scales (Goodman, Rasmussen, Price, Mazure, Heninger & Charney, 1986). A specific TS-related OC scale may be developed when, and if, specific OC symptoms associated with TS are identified as being characteristic of TS related forms of OCD.

There are no clinician-rated scales to assess ADD symptoms currently available. This may be a result of clinical experience that suggests that in the relaxed, structured confines of the consultation room children with ADDH may appear asymptomatic.

Table 4.4. *Agreement Between Frequency and Disruption for Simple and Complex Motor and Phonic Tics of the TSGS (N = 63)*

TSGS Variables	Pearson Correlation (r)
Simple motor frequency vs. disruption	.69
Complex motor frequency vs. disruption	.79
Simple phonic frequency vs. disruption	.81
Complex phonic frequency vs. disruption	.92

FUTURE DIRECTIONS

Efforts to refine existing tic scales for use in clinical trials and in studies of phenomenology have led to the development of ordinal scales that address the various dimensions of tic behavior including number, frequency, intensity, complexity, interference, and impairment. These scales (Appendix 4.4) are designed to be completed by the clinician after an interview during which the tic behaviors present during the past week are reviewed in some detail. The scales work best when multiple informants are available, as unintentional biases in reporting are frequent. Explicit anchor points for these 6-point ordinal scales have also been drafted and piloted and are included in the Appendix 4.4. Data on the reliability and validity of these measures are currently being collected.

Similar efforts have resulted in anchored Global Clinical Impression Scales for use in tic disorder patients that focus explicitly on tic disorders, obsessive–compulsive disorder, and attention deficit disorder. These 7-point ordinal scales were developed for use in an ongoing clinical trial and have performed reasonably well in that setting (Appendix 4.5). These newly developed scales have not been fully assessed at the present time. In particular, their reliability in large samples with multiple raters has yet to be determined fully.

SUMMARY

Despite the audible and visible nature of most tics, formidable methodological problems arise in attempting to assess rigorously the severity of tic disorders, including problems of definition and comparison. The variability of tics and impact of environmental changes also require that the clinician rely on more than his or her own observations by eliciting information from multiple informants.

Although a number of self-report instruments have been developed, their accuracy is limited by the respondent's awareness of his or her symptoms. They can be valuable adjuncts when efforts are made to educate patients and families about TS.

Valid and reliable clinician rating instruments for the assessment of tic disorders have been developed. Although originally designed as research instruments, several (See Appendixes) may be useful in clinical practice. New instruments are currently being developed.

Preliminary studies suggest that rating the number, frequency, intensity, complexity, and interference of motor and phonic tics as discrete dimensions is valid and useful. These studies also suggest that these dimensions per se do not solely determine the level of impairment.

Other factors such as premorbid social functioning, duration of illness, presence of specific development disorders, ADD, OCD, other psychiatric disorders, and family dysfunction can influence the level of impairment associated with TS.

Further development and revision of the existing instruments are needed, including the validation of psychometric weightings and standardization for populations of patients with varying tic syndromes.

Validation of some of the clinical distinctions explicit in some of the rating instruments may follow in the wake of phenomenologic studies performed in conjunction with neurophysiologic investigations.

REFERENCES

Asberg, M., Montgomery, S.A. & Perris, C., (1977). A comprehensive psychopathological rating scale. *Acta Psychiatrica Scandanavia, 1271,* 5–27.

Berg, C., Rapoport, J.L., & Flament, M. (1986). The Leyton Obsessional Inventory—Child Version. *Journal of the American Academy of Child Psychiatry, 25*(1), 84–91.

Cohen, D.J., Leckman, J.F., & Shaywitz, B.A. (1984). The Tourette syndrome and other tics. In D. Shaffer, A.A. Ehrhardt, & L. Greenwill (Eds.), *The clinical guide to child psychiatry.* New York: Free Press.

Endicott, J., Spitzer, R.L., Fleiss, J.L., et al. (1976). The Clinical Global Scale: A procedure for measuring overall severity of psychiatric disturbance. *Archives of General Psychiatry, 33,* 766–771.

Gilles de la Tourette, G. (1885). Étude sur une affection nerveuse caractérisée par de l'incoordination motrice accompagnée d'echolalie et de coprolalie. *Archives de Neurologie, 9,* 19–42, 158–200.

Goodman WK, Rasmussen SA, Price LH, Mazure C, Heninger GR, and Charney DS. (1986) *Yale-Brown Obsessive Compulsive Scale,* First Edition. Connecticut Mental Health Center, New Haven, CT.

Goyette, C.H., Connors, C.K., & Ulrich, R.F. (1978). Normative data on Revised Connors Parent and Teacher Rating Scales. *Journal of Abnormal Child Psychology, 6,* 221–236.

Harcherick, D.F., Leckman, J.F., Detlor, J. & Cohen D.J. (1984). A new instrument for clinical studies of Tourette's syndrome. *Journal of the American Academy of Child Psychiatry, 23*(2), 153–160.

Insel, T., Murphy, D.L., Cohen, R.M., Alterman, I., Kilts, C., & Linnoila, M. (1983). Obsessive-compulsive disorder. *Archives of General Psychiatry, 40,* 605–612.

Jagger, J., Prusoff, B.A., Cohen, D.J., Kidd, K.K., Carbonari, C.M., & John, K. (1982). The epidemiology of Tourette's syndrome. *Schizophrenia Bulletin, 8*(2), 267–278.

Leckman, J.F., Walkup, J.T., Riddle, M.A., Towbin, K.E., & Cohen, D.J. (1987). Tic Disorders. In H.Y. Meltzer, W. Bunney, J. Coyle, J. David, I. Kopin, C. Schuster,

R. Shader, & G. Simpson, (Eds.), *Psychopharmacology, the Third Generation of Progress.* New York: Raven.

Meige, H., & Feindel, F. (1907). *Tics and Their Ttreatment.* London: Sidney Appleton.

Pauls, D.L., Kruger, S.D., Leckman, J.F., Cohen, D.J., & Kidd, K.K. (1984). The risk of Tourette's syndrome and chronic multiple tics among relatives of Tourette's syndrome patients obtained by direct interview. *Journal of the American Academy of Child Psychiatry, 23*(2), 134–137.

Pauls, D.L., Leckman, J.F., Towbin, K.E., Zahner, G.E.P. & Cohen, D.J. (1986). A possible genetic relationship exists between Tourette's syndrome and obsessive-compulsive disorder. *Psychopharmacology Bulletin, 22,* 730–733.

Shaffer, D., Gould, M.S., Brasic, J., Ambrosini, P., Fisher, P., Bird, H., & Aluwahalia, S. (1983). A children's global assessment scale. *Archives of General Psychiatry, 40,* 1228–1231.

Shapiro, A.K., Shapiro, E., & Eisenkraft, G.J. (1983). Treatment of Gilles de la Tourette syndrome with pimozide. *American Journal of Psychiatry, 140,* 1183–1186.

Shapiro, A.K., Shapiro, E. (1984). Controlled study of pimozide vs. placebo in Tourette's syndrome. *Journal of the American Academy of Child Psychiatry, 23*(2), 161–173.

Stefl, M.E. (1983). *The Ohio Tourette Study.* School of Planning, University of Cincinnati.

Tanner, C.M., Goetz, G.G., & Klawans, H.L. (1982). Cholinergic mechanisms in Tourette syndrome. *Neurology, 32,* 1315–1317.

Thoren, P., Asberg, M., Cronholm, B., & Bertilisson, L. (1980). Clomipramine treatment of obsessive compulsive disorder. *Archives of General Psychiatry, 37,* 1281–1295.

Appendix 4.1. Tourette Syndrome Symptom List (Revised - TSSL)

Name of patient _____   ID# _____

Date _____

Rate each symptom by putting the appropriate number in the box each day. (Use the reverse side for any detailed comments).

0 = Not at all or symptom free.	3 = Very much.
1 = Just a little.	4 = Extreme.
2 = Pretty much.	5 = Almost always.

Rater: _____

☐ Patient ☐ Father
☐ Mother   ☐ Other

Date	MON	TUE	WED	THU	FRI	SAT	SUN	SUM OF 1–11 MON – SUN		
SIMPLE MOTOR 1. Eyeblinking										
2. Other facial tics										
3. Head jerks								# OF SYMPTOMS 1–11 MON – SUN		
4. Shoulder jerks										
5. Arm movements										
6. Finger or hand movements										
7. Stomach jerks										
8. Kicking leg movements										
9. Tense parts of body										
10. Other:										
11. Other:										

(continued)

Appendix 4.1. *Tourette Syndrome Symptom List* (Continued)

Date	MON	TUE	WED	THU	FRI	SAT	SUN	
COMPLEX MOTOR 12. Touching part of body								
13. Touching other people								
14. Touching objects								
15. Can't start actions								
16. Hurts self								
17. Finger or hand tapping								
18. Hopping								
19. Picks at things (clothing, etc.)								
20. Copropraxia								
21. Other:								SUM OF 12–22 MON – SUN
22. Other:								# OF SYMPTOMS 12–22 MON – SUN
SIMPLE PHONIC 23. Noises								
24. Grunting								
25. Throat clearing								
26. Coughing								SUM OF 23–28 MON – SUN
27. Other:								# OF SYMPTOMS 23–28 MON – SUN
28. Other:								

66

								SUM OF 29–35 MON – SUN	
COMPLEX PHONIC									
29. Words									
30. Repeats own words/sentences									
31. Repeats others' speech									
32. Coprolalia (obscene words)								# OF SYMPTOMS 29–35 MON – SUN	
33. Insults (lack of inhibition)									
34. Other:									
35. Other:									
BEHAVIOR								SUM OF 36–41 MON – SUN	
36. Argumentative									
37. Poor frustration tolerance									
38. Anger, temper fits								# OF SYMPTOMS 36–41 MON – SUN	
39. Provocative									
40. Other:									
41. Other:									

Appendix 4.2.   Shapiro TS Severity Scale

RATINGS

TICS NOTICEABLE TO OTHERS	TICS ELICIT COMMENTS OR CURIOSITY	PATIENT CONSIDERED ODD OR BIZARRE	TICS INTERFERE WITH FUNCTIONING	INCAPACITATED, HOMEBOUND OR HOSPITALIZED
no (0)	no (0)	no (0)	no (0)	no (0)
very few (.5)	no (0)	no (0)	no (0)	no (0)
some (1)	no (0)	no (0)	no (0)	no (0)
most (2)	possibly (0.5)	no (0)	no (0)	no (0)
all (3)	yes (1)	possibly (1)	occasionally (1)	no (0)
all (3)	yes (1)	yes (2)	yes (2)	no (0)
all (3)	yes (1)	yes (2)	yes (2)	yes (1)

SUM OF RATINGS ———

GLOBAL SEVERITY RATING

0) NONE = 0
1) VERY MILD = 0 to < 1
2) MILD = 1 to < 2
3) MODERATE = 2 to < 4
4) MARKED = 4 to < 6
5) SEVERE = 6 to 8
6) VERY SEVERE = > 8

Variables

The TS Severity Scale yields seven variables that can be used for different clinical and research purposes: Tics Noticeable to Others; Tics Elicit Comments or Curiosity; Patient Considered Odd or Bizarre; Tics Interfere with Functioning; Incapacitated, Homebound or Hospitalized; Total Sum of Ratings; and Global Severity Rating.

Tics Noticeable to Others
0   Tics are not present.
0.5 Tics are infrequent or mild and usually are not noticed by employers, teachers, friends or strangers, although some family members or very close friends may be aware of the presence of tics. Symptoms can be diminished significantly or controlled completely in public places.
1   Same as above, except tics are noticed by most friends and occasionally by some employers, teachers, or strangers.
2   Same as above, except tics are noticed by many or most employers, teachers, and strangers.
3   Same as above, except tics are noticed by all individuals.

Tics Elicit Comments or Curiosity
0   Tics are not present or are so infrequent and mild that they are not noticed and do not elicit comments and curiosity from employers, teachers, and friends, although they may be apparent to close family members.
0.5 Tics are more frequent and apparent and possibly elicit comments or curiosity by some individuals.
1   Tics are frequent and apparent and elicit comments or curiosity by all individuals.

Patient Considered Odd or Bizarre
0   Tics are not present or are infrequent and mild and other individuals would not consider the patient odd or bizarre.
1   Tics are more frequent, startling, or distort the appearance of the patient, and some observers consider the patient odd or bizarre.
2   Tics are frequent, startling, or distort the appearance of the patient, and most or all observers consider the patient odd or bizarre.

Tics Interfere with Functioning
0   Tics are absent or are present but do not interfere with academic, vocational, social, or psychological functioning and coordination.
1   Tics occasionally or somewhat interfere with academic, vocational, social, or psychological functioning or coordination.
2   Tics frequently, usually or always interfere with academic, vocational, social or psychological functioning or coordination.

Total Sum of Ratings
   The Total Sum of Ratings is the sum of the ratings of the five factors listed above. The rater has the option of assigning half scores on all factors, e.g., 0.5 for ratings that fall between values.

Global Severity Rating
   The Total Sum of Ratings is assigned a Global Severity Rating using the ranges (listed in parentheses) in the last column.

Appendix 4.3.   Tourette's Syndrome Global Scale (TSGS)

Name _____   Date _____   Rater _____

CODE FOR FREQUENCY

1 = 1 or less in 5 min
2 = 1 in 2–4.9 min
3 = from 1 in 1.9 min to 4 in 1 min
4 = 5 or more in 1 min
5 = virtually uncountable

	FREQUENCY (F)						DISRUPTION (D)					
	None	Rarely	Occasionally	Frequently	Almost Always	Always	Camouflaged	Audible or Visible No Problem	Some Problem	Impaired Functioning	Cannot Function	
SIMPLE MOTOR (SM): Nonpurposeful, tics, jerks and/or movements	0	1	2	3	4	5	1	2	3	4	5	F × D = _____
COMPLEX MOTOR (CM): Purposeful, thoughtful actions (systematic actions), rituals, touching self, others, or objects	0	1	2	3	4	5	1	2	3	4	5	F × D = _____
SIMPLE PHONIC (SP): Nonpurposeful noises, throat clearing, coughing	0	1	2	3	4	5	1	2	3	4	5	F × D = _____
COMPLEX PHONIC (CP): Purposeful, insults, coprolalia, words, distinguishable speech	0	1	2	3	4	5	1	2	3	4	5	F × D = _____

BEHAVIOR (B) (conduct)
0 No problem
5 Subtle problems, normal peer, school, and family relations
10 Some problems, at least one relationship area impaired
15 Clear impairment in more than one area
20 Serious impairment, affects all areas
25 Unacceptable social behavior, constant supervision

MOTOR RESTLESSNESS (MR)
0 Normal movement
5 Adventitial movements, visible, no problem
10 Increased motor restlessness, clearly visible, some problem
15 Clear motor restlessness, moderate problem
20 Mostly in motion but occasionally stops, impaired functioning
25 Nonstop motion, clearly cannot function

SCHOOL AND LEARNING PROBLEMS
0 No problem
5 Low grades
10 Should be or in some special classes, or repeated
15 All special classes
20 Special School
25 Unable to remain in school, home bound

WORK AND OCCUPATION PROBLEMS
0 No problem
5 Stable job, some difficulty
10 Serious problems
15 Lost lots of jobs
20 Almost never employed
25 Unemployed

$$((SM + CM)/2) + ((SP + CP)/2) + ((B + MR + SCHOOL \text{ OR } WORK \text{ PROBLEMS}) \times \tfrac{2}{3}) = GLOBAL \text{ } SCORE$$

71

Appendix 4.4. Yale Global Tic Severity Scale

	Number	Frequency	Intensity	Complexity	Interference
A. Motor Tics	_____	_____	_____	_____	_____

	Number	Frequency	Intensity	Complexity	Interference
B. Phonic Tics	_____	_____	_____	_____	_____

	Number	Frequency	Intensity	Complexity	Interference
C. Total for All Tics	_____	_____	_____	_____	_____

D. Global Severity Ratings
   Motor Tic Score =
   Sum Motor Tics   (Number + Frequency + Intensity
                                        + Complexity + Interference)   = _____
   Phonic Tic Score =
   Sum Phonic Tics   (Number + Frequency + Intensity
                                        + Complexity + Interference)   = _____
   Total Tic score,
                              (Number + Frequency + Intensity
                                        + Complexity + Interference)   = _____

   Overall TS Impairment Rating   = _____
   Global Severity   (Total Tic score + TS impairment) = _____

Description of Motor Symptoms (Check motor tics present during past week)

   Simple Motor Tics: (rapid, darting, "meaningless")

   _____   Eye blinking
   _____   Eye movements
   _____   Nose movements
   _____   Mouth movements
   _____   Facial grimace
   _____   Head jerks/movements
   _____   Shoulder shrugs
   _____   Arm movements
   _____   Hand movements
   _____   Abdominal tensing
   _____   Leg or foot or toe movements
   _____   Other _____

   Complex Motor Tics (slower, "purposeful")

   _____   Eye movements
   _____   Mouth movements
   _____   Facial movements or expressions
   _____   Head gestures or movements

Appendix 4.4.   *Yale Global Tic Severity Scale* (Continued)

_____	Shoulder movements
_____	Arm movements
_____	Hand movements
_____	Blocking
_____	Writing tics
_____	Dystonic postures
_____	Bending or gyrating
_____	Rotating
_____	Leg or foot or toe movements
_____	Blocking
_____	Tic-related compulsive behaviors (touching, tapping, grooming, evening up)
_____	Copropraxia
_____	Self-abusive behavior
_____	Paroxysms of tics (displays), duration _____ seconds
_____	Disinhibited behavior (describe)* _____
_____	Other _____

Description of Phonic Symptoms (Check phonic tics present over the past week)

Simple Phonic Symptoms (fast, "meaningless" sounds)

_____	Sounds, noises (circle: coughing, throat clearing, sniffing, grunting, whistling, animal or bird noises)
_____	Other (list) _____

Complex Phonic Symptoms (language: words, phrases, statements)

_____	Syllables (list) _____
_____	Words (list) _____
_____	Coprolalia (list) _____
_____	Echolalia
_____	Palilalia
_____	Blocking
_____	Speech atypicalities (describe) _____
_____	Disinhibited speech (describe)* _____

Number

  0 *None*

  1 *Single tic*

(*continued*)

Appendix 4.4. Yale Global Tic Severity Scale **(Continued)**

Number

   2 *Multiple discrete tics (2–5)*

   3 *Multiple discrete tics (>5)*

   4 *Multiple discrete tics plus at least one orchestrated pattern of multiple simultaneous or sequential tics where it is difficult to distinguish discrete tics.*

   5 *Multiple discrete tics plus several (>2) orchestrated pattern of multiple simultaneous or sequential tics where it is difficult to distinguish discrete tics.*

Frequency

   0 *None*   No evidence of specific tic behaviors

   1 *Rarely*   Specific tic behaviors have been present during previous week. These behaviors occur infrequently, often not on a daily basis. If bouts of tics occur, they are brief and uncommon.

   2 *Occasionally*   Specific tic behaviors are usually present on a daily basis, but there are long tic-free intervals during the day. Bouts of tics may occur on occasion and are not sustained for more than a few minutes at a time.

   3 *Frequently*   Specific tic behaviors are present on a daily basis. Tic-free intervals as long as an hour are not uncommon. Bouts of tics occur regularly but may be limited to a single setting.

   4 *Almost always*   Specific tic behaviors are present virtually every waking hour of every day, and periods of sustained tic behaviors occur regularly. Tic-free intervals of 5 to 10 minutes can occur. Bouts of tics are common and are not limited to a single setting.

   5 *Always*   Specific tic behaviors are present virtually all the time. Tic-free intervals are difficult to identify and do not last more than 1 or 2 minutes at most.

Intensity

   0 *Absent*

   1 *Minimal intensity*   Tics not visible or audible (based solely on patient's private experience) or tics are less forceful than comparable voluntary actions and are typically not noticed because of their intensity.

   2 *Mild intensity*   Tics are not more forceful than comparable voluntary actions or utterances and are typically not noticed because of their intensity.

   3 *Moderate intensity*   Tics are more forceful than comparable voluntary actions, but are not outside the range of normal expression for comparable voluntary actions or utterances. They may call attention to the individual because of their forceful character.

   4 *Marked intensity*   Tics are more forceful than comparable voluntary actions or utterances and typically have an "exaggerated" character. Such tics frequently call attention to the individual because of their forceful and exaggerated character.

Appendix 4.4.   Yale Global Tic Severity Scale (Continued)

5 *Severe intensity*   Tics are extremely forceful and exaggerated in expression. These tics call attention to the individual and may result in risk of physical injury (accidental, provoked, or self-inflicted) because of their forceful expression.

Complexity

0 *None*   If present, all tics are clearly "simple" (sudden, brief, purposeless) in character.

1 *Borderline*   Some tics are not clearly "simple" in character.

2 *Mild*   Some tics are clearly "complex" (purposive in appearance) and mimic brief "automatic" behaviors, such as grooming, syllables or brief meaningful utterances such as "ah huh," "hi," that could be readily camouflaged.

3 *Moderate*   Some tics are more "complex" (more purposive and sustained in appearance) and may occur in orchestrated bouts that would be difficult to camouflage but could be rationalized or "explained" as normal behavior or speech (picking, tapping, saying "you bet" or "honey," brief echolalia).

4 *Marked*   Some tics are very "complex" in character and tend to occur in sustained orchestrated bouts that would be difficult to camouflage and could not be easily rationalized as normal behavior or speech because of their duration and/or their unusual, inappropriate, bizzare, or obscene character (a lengthy facial contortion, touching genitals, echolalia, speech atypicalities, longer bouts of saying "what do you mean" repeatedly, or saying "fu" or "sh").

5 *Severe*   Some tics involve lengthy bouts of orchestrated behavior or speech that would be impossible to camouflage or successfully rationalize as normal because of their duration and/or extremely unusual, inappropriate, bizarre, or obscene character (lengthy displays or utterances often involving copropraxia, self-abusive behavior, or coprolalia).

Interference

0 *None*

1 *Minimal*   When tics are present, they rarely interrupt the flow of behavior or speech.

2 *Mild*   When tics are present, they occasionally interrupt the flow of behavior or speech.

3 *Moderate*   When tics are present, they frequently interrupt the flow of behavior or speech.

4 *Marked*   When tics are present, they frequently interrupt the flow of behavior or speech, and they occasionally disrupt entirely the intended action or communication.

5 *Severe*   When tics are present, they frequently disrupt intended action or communication.

(continued)

Appendix 4.4.   Yale Global Tic Severity Scale **(Continued)**

Overall TS Impairment

  0 None

  10 *Minimal*   Tics associated with subtle difficulties in self-esteem, family life, social acceptance, or school or job functioning (infrequent upset or concern about tics vis-à-vis the future; periodic, slight increase in family tensions because of tics; friends or acquaintances may occasionally notice or comment about tics in an upsetting way).

  20 *Mild*   Tics associated with minor difficulties in self-esteem, family life, social acceptance, or school or job functioning.

  30 *Moderate*   Tics associated with some clear problems in self-esteem, family life, social acceptance, or school or job functioning (episodes of dysphoria; periodic distress and upheaval in the family; frequent teasing by peers or episodic social avoidance; periodic interference in school or job performance because of tics).

  40 *Marked*   Tics associated with major difficulties in self-esteem, family life, social acceptance, or school or job functioning.

  50 *Severe*   Tics associated with extreme difficulties in self-esteem, family life, social acceptance, or school or job functioning (severe depression with suicidal ideation); disruption of the family (separation/divorce, residential placement); disruption of social ties (severely restricted life because of social stigma and social avoidance; removal from school or loss of job).

*Do not include in ratings of tic behaviors

Appendix 4.5.   Clinical Global Impression Scales for TS, OCD, and ADD

A. TS–Clinical Global Impression Scale

   This scale is based on all available information concerning the adverse impact of clearly defined *tic* behaviors on the individual's life.

Normal	No tic symptoms.
Borderline	Questionable tic symptoms. Does not satisfy criteria for a diagnosis of a definite chronic tic disorder.
Mild	Satisfies DSM-III criteria for a chronic tic disorder. Symptoms do not interfere and are not noticeable to most people.
Moderate	Tic symptoms cause some problems in some areas of functioning and are noticeable to some* people some of the time.
Marked	Tic symptoms cause clear problems in more than one area of functioning. Tics are usually frequent and quite noticeable in most situations most of the time.

Appendix 4.5.   *Clinical Global Impression Scales for TS, OCD, and ADD* (Cont.)

Severe	Tic symptoms cause significant impairment in primary social role such that functioning in "usual" settings is impossible or in serious jeopardy.
Extremely Severe	Tic symptoms are incapacitating and/or have caused serious physical injury.

B. OCD—Clinical Global Impression Scale

B. Overall level of obsessive–compulsive (OC) symptomatology based on all available information.

Normal	No OC symptoms or OC behaviors are developmentally appropriate.
Borderline	Clear symptoms, but they do not impair school, social, or occupational function.
Mild	Mild disturbance in school, social, or occupational function. Meets DSM-III for OCD. Not obvious to those who do not know the patient.
Moderate	Some disturbance in school, social, or occupational function that is noticeable to those who do not know the patient. Patient still able to sustain fair degree of function.
Marked	Impairment of school, social, or occupational functioning to a degree that causes serious concern at home and school or on the job. Ability to continue in full-time employment or study is threatened by OC symptoms.
Severe	At least two areas of function are clearly impaired because of symptoms. School or work function has been reduced because of the inability to carry a full load.
Extremely Severe	Disruption in multiple areas of function including home, school/work, and peer relationships. Patient is or nearly is incapacitated by symptoms. Spends virtually all day engaged in symptom-related behavior.

C. ADD—Clinical Global Impression Scale

Rate on basis of all clinical information available, including interview observations and teacher reports.

Normal, not at all	No reported symptoms of inattention, impulsivity, or hyperactivity.
Borderline	Transient, intermittent, and infrequent symptoms of inattention and/or impulsivity and/or hyperactivity causing no impairment. Does not meet DSM-III criteria for ADDH.

(continued)

Appendix 4.5.   Clinical Global Impression Scales for TS, OCD, and ADD (Cont.)

C. ADD—Clinical Global Impression Scale (Cont.)

Mild	Symptoms sufficient to meet DSM-III criteria for ADDH. Behavior organized and appropriate in environment *not* highly structured. Could function in average home or regular classroom with minimal disruption.
Moderate	Symptoms vary with situation and time. Requires some structuring of environment for behavior to be organized and appropriate, but rarely requires one-to-one supervision.
Marked	Requires considerable structuring of environment to be well organized and appropriate. If supervised at home, has symptoms but is generally well organized and appropriate.
Severe	Pervasive and frequent symptoms of inattention, impulsivity, and hyperactivity. Often requires one-to-one supervision.
Extremely Severe	Unable to function in home or school because of constant, pervasive symptoms of inattention, impulsivity, and hyperactivity. Needs constant supervision (24-hour care).

*NB *Some* refers to those people who come into close contact with the patient.

CHAPTER FIVE

The Epidemiology
of Tourette's Syndrome

Gwendolyn E.P. Zahner
Mariann M. Clubb
James F. Leckman
David L. Pauls

Descriptive epidemiologic studies employing data from population surveys, vital statistics, and public health surveillance systems provide information on the occurrence of disease across time and place. This descriptive information quantifies the impact of a disease in a population, typically reported as the proportion of existing cases in a population (the prevalence rate); the proportion of new cases arising in a specified time period (the cumulative incidence rate); and the proportion of individuals in a population dying from the condition (mortality and case fatality rates).

Epidemiologic rates can provide useful clinical and programmatic information. Prevalence and incidence rates inform clinicians, service planners, and policymakers of the magnitude of the public health problem presented by various disorders. These rates also indicate the level of services needed by different segments of the population. Geographic or demographic variation in disease rates within and across regions may help to identify possible environmental or genetic bases for a disorder. Time trends in disease morbidity and mortality can suggest mechanisms of disease causation and are also important for projecting a population's future service needs.

Modern chronic disease epidemiology examines disease course and etiology by a number of observational and experimental study designs, (e.g., case-control studies, prospective and retrospective cohort studies, and clinical trials). With the exception of clinical trials of treatment efficacy, these analytic research designs have not been employed in the study of Tourette's syndrome, and will not be covered in this chapter. Our discussion will be restricted to descriptive information on population rates, and will critically examine methodological limitations of previous research in this area.

RATES OF TOURETTE'S SYNDROME
IN TREATMENT POPULATIONS

Since the early description of Tourette's syndrome at the Saltpetriere, the rate of this disorder in the general population has been an area of clinical speculation, but not an active area of systematic research. Prior to 1960 there were no reports on the population incidence or prevalence of this disorder, and published rates were based on cases seen in treatment.

Reported rates of Tourette's syndrome within treatment populations are highly variable, although all indicate that it is a rare syndrome. Four studies of the proportion of Tourette's patients among psychiatric patient caseloads reported rates to be 10 per 10,000 child psychiatric clinic outpatients (Lucas, Kauffman, & Morris, 1967), 1.9 in 10,000 children at an educational guidance clinic (Salmi, 1961), and 0.7 in 10,000 in- and outpatients at a child psychiatric clinic and at the Mayo Clinic (Ascher, 1948; Feild, Corbin, Goldstein, & Klass, 1966). Although the rates reported in these studies have been described as "incidence" rates, it should be noted that they do not represent incidence in an epidemiologic sense, that is, the number of new cases occurring in a defined geographic population within a discrete interval of time. These figures should be interpreted as the frequency with which a clinician should expect to see a Tourette's patient in a clinic setting, taking patient characteristics and the time and location of the study into consideration.

There also has been a dramatic shift in the rate at which Tourette's syndrome cases have been reported over time. In the 15 years following Tourette's 1885 report, approximately 50 case descriptions appeared in the clinical literature (Lucas, 1970). A marked decline occurred in the twentieth century, with few new cases reported until the 1960s (Shapiro & Shapiro, 1982).

RATES OF TOURETTE'S SYNDROME IN GEOGRAPHICALLY DEFINED POPULATIONS

Because of the selective nature of clinic populations, rates based on cases arising in defined geographic regions are preferred for describing the population distribution and characteristics of most diseases. The types of surveys required to provide accurate estimates of population rates are difficult to undertake and are not without methodological limitations. Population-based surveys are costly to undertake with rare disorders. Extremely large regions must be surveyed in order to identify enough cases for meaningful research. As an example, a population of 100,000 may only include 10 cases of a rare syndrome, and a sample of 1000 surveyed in that population may not include any cases.

Also, because the cost of direct clinical assessment of subjects in large population surveys is prohibitive, the population is usually screened for the condition under study with comparatively inexpensive, but less accurate, case identification procedures. Some of the typical screening procedures employed to identify Tourette's syndrome cases in a region have included use of medical registries, surveys of clinics and practitioners serving a region, or self-report survey indices administered to a population sample. Thus population surveys of Tourette's syndrome vary in the comprehensiveness and accuracy of the initial screen, and also in the thoroughness of the subsequent clinical diagnostic evaluation.

Only two major surveys of Tourette's syndrome in geographically defined populations have been undertaken in the United States, and a third is in progress. These studies include (1) a survey conducted in Rochester, Minnesota, (Lucas, Beard, Rajput, & Kurland, 1982), (2) a study of Tourette's syndrome in North Dakota (Burd, Kerbeshian, Wikenheiser, & Fisher, 1986), and (3) a survey of Tourette's syndrome in Rochester, New York (Caine, McBride, Chiverton, Bamford, Rediess & Shiao, 1987).

To estimate annual incidence of Tourette's syndrome in Rochester, Minnesota, cases were identified from a computerized index maintained by the Mayo Clinic containing diagnostic information on patients seen at all medical facilities in the surrounding county. Three Tourette's cases, all male, were diagnosed in Rochester in a 12-year period. The annual incidence of Tourette's syndrome in the Rochester population was estimated as .05 per 10,000 (95 percent confidence interval .01 to .12 per 10,000). This rate roughly represents the number of newly diagnosed cases arising in the Rochester population each year. Based on this rate, the authors estimated that 1000 new cases would be diagnosed each year in the United States.

Whereas incidence measures the rate at which *new* cases develop over time, prevalence rates measure the proportion of *all* cases, new and old, in the population. In order to determine the prevalence of Tourette's syndrome in the state of North Dakota, Burd and colleagues (1986) sent questionnaires to all North Dakota pediatricians, psychiatrists, neurologists, family practitioners, mental health centers and psychiatric hospitals, state institutions for the mentally retarded, and the state comprehensive evaluation center. Care providers were instructed to provide age and sex information on all individuals meeting DSM-III criteria for Tourette's syndrome. A very high response rate was obtained. Questionnaires were returned by 72 percent of the care providers contacted; all but two of the remaining physicians provided information by telephone. Symptom information was gathered for most of the cases identified by the participating physicians and centers, and individuals failing to meet DSM-III criteria on the basis of this symptom information were excluded.

The prevalence of Tourette's syndrome among North Dakota children aged 18 and younger was 9.3 and 1.0 per 10,000 for boys and girls, respectively. The prevalence rate among adults was significantly lower: .77 per 10,000 for men, and .22 per 10,000 among women. The male-female ratio also diminished with age, from approximately 9–1 in children to 3–1 in adults. Projecting the North Dakota estimates to the United States population at the 1980 census, there are approximately 6000 men, 2000 women, 30,000 boys, and 3000 girls with Tourette's syndrome. These figures strongly suggest that many TS patients experience a marked reduction in symptomatology during late adolescence, as suggested by Bruun (Chapter 2, this volume). These estimates also assume that Tourette's syndrome does not vary geographically.

Both the Minnesota and North Dakota surveys used cases previously identified in the treatment system for calculating population rates of Tourette's syndrome. In a recent survey of Tourette's syndrome among school-age children in Monroe County, New York, investigators at the University of Rochester attempted to identify all treated and untreated cases in the population by using public media, contacting school health personnel, as well as requesting referrals from physicians and medical centers (Caine, McBride, Chiverton, Bamford, Rediess & Shiao, 1987). All referrals were examined individually by physicians at the university. Most of the children identified with Tourette's syndrome in this survey had a milder form of the disorder than characteristically seen in treatment, less than half requiring pharmacotherapy. Although this survey included many subclinical cases and referrals from sources outside of the medical treatment system, the overall prevalence rate was not higher than observed in the North Dakota survey. Forty-one children were identified with Tourette's syndrome out of a population of 142,636, a prevalence rate of 2.87 per 10,000.

RATES OF TICS IN POPULATION SURVEYS: AN UPPER BOUND FOR PREVALENCE OF TOURETTE'S SYNDROME

To date, there has not been an epidemiologic survey of Tourette's syndrome in which all members of a population, or a representative sample thereof, are evaluated directly for Tourette's syndrome. The aforementioned surveys utilized referrals from care providers in the medical or school systems. Because many Tourette's sufferers do not seek treatment for their condition, the rates based on cases seen in treatment systems are likely to be underestimates. In addition, these studies have revealed comparatively little about the social and demographic characteristics of individuals with Tourette's syndrome, largely because the numbers of cases yielded in population screening were too small to perform extensive analysis.

As an upper limit for an estimate of the population prevalence of Tourette's syndrome, we can turn to information from a number of community surveys of childhood psychiatric disorders that have measured prevalence of tics, twitches, or nervous movements as reported by parents and/or teachers. Symptom inventories such as the Child Behavior Checklist (Achenbach & Edelbrock, 1981), the parent or teacher Child Behavior Questionnaires developed by Rutter, Tizard, and Whitmore (1970) in the Isle of Wight study, or the Vineland Adaptive Behavior Scales (Sparrow, Balla, & Cicchetti, 1984) include an item measuring presence of tics. Few investigators using these measures in community surveys, however, have published prevalence rates for characteristics measured by individual items. Table 5.1 summarizes the

Table 5.1. Frequency of Tics Reported in 5 Major Child Psychiatric Epidemiologic Surveys

Study	Location	Study Design	Description of Tic Measure	% Boys	% Girls
Achenbach & Edelbrock (1981)	Washington, D.C., Maryland, No. Virginia	Probability sample of 1300 children ages 6–18; parent report.	Nervous movements, including twitches	18%*	11%*
Lapouse & Monk (1964)	Buffalo, N.Y.	Systematic sample of households, 482 children ages 6–12; parent report.	Tics	13%	11%
Rutter et al., (1970)	Isle of Wight, Great Britain	Census of 3316 10–11 year olds; parent & teacher report.	Has twitches, mannerisms, tics of face or body	*Parent report:* 5.9% *Teacher report:* 5.4%	2.9% 1.1%
Rutter et al., (1974)	Inner London Borough, Great Britain	Census of 1045 10 year olds; teacher report	Has twitches, mannerisms, tics of face or body	*Non-immigrant:* 8.3% *West-Indian immigrant:* 7.0%	3.6% 5.5%
Verhulst et al., (1985)	Zuid Holland Province	Probability sample of 2600 children ages 4–16; parent report	Nervous movements, including twitches	10%*	9%*

*Rates for children ages 10–11 estimated from author's graphical presentations.

prevalence of tics reported in five major community surveys of child psychiatric disorders. These epidemiologic surveys measure prevalence of tics in probability samples or censuses of geographically defined populations. A description of the sample and the wording of items assessing tics are also denoted in this table. It should be noted that these do not measure chronic, multiple, or severe tics. They are overly inclusive measures of tic behaviors and should not be considered as indices of Tourette's syndrome "caseness."

The prevalence of tics reported in these community surveys is approximately 100 to 1000 times more common than the prevalence of Tourette's syndrome measured in surveys of cases known to the treatment system. The range of prevalence rates in these community surveys itself is quite broad, and to some degree reflects the spectrum of behaviors measured by the item assessing "tics." The highest rates (9 to 18 percent) are observed in surveys utilizing the Child Behavior Checklist (Achenbach & Edelbrock, 1981; Verhulst, Akkerhuis & Althaus, 1985), which measures presence of tics in an item labeled "nervous movements, including twitches." However, Lapouse and Monk's (1964) Buffalo survey, using an item more narrowly defined as "tics," also detected a high prevalence rate: 13 percent of boys and 11 percent of girls.

DEMOGRAPHIC PATTERNS OF TICS OBSERVED IN COMMUNITY SURVEYS

In addition to apparent age effect, a number of demographic patterns for tics are suggested by the five community surveys of childhood psychiatric disorders. One important demographic characteristic is that the gender differences in rates of tics appear to be lower than for Tourette's patients. Male–female ratios for Tourette's syndrome are commonly reported in the range of 3–1, and in the case of Burd and colleagues' North Dakota survey, have been as high as 9–1. By comparison, most community surveys of tics reported male–female ratios as less than 2–1.

Tics have not been shown to vary by *race*. In Rutter and colleagues' (1974) inner London survey, West Indian immigrants reported rates of tics similar to those of British-born respondents. No statistically significant differences in prevalence of tics were observed by race or social class in LaPouse's Buffalo survey. When the analyses were restricted to the lower-class residents of Buffalo, there was a nonsignificant trend toward higher rates among non-Whites (18 percent) than among Whites (10 percent).

Urbanicity may be associated with higher rates of tics: Rutter's inner

London sample reported higher rates of tics than observed in the Isle of Wight, although the difference may not be significant.

METHODOLOGIC PROBLEMS IN ASSESSING THE PREVALENCE OF TOURETTE'S SYNDROME

The instability in reported rates of Tourette's syndrome is perplexing, and is probably more artifact than truth. Since onset of Tourette's syndrome does not appear to have a significant infectious or environmental component, and since no changes have been made in the rate of case fatality or recovery over time, a greater stability in rates is expected than has been reported in the literature.

There are a number of factors that can be implicated in the fluctuating rates of Tourette's syndrome. One determinant appears to be the changing level of clinical and public recognition that this constellation of motor and phonic tics, ranging broadly in severity, frequency, and degree of impact on social functioning, constitutes a clinical entity. This effect can be pronounced, as described in an informal account by the neurologist Oliver Sacks (1985) in his collection of clinical tales.

> *Early in 1971, the* Washington Post, *which had taken an interest in the awakening of my post-encephalitic patients, asked me how they were getting on. I replied, "they are ticcing," which prompted them to publish an article on "Tics." After the publication of this article, I received countless letters, the majority of which I passed on to my colleagues. But there was one patient I did consent to see—Ray.*
>
> *The day after seeing Ray, it seemed to me that I noticed three Touretters in the street in downtown New York. I was confounded, for Tourette's syndrome was said to be excessively rare. It had an incidence, I had read, of one in a million, yet I had apparently seen three examples in an hour. I was thrown into a turmoil of bewilderment and wonder: was it possible that I had been overlooking this all the time, either not seeing such patients or vaguely dismissing them as "nervous," "cracked," "twitchy"? Was it possible that everyone had been overlooking them? Was it possible that Tourette's was not a rarity, but rather common—a thousand times more common, say, than previously exposed. At this point I conceived a whimsical fantasy or private joke: suppose (I said to myself) that Tourette's is very common but fails to be recognized but once recognized is easily and constantly seen. (p. 89)*

Sacks describes a similar situation observed with muscular dystrophy, where hundreds of cases were reported shortly after the syndrome was described by Duchenne in 1950, none of which had been recognized before Duchenne's report. It is clear that case identification is highly dependent on clinical and public awareness of the syndrome. The geographic and chronological variations in rates probably reflect changing patterns of clinical awareness of the syndrome more than any real change in rates. The role of the Tourette Syndrome Association in educating the public about the signs and symptoms of this disorder cannot be discounted in the significant increase in reported cases in the last two decades.

An increased level of awareness among medical professionals should lead to more accurate case identification. Unfortunately, there may also be a tendency for professionals who have limited experience with Tourette's syndrome to overdiagnose the condition, exposing some children with mild and self-limiting tic disorders to unnecessary trials with potent psychoactive medications. Children with tics and comorbid emotional or learning problems may be particularly vulnerable to an incorrect or premature diagnosis of Tourette's syndrome as parents and mental health professionals struggle to make the one diagnosis that will account for all of the child's difficulties.

Lack of specificity in diagnostic criteria, the presence of mild, subclinical cases that satisfy the existing criteria for Tourette's syndrome but are not severe enough to warrant intervention, and the low percentage of cases presenting for treatment represent other major factors limiting accurate determination of the rates of this condition. In this regard, Tourette's syndrome shares many of the problems in epidemiologic investigations of most psychiatric disorders.

Clearly defined diagnostic criteria are a prerequisite for a meaningful and replicable process of counting the number of cases in a population. Some of the major points of disagreement about inclusion and exclusion criteria for diagnosis of Tourette's syndrome are described elsewhere in this volume (Leckman and Cohen, Chapter 1). Several of the areas of controversy will have predictable effects upon reported rates of Tourette's syndrome. One salient area of diagnostic uncertainty is whether Tourette's symptomatology must be sustained until adulthood in order to establish a diagnosis. The higher rates of Tourette's syndrome reported for cohorts of children than cohorts of adults has been attributed in part of the failure to discount transient disorders that do not persist into adulthood (Burd, Kerbeshian, Wikenheiser, & Fisher, 1986).

Similarly, genetic studies suggest that the presence of chronic tics may also be a milder but more prevalent expression of the putative Tourette's gene. Inclusion of individuals with these more limited symptoms in epidemiologic studies can be expected to increase the population rates for this disorder. Thus rates and demographic features of tics reported by epidemiologic surveys of childhood psychiatric disorders, particularly if chronicity can be demonstrated, may provide useful information about the distribution of the Tourette's syndrome phenotype in the population.

Although the accuracy of population rates based on epidemiologic measures shares the limitations of the diagnostic criteria on which they are founded, population surveys can also help advance nosology by describing the natural distribution of component symptomatology and the degree of overlap with other disorders. In order for epidemiologic information to be useful, however, replicable diagnostic procedures must be employed. Ideally, information on symptoms, severity, and certainty of diagnosis should be collected in addition to a DSM-III diagnosis of the syndrome. Although a number of patient and family studies have used structured interview protocols or symptom checklists yielding detailed diagnostic information on frequency of motor and phonic tics and associated features, no clinic- or population-based epidemiologic survey has reported the case diagnostic features on this atomistic level.

There is increasing scientific interest in the field of childhood psychiatric epidemiology in the United States, and it is likely that a number of community surveys of childhood neuropsychiatric disorders will be undertaken in the next decade. Surveys using structured interview schedules with coverage of Tourette's symptomatology (e.g., the National Institute of Mental Health Diagnostic Interview Schedule for Children) have the potential to advance significantly our knowledge of the natural distribution of symptoms, severity, and population characteristics of this disorder. This information, in turn, should provide a scientifically sound body of data for refining diagnostic criteria, for generating hypotheses about factors influencing onset and course, and for planning better services for victims of Tourette's syndrome.

BIBLIOGRAPHY

Achenbach, T.M., & Edelbrock, C.S. (1981). Behavioral problems and competencies reported by parents of normal and disturbed children aged four through sixteen. *Monographs of the Society for Research in Child Development, 46.*

Ascher, E. (1948). Psychodynamic considerations in Gilles de la Tourette's disease (maladie des tics): With a report of 5 cases and discussion of the literature. *American Journal of Psychiatry, 105,* 267–276.

Burd, L., Kerbeshian, J., Wikenheiser, M., & Fisher, W. (1986). Prevalence of Gilles de la Tourette's syndrome in North Dakota adults. *American Journal of Psychiatry, 143,* 787–788.

Caine, E.D., McBride, M.C., Chiverton, P., Bamford, K.A., Rediess, S., & Shiao, S. (1988). Tourette syndrome in Monroe County school children. *Neurology,* (in press).

Field, J.R., Corbin, K.B., Goldstein, N.P., & Klauss, D.W. (1966). Gilles de la Tourette's syndrome. *Neurology, 16,* 453–462.

Lapouse, R., & Monk, M.A. (1964). Behavior deviations in a representative sample of children: Variation between sex, age, race, social class, and family size. *American Journal of Orthopsychiatry, 34,* 436–446.

Lucas, A.R. (1970). Gilles de la Tourette syndrome: An overview. *New York State Journal of Medicine, 70,* 2197–2200.

Lucas, A.R., Beard, C.M., Rajput, A.H., & Kurland, L.T. (1982). Tourette syndrome in Rochester, Minnesota, 1968–1979. In A.J. Friedhoff & T.N. Chase (Eds.), *Gilles de la Tourette Syndrome.* New York: Raven.

Lucas, A.R., Kauffman, P.E., & Morris, E.M. (1967). Gilles de la Tourette's disease: A clinical study of fifteen cases. *Journal of the American Academy of Child Psychiatry, 6,* 700–722.

Rutter, M., Tizard, J., & Whitmore, K. (Eds.). (1970). *Education, Health and Behavior.* London: Longman.

Rutter, M., Yule, W., Berger, M., Yule, B., Morton, J., & Bagley, C. (1974). Children of West Indian immigrants—I. Rates of behavioral deviance and psychiatric disorder. *Journal of Child Psychology & Psychiatry, 15,* 241–262.

Sacks, O. (1985). *The Man Who Mistook his Wife for a Hat and Other Clinical Tales.* New York: Summit.

Salmi, K. (1961). Gilles de la Tourette's disease: The report of a case and its treatment. *Acta Psychiatrica et Neurologica Scandinavia, 36,* 157–162.

Shapiro, A.K., & Shapiro, E. (1982). Tourette syndrome: History and present status. In A.J. Friedhoff & T.N. Chase (Eds.), *Gilles de la Tourette Syndrome.* New York: Raven.

Sparrow, S.S., Balla, D.A., & Cicchetti, D.V. (1984). *Vineland Adaptive Behavior Scales.* Circle Pines, MN: American Guidance Clinic.

Verhulst, F.C., Akkerhuis, G.W., & Althaus, M. (1985). Mental health in Dutch children: (1) A cross-cultural comparison. *Acta Psychiatrica Scandenavica, 72,* Suppl. 323.

CHAPTER SIX

The Genetics of Tourette's Syndrome

David L. Pauls
James F. Leckman

Recent advances in molecular biology hold enormous promise for the elucidation of the fundamental mechanisms responsible for a number of genetically determined human disorders including some forms of bipolar affective disorder, Huntington's Chorea, and Alzheimer's disease. Available data on the pattern of transmission of Tourette's syndrome (TS) and related conditions suggest that the vulnerability to develop TS may be inherited as an autosomal dominant trait in some families. If this can be confirmed through genetic linkage studies (which have the potential to identify the chromosomal location of the putative TS gene), a new era of TS research will commence. Knowledge of the genetic mechanisms can be anticipated to lead to improved diagnostic techniques, a more thoroughgoing knowledge of the pathophysiology of the disorder and the mediating role of non-genetic factors, and more rational treatment and prevention strategies. It will also be possible to greatly improve the counselling of families concerning the risk to offspring. This chapter provides a brief overview of the current status of genetic research in TS and guidelines for the genetic counselling of TS families (given our current state of knowledge).

FAMILY HISTORY STUDIES

The familial aggregation of TS and other chronic tic disorders has long been recognized. It is noteworthy that in his seminal report published a century ago Gilles de la Tourette considered the disorder to be hereditary, particularly if chronic tics (CT) were considered to be related to TS. Even so, only a modest literature on the familial nature of TS and CT has emerged. Over the past decade empirical studies have demonstrated that TS and CT show a familial concentration (Comings, Comings, Devor, & Cloninger, 1984; Elridge, Sweet, Lake, Ziegler, & Shapiro, 1977; Golden, 1978; Kidd, Prusoff, & Cohen, 1980; Nee, Caine, Polinsky, Eldridge, & Ebert, 1980; Pauls, Kruger, Leckman, Cohen, & Kidd, 1984; Shapiro, Shapiro, Bruun, & Sweet, 1978), and, in families of TS patients, CT occurs as a milder manifestation of the same etiologic factors (Pauls, Cohen, Heimbuch, Detlor, & Kidd, 1981).

TWIN STUDIES

In contrast to studies of the recurrence risk to first degree family members (which may be confounded by forms of "cultural" or non-genetic transmission), studies of identical (monozygotic, MZ) and fraternal (dizygotic, DZ) twin pairs provide direct evidence for the importance of genetic factors in the pathogenesis of TS (Price, Kidd, Cohen, Pauls & Leckmann, 1985). In a study of 43 pairs of same sex twins, Price and coworkers reported a concordance of 53% for MZ twin pairs and 8% for DZ pairs. When the criteria were broadened to include chronic tic disorders as well as TS, the concordance increased to 77% and 23% for MZ and DZ pairs respectively. Differences in the concordance of the MZ and DZ pairs are suggestive of a substantial genetic etiology. The high incidence of chronic tic disorders in the co-twins also supports the view that these more prevalent tic disorders are etiologically related to TS. The MZ twin data also indicate that non-genetic factors also influence the expression of the inherited TS diathesis. These twin data were obtained from the parents of the twins. More recent unpublished data, collected by direct interview with the twins, suggests that the concordance rate for MZ twins is substantially higher.

RANGE OF PHENOTYPIC EXPRESSION

A critical question in TS genetic research concerns the definition of alternate phenotypes. Do these disorders arise from the same underlying genetic diathesis? Family and twin studies strongly suggest that chronic tic disorders may be one such alternate phenotype, but are there others? Cohen, Detlor, Shaywitz and Leckman (1982) and Comings and Comings (1984) have suggested that attention deficit disorder occurring in the families of TS patients is related genetically to TS. This is a reasonable hypothesis since many investigators have demonstrated a much higher frequency of ADD among TS clinical patients than would be expected by chance (A. Shapiro, E. Shapiro, Bruun & Sweet, 1978; Comings and Comings, 1985). However, Pauls et al. (1986) examined data from a family study and found no evidence to support the hypothesis that TS and ADD are related genetically. Although there was an increased rate of ADD among TS probands, the patterns within families were consistent with the hypothesis that assumed the two disorders to be etiologically independent. The high co-occurrence of TS and ADD in clinical populations may be due to a bias of the type described by Berkson (1946). Comings and Comings (chapter 8, this volume), however, also review these data and arrive at a sharply contrasting conclusion.

Other investigators (Fernando, 1967; Montgomery, Clayton & Friedhoff, 1982; Nee, Caine, Polinsky, Eldridge & Ebert, 1980; Nee, Polinsky & Ebert, 1982; Yaryura-Tobias, Neziroglu, Howard & Fuller, 1981) have suggested that obsessive-compulsive (OC) illness may be associated with the syndrome since increased rates of OC symptoms have been observed in TS patients. In addition, the results of a family study (Pauls,

Towbin, Leckman, Zahner & Cohen, 1986) show that rates of OC symptoms are elevated significantly in the families of TS probands, giving additional evidence that OC symptoms are a part of the spectrum of behaviors associated with TS. However, questions remain about whether the OC symptoms observed in association with TS represent the same disorder as when these are found in isolation or in families without any evidence of tic disorders (See Towbin, chapter 9, this volume).

SEX DIFFERENCES

Early family history studies suggested that the sex difference observed for the frequency of TS was related to the transmission of the disorder (Kidd, Prusoff & Cohen, 1980; Pauls, Cohen, Heimbuch, Detlor & Kidd, 1981; A. Shapiro, E. Shapiro, Bruun & Sweet, 1978), with relatives of females being at higher risk than relatives of males. Data from a family study suggest that this sex difference may not be real. Table 6.1 shows the morbid risks obtained from the ongoing family study at the Yale Child Study Center (Pauls, Kruger, Leckman, Cohen & Kidd, 1984). There clearly is no significant difference between relatives of males and relatives of females. Nevertheless, the difference in frequency between males and females is still observed (i.e., males are more likely than females to manifest motor and/or phonic tics). It is interesting to note that this difference in frequency diminishes when relatives with OCD are included as affected, since more female relatives than male relatives have OCD (see Table 6.2). Thus there may be a sex-specific expression of symptoms, rather than a difference in frequency of affected status between the sexes.

GENETIC MECHANISMS

Five studies have been done to test whether specific genetic hypotheses could account for the pattern of transmission observed in families of

Table 6.1. Recurrence Risks of TS/CT in the Relatives of TS Probands

Diagnosis	Sex of Proband		Total
	Male	Female	
TS	6/57 (10.5%)	5/46 (10.9%)	11/103 (10.7%)
CT	10/57 (17.5%)	9/46 (19.6%)	19/103 (18.4%)
Total	16/57 (28.1%)	14/46 (30.4%)	30/103 (29.1%)

Table 6.2.   Comparison of Risks of Diagnosis Among First-Degree Relatives

Sex of Relative	Diagnosis			Total
	TS	CT	OCD	
Male	8/45 (17.7%)	14/45 (31.1%)	3/45 (6.7%)	25/45 (55.5%)
Female	3/58 (5.2%)	5/58 (8.6%)	10/58 (17.2%)	18/58 (31.0%)
Total	11/103 (10.7%)	19/103 (18.4%)	13/103 (12.6%)	43/103 (41.7%)

TS patients. Baron, Shapiro, Shapiro, and Rainer (1981) demonstrated that a simple genetic threshold model could explain their family history data; however, the genetic model parameters obtained predicted that approximately 71 percent of all cases in the families were phenocopies. Kidd and Pauls (1982) tested several alternative hypotheses incorporating both sex and severity difference. Thus, rather than assuming TS and CT were equivalent forms of the disorder, they assumed that CT was a genetically milder form and incorporated that information into the analyses. They were unable to reject either a single-locus or a multifactorial–polygenic hypothesis; however, a single-locus model gave the best fit to the data. Their solution predicted a very low rate (less than 1.0 percent) of phenocopies.

Comings and colleagues (1984) and Devor (1984) reported results of segregation analyses based on family history data. Both of these studies assumed that TS and CT were equivalent. The results suggested that a single major gene contributes to the expression of the syndrome. However, the specific mode of inheritance suggested differed from study to study. Comings and colleagues (1984) suggested that the mode of transmission was consistent with a dominant model where the penetrance of the heterozygote was estimated at .68 for males and .30 for females. Their solution predicted that approximately 35 percent of cases would be phenocopies. Devor (1984) suggested that his results also were consistent with a semidominant gene. However, the estimates of penetrance were quite different than those reported by Comings and colleagues (1984). Devor estimated the penetrance for male heterozygotes to be .125 and for female heterozygotes to be .015. The penetrance for the homozygotes was .999 for both males and females. Devor implies that a dominant model can be rejected. Thus, the mode of transmission, while consistent with a single gene, is quite different than the solution obtained by Comings and colleagues (1984).

This variability in results may be due in part to the fact that all of these studies relied on family history data for diagnoses of relatives. That is, only one or two informants gave information about all other relatives, and, on the basis of that information, a diagnostic estimate was made. Pauls and colleagues (1984) showed that, when relatives are interviewed directly, the recurrence risks and patterns within families can change when compared to family history data. Thus it is imperative that family study data be used to examine genetic hypotheses for TS.

Pauls and Leckman (1986) have reported the results of segregation analyses of family data collected by direct interview of all relatives. The analyses were done using three diagnostic classifications. First, only relatives with a DSM-III diagnosis of TS were included as "affected." Next, relatives with CT also were included. Finally, relatives with OCD were included. All results are consistent with an autosomal dominant hypothesis. In all cases the multifactorial–polygenic hypothesis can be rejected, and the dominant hypothesis is not significantly different from other more general Mendelian hypotheses. A summary of the results obtained under the autosomal dominant hypothesis is presented in Table 6.3.

It is noteworthy that the analyses that included only relatives with TS gave results consistent with an autosomal dominant hypothesis. Of course, the penetrance estimates are quite low, but the results, nevertheless, are consistent with a dominant mode of transmission.

Penetrance estimates increase substantially when individuals with CT are included in the analyses. This is to be expected since a large percentage of the relatives manifested some chronic tics. There still is a substantial difference between males and females in the probability of being affected. The penetrance for males is estimated at .999, and the penetrance for females is estimated at .560.

Finally, when individuals with OCD were included in the analyses, the results again were consistent with an autosomal dominant model. This suggests that OCD is part of the spectrum of behaviors associated with TS. The penetrances estimated for these analyses were 1.00 and .71 for males and females, respectively. It should be noted that, although the estimate of penetrance for males is 1.00, this is a statistical estimate with a standard error. Therefore, it is still possible to observe situations within families where males appear to carry the gene without expressing any form of the syndrome.

The results suggesting a genetic relationship between OCD and TS do not imply that all individuals with OCD have a form that is genetically related to TS. What seems to be the case is that within families of TS patients individuals may exhibit OC symptoms and those individuals appear to have a form of OCD genetically related to TS. It is not clear what percentage of OCD patients seen in a medical practice have the form related to TS. Much additional research needs to be done so that it will be possible to understand more clearly the relationship between these two groups of disorders.

In summary, it appears that the syndrome (TS and associated behaviors) is transmitted as an autosomal dominant trait and that there may

Table 6.3. Sex-Specific Genetic Parameter Estimates for an Autosomal Dominant Model Using Three Diagnostic Classification Schemes

Diagnostic Scheme	Males		Females
TS only	$K_{pm} = .0005$		$K_{pf} = .00015$
		$q = .0004$	
	$f_2 = .45$		$f_2 = .17$
	$f_1 = .45$		$f_1 = .17$
	$f_0 = .00$		$f_0 = .00$
TS or CT	$K_{pm} = 0.010$		$K_{pf} = .003$
		$q = 0.003$	
	$f_2 = .99$		$f_2 = .56$
	$f_1 = .99$		$f_1 = .56$
	$f_0 = .01$		$f_0 = .00$
TS, CT, or OCD	$K_{pm} = .0125$		$K_{pf} = .0075$
		$q = .006$	
	$f_2 = 1.00$		$f_2 = .71$
	$f_1 = 1.00$		$f_1 = .71$
	$f_0 = .00$		$f_0 = .00$

Note: K_{pm} = male population prevalence; K_{pf} = female population prevalence; q = frequency of the suceptibility allele S_s; f_2 = penetrance for genotype with two susceptibility alleles, S_2S_2; f_1 = penetrance for genotype with one susceptibility allele, S_2S_1; f_0 = penetrance for genotype with no susceptibility alleles, S_1S_1.

be a sex-specific expression of specific types of symptoms. More data are needed to characterize more fully the difference between males and females. What appears to be the case is that there is *not* a difference in the risk to relatives of male or female patients, but there may be a difference in the risk to male and female relatives with respect to the specific symptoms they will exhibit.

FUTURE DIRECTIONS IN GENETIC RESEARCH

The suggestion that an autosomal dominant trait is responsible for the vulnerability to develop TS or a related disorder has lead several groups of investigators to study large, multigenerational TS families that are suitable for genetic linkage studies (Kurlan, Behr, Medred, Shoulson, Pauls, & Kidd, 1987). Genetic linkage has long been recognized as a way of demonstrating that a specific genetic factor is involved in the transmission of a particular disorder. Until a few years ago this method had limited applicability to human disorders because of the small number of polymorphic genetic markers of known location in man. Over the past few years the field of human molecular genetics has changed dramatically. Using recombinant DNA techniques, investigators are identifying a growing number of highly polymorphic markers. Since these markers are now being identified at an ever increasing rate, it should be possible to construct a saturated map of the human genome in the next few years. As a result it is anticipated that it will be possible to establish the chromosomal location of the putative TS gene in the next two to five years.

If linkage can be demonstrated it should eventually also be possible to isolate the specific gene and gain insight into the basic constitutional events that may predispose an individual to TS. Equally exciting is the possibility that by ascertaining which individuals are at risk in a particular family, it will be possible through the use of appropriate longitudinal research designs to identify those risk and protective factors which mediate the expression of the disorder. Important and rational strategies for treatment and possible prevention can also be anticipated as well as improved diagnostic methods.

GENETIC COUNSELING

A commonly asked question is: "What is the chance that a person with TS will have an affected child?" The answer to that question depends on the understanding that chronic tics and obsessive–compulsive behaviors are related to TS. The results from several of our family studies indicate that the TS spectrum of behaviors is inherited as a dominant gene. This means that a person with TS who has a positive family history has a 50 percent chance of passing the gene on to one of his or her children. Once a child has inherited the gene, there is a difference in the probability of expression of these behaviors that depends on the sex of the child. If a son receives the gene from his parent, it is almost certain that he will have some of these behaviors (either TS, chronic tics, or obsessive–compulsive symptoms). If a daughter receives the gene, her chance is approximately 70 percent that she will have some form of the disorder. Thus if an individual with TS and a positive family history marries someone without TS, the chance that this couple will have an affected son approaches 50 percent; the chance that a daughter will be affected is approximately 35 percent.

Another common situation is one in which neither parent is apparently affected but they have had a child with TS. This couple wants to know what the chance is that a second or subsequent child will also have the disorder. To answer such a question requires a careful documentation of whether other family members are affected. Once all relevant family information has been collected, Bayesian probabilities can be calculated for each family. If there is an affected grandparent or aunt or uncle, then the situation is essentially the same as for the case described above for affected parents. If after careful assessment there does not appear to be a family history, then unfortunately it is not possible to give a precise estimate for recurrence. Current data suggest that approximately 10 to 35 percent of all cases are sporadic (i.e., there are no affected relatives). More data are needed before accurate recurrence risks can be determined for couples in this situation.

At the present time there is no test that allows carrier detection. Thus it is not possible to perform prenatal tests or to determine whether an unaffected person who has an affected relative is carrying the gene. It is hoped that in the future such a test will become available. Until that time it will be necessary to rely on careful assessment of all family members to determine the best estimates of recurrence risks.

It must be stressed that in most instances children of parents with TS will be mildly affected. However, it is not possible at this time to predict severity of the symptoms. Data from the ongoing family study at Yale suggest that only about 10 percent of affected relatives have symptoms severe enough for their lives to be affected significantly. Thus the overwhelming majority of affected relatives, while having enough symptoms to meet criteria for a diagnosis, may find their symptoms not severe enough to cause significant difficulty in their everyday lives. In other words, while the chance of having a child with symptoms approaches 50 percent, the chance that that child will have a severe case of TS is considerably smaller.

REFERENCES

Baron, M., Shapiro, E., Shapiro, A., & Rainer, J.D. (1981). Genetic analysis of Tourette syndrome suggesting major gene affect. *American Journal of Human Genetics, 33,* 767–775.

Berkson, J. (1946). Limitations of the application of fourfold table analysis to hospital data. *Biometrics, 2,* 47–51.

Cohen, D.J., Detlor, J., Shaywitz, B.A., & Leckman, J.F. (1982). Interaction of biological and psychological factors in the natural history of Tourette's syndrome. In A.J. Friedhoff & T.N. Chase (Eds.). *Gilles de la Tourette Syndrome.* New York: Raven Press, pp. 32–40.

Comings, D.E., & Comings, B.G. (1984). Tourette syndrome and attention deficit disorder with hyperactivity: Are they genetically related? *Journal of the American Academy of Child Psychiatry, 23,* 138–146.

Comings, D.E., & Comings, B.G. (1985). Tourette syndrome: Clinical and psychological aspects of 250 cases. *American Jounal of Human Genetics, 37,* 435–450.

Comings, D.E., Comings, B.G., Devor, E.J., & Cloninger, C.R. (1984). Detection of a major gene for Gilles de la Tourette syndrome. *American Journal of Human Genetics, 36,* 586–600.

Devor, E.J. (1984). Complex segregation analysis of Gilles de la Tourette syndrome: Further evidence for a major locus mode of transmission. *American Journal of Human Genetics, 36,* 704–709.

Eldridge, R., Sweet, R., Lake, C.R., Ziegler, M., & Shapiro, A.K. (1977). Gilles de la Tourette's syndrome: Clinical, genetic, psychologic and biochemical aspects in 21 selected families. *Neurology, 27,* 115–124.

Fernando, S.J.M. (1967). Gilles de la Tourette's syndrome. *British Journal of Psychiatry, 113,* 607–617.

Golden, G.S. (1978). Tics and Tourette's: A continuum of symptoms? *Annals of Neurology, 4,* 145–148.

Kidd, K.K., & Pauls, D.L. (1982). Genetic hypotheses for Tourette syndrome. In T.N. Chase & A.J. Friedhoff (Eds.), *Gilles de la Tourette Syndrome.* New York: Raven. 243–249.

Kidd, K.K., Prusoff, B.A., & Cohen, D.J. (1980). The familial pattern of Gilles de la Tourette syndrome. *Archives of General Psychiatry, 37,* 1336–1339.

Kurlan, R., Behr, J., Medved, L., Shoulson, I., Behr, J., Pauls, D.L., Kidd, K.K. (1987). Severity of Tourette's syndrome in one large kindred: Significance for determination of disease prevalence rate. *Archives of Neurology.* 44; 268–269.

Montgomery, M.A., Clayton, P.J., & Friedhoff, A.J. (1982). Psychiatric illness in Tourette syndrome patients and first degree relatives. In T.N. Chase & A.J. Friedhoff (Eds.), *Gilles de la Tourette Syndrome.* New York: Raven.

Nee, L.E., Caine, E.D., Polinsky, R.J., Eldridge, R., & Ebert, M.H. (1980). Gilles de la Tourette syndrome: Clinical and family study of 50 cases. *Ann Neurol, 7,* 41–49.

Nee, L.E., Polinsky, R.J., & Ebert, M.H. (1982). Tourette syndrome: Clinical and family studies. In T.N. Chase & A.J. Friedhoff (Eds.), *Gilles de la Tourette Syndrome.* New York: Raven.

Pauls, D.L., Cohen, D.J., Heimbuch, R., Detlor, J., & Kidd, K.K. (1981). Familial pattern and transmission of Gilles de la Tourette syndrome and multiple tics. *Archives of General Psychiatry, 38,* 1091–1093.

Pauls, D.L., Hurst, C.R., Kidd, K.K., Kruger, S.D., Leckman, J.F., & Cohen, D.J. (1986). Tourette syndrome and attention deficit disorder: Evidence against a genetic relationship. *Archives of General Psychiatry, 43,* 1177–1179.

Pauls, D.L., Kruger, S.D., Leckman, J.F., Cohen, D.J., & Kidd, K.K. (1984). The risk of Tourette's syndrome and chronic multiple tics among relatives of Tourette's syndrome patients obtained by direct interview. *Journal of the American Academy of Child Psychiatry, 23,* 134–137.

Pauls, D.L., & Leckman, J.F. (1986). The inheritance of Gilles de la Tourette's syndrome and associated behaviors: Evidence for autosomal dominant transmission. *New England Journal of Medicine, 315,* 993–997.

Pauls, D.L., Towbin, K.E., Leckman, J.F., Zahner, G.E.P., & Cohen, D.J. (1986). Gilles de la Tourette syndrome and obsessive compulsive disorder: Evidence supporting an etiological relationship. *Archives of General Psychiatry, 43,* 1180–1182.

Price, R.A., Kidd, K.K., Cohen, D.J., & Pauls, D.L., Leckman, J.F., Cohen, D.J. & Kidd, K.K. A twin study of Gilles de la Tourette's syndrome. *Archives of General Psychiatry,* 42; 815–820.

Shapiro, A., Shapiro, E., Bruun, R., & Sweet, R. (1978). *Gilles de la Tourette syndrome.* New York: Raven.

Yaryura-Tobias, J.A., Neziroglu, F., Howard, S., & Fuller, B. (1981). Clinical aspects of Gilles de la Tourette syndrome. *Orthomolecular Psychiatry, 10,* 263–268.

CHAPTER SEVEN

Pathobiology of Tourette's Syndrome

James F. Leckman
Mark A. Riddle
Donald J. Cohen

Despite major advances in the treatment of Tourette's syndrome (TS) over the past 25 years, the pathophysiology of TS and related disorders is unknown. Treatment regimens continue to be established and refined on solely empirical grounds, and there are no objective, biologically sound means presently available to monitor or guide treatment. Although nigrostriatal, mesolimbic, and mesocortical dopaminergic systems located in the midbrain with projections to the prefrontal cortex remain a major focus of research interest, our rapidly expanding knowledge of the modulatory role of these systems and their intimate association with other compensatory neurotransmitter and neuromodulator systems has made a unitary dopaminergic hypothesis increasingly untenable. A number of the other brain neurochemical, neuropeptide, and neuroendocrine systems that interact with brain dopaminergic systems have also been implicated in the expression of these disorders, but no direct evidence has been presented that establishes unequivocally the etiological significance, if any, of these systems. Evidence supporting an etiological association between TS and some forms of obsessive–compulsive disorder (OCD) has led to a renewed interest in the possible role of serotonergic mechanisms in TS as well as a full appreciation of encephalitis lethargica as a useful neuropathological model. Other recent data have led to intriguing hypotheses concerning the involvement of gender-specific neuroendocrine and endogenous opioid systems.

Given the expanding interest in TS and related conditions, steady progress in this area can be expected over the next decades. Despite initial disappointments, newer brain-imaging techniques may provide important clues. If TS is in part the result of a single major autosomal gene, recent advances in molecular genetics hold considerable promise for the eventual explication of the pathophysiological processes responsible for TS and related disorders including some forms of OCD. The identification of these mechanisms can be expected to improve dramatically our chances to develop more specific and effective treatments for these disorders and to establish sound means to monitor an individual's course and response to treatment. In addition, it will likely provide new insights into the basic mechanisms of gender-specific aspects of brain development and lead to an increased awareness of how environmental stress, specific comorbid conditions (including attention deficit disorder, migraine, and asthma), and toxic exposures can affect the natural history of TS and influence its onset, character, and severity.

NEUROANATOMICAL SITES

The basal ganglia and the substantia nigra are widely considered to be the neuroanatomical regions associated with a variety of movement disorders including Parkinson's disease, encephalitis lethargica, Huntington's disease, and tardive dyskinesia. Although the neuropathological correlates of TS remain to be fully established, the presence of abnormal movements in TS, suggestive neuropathological data, and a substantial body of pharmacological and metabolic data implicating neurochemical systems localized in these regions have led to the hypothesis that the pathophysiology of TS and related disorders may involve some dysfunction in these areas.

Based largely on parallels between the tics, vocalizations, and obsessive–compulsive behaviors seen in some patients with encephalitis lethargica, Devinsky (1983) has suggested that TS is the result of altered dopaminergic function in the midbrain. Almost all central dopamine is produced in the midbrain. The substantia nigra and the ventral tegmental area (VTA) are adjacent midbrain sites unusually rich in dopamine neurons. The dopamine cell bodies in the substantia nigra give rise to the ascending nigrostriatal dopamine pathway. The dopamine neurons of the VTA send ascending projections to the anterior cingulate gyrus, various limbic structures, and certain thalamic nuclei (Iversen & Alpert, 1982). The dopamine neurons in the substantia nigra and those of the VTA also give rise to descending pathways projecting to the dorsal pontine tegmentum in the region of the adrenergic locus coeruleus (Deutch, Goldstein, & Roth, 1986).

In addition, GABA and substance P containing neurons have been identified in the striatum. Their projections form a descending striatonigral pathway (Javoy-Agid et al., 1982). Serotonergic inputs from the dorsal raphe to both the substantia nigra and striatum have also been identified and partially characterized (Bunney & DeRiemer, 1982). Numerous other actual and putative neurotransmitters and neuromodulators have also been localized in these regions including: cholecystokinin, norepinephrine, met-enkephalin, dynorphin, substance K, thyrotropin releasing hormone, glycine, vasoactive intestinal peptide, somatostatin, neurotensin, and histamine (Buck & Yamamura, 1982; Javoy-Agid et al., 1982; Quirion, Gaudreau, Martel, St-Pierre & Zamir, 1985). Although the functional significance of these systems is not completely understood, a more comprehensive picture is gradually taking shape of a tightly regulated subcortical system involved with the control of voluntary movement that displays a distinctive ontogenic progression, is sensitive to stress (Bannon et al., 1983) and gender-specific hormonal influences (Hruska, 1986), and interconnects with a large number of other brain regions including limbic and prefrontal cortical areas.

PATHOPHYSIOLOGICAL MECHANISMS

Dopaminergic Mechanisms

Clinical trials first performed by Seignot (1961) over two decades ago that indicated that haloperidol, a dopaminergic blocking agent, was effective in the suppression of motor and phonic tics had a revolutionary impact on the field. The position that TS was determined solely by psychogenic factors was no longer tenable, and the search for biological determinants gained new impetus. Although a number of brain neurochemical systems have subsequently been implicated in the pathophysiology of tic disorders, the most developed data remain those concerning central dopaminergic mechanisms. These data include pharmacological trials in which other agents that block dopaminergic receptors, such as fluphenazine, pimozide, and penfluridol, have also been found to be effective in the suppression of tics in a majority of TS patients (Moldofsky & Sandor, Chapter 19; Shapiro & Shapiro, Chapter 18; Singer, Trifiletti, & Gammon, Chapter 21, this volume). Tic suppression has also been reported following administration of alphamethylparatyrosine, an agent that blocks dopamine synthesis (Sweet, Bruun, Shapiro, & Shapiro, 1974), and following trials of tetrabenazine, an agent that blocks the accumulation of dopamine in presynaptic storage vesicles (Jankovic, Glaze, & Frost, 1984). In contrast, TS-like syndromes have appeared following withdrawal of neuroleptics (Klawans, Falk, Nausieda, & Weiner, 1978), and tics are often exacerbated following exposure to agents that increase central dopaminergic activity such as L-dopa, amphetamine, methylphenidate, and pemoline (Golden, Chapter 22, this volume).

These pharmacological data, taken together with reports of lowered baseline and post-probenicid mean CSF levels of homovanillic acid (HVA), a major metabolite of brain dopamine, in TS patients compared to available contrast groups (Butler, Koslow, Seifert, Caprioli, & Singer, 1979; Cohen, Shaywitz, Caparulo, Young, & Bowers, 1978; Cohen et al., 1979), have led several groups of investigators to suggest that TS is a disorder in which postsynaptic dopaminergic receptors are hypersensitive (Butler et al., 1979; Cohen et al., 1978). Friedhoff and coworkers (1982) have sought to test this hypothesis by administering gradually increasing amounts of L-dopa in an attempt to down-regulate the putative hypersensitive dopamine receptors. This strategy has met with only limited success.

Stahl and Berger (1982) have used rank-order correlations of neuroleptic efficacy in TS versus the effect of neuroleptics on a number of in vitro tests of dopamine receptor function to frame the hypothesis that the agents that either inhibit the presynaptic release of dopamine or specifically block D-2 dopaminergic receptors would be particularly effective in the suppression of tic symptoms. Preliminary evidence suggests there may be a reduction of TS symptoms following low doses of dopamine receptor agonists, such as apomorphine, which presumably act via presynaptic dopaminergic receptors and produce a net reduction in activity in those dopaminergic systems with autoreceptors

(Feinberg & Carroll, 1979). Trials of specific dopamine autoreceptor agonists, as they become available, will therefore be of theoretical and practical interest. Similarly, ongoing European experience with substituted benzamides that selectively block D-2 dopaminergic receptors, including tiapride and sulpiride, show promise in the treatment of TS (Rothenberger, 1984). Preliminary studies with RO22-1319, a water-soluble pyroloisoquinoline derivative with selective D-2 dopaminergic blocking activity, are also encouraging (Uhr, Berger, Pruitt, & Stahl, 1985). Additional clinical trials are needed to confirm these optimistic results.

Although much of these data support the view that central dopaminergic mechanisms, localized in the basal ganglia, are involved in the pathophysiology of tic disorders, unequivocal evidence for dopamine systems playing a primary role is lacking. Indeed, recent preliminary PET imaging studies of brain dopamine receptors do not support the view that there are increased numbers of these receptors in the few TS patients that have been studied (Chase et al., 1984; Sedvall, unpublished data). It is also important to keep in mind that the reported pharmacological effects are partial. Dopamine receptor blocking agents suppress tics; they do not eliminate them. There is also a significant minority of patients who do not respond to these agents. With few exceptions, the clinical trials involve small numbers of patients treated over relatively brief periods of time without adequate controls. The effect of stimulant medications in exacerbating tic behaviors is also problematic, with recent surveys indicating that there are many tic patients who have had long-term exposure to these agents without experiencing significant difficulty (Price, Leckman, Pauls, Cohen, & Kidd, 1986). Taken together these data suggest that the inferred dysfunction in brain dopaminergic systems may not be the primary pathophysiologic mechanism in all tic disorder patients.

The hypothesis that abnormalities in central dopaminergic systems predispose genetically vulnerable individuals to a more severe expression of the disorder may be an attractive alternative (Leckman, et al., 1986). This interactive model might account for the variable phenotypic expression of the TS trait as observed in the study of MZ twins and first-degree relatives and open the door to prospective longitudinal studies that focus in part on those events that can affect the development of central dopaminergic systems (Price, Kidd, Cohen, Pauls, & Leckman 1985). Such events would include pre- and post-natal exposure to specific pharmacologic and endocrine agents, for example, anti-emetics and CNS stimulants, and exposure to specific sex steroids, as well as the occurrence of pre- and postnatal stresses and comorbid conditions that may be associated with endogenous processes that activate central dopaminergic systems.

Another model that tic disorders are etiologically heterogenous with dopaminergic mechanisms having a more central role in some but not all forms of the disorder also merits attention. Reports suggesting that a positive response to haloperidol is associated with a positive family history of tics and TS are consistent with this view (Price, Pauls, & Caine, 1984). A third hypothesis, that abnormalities in central dopaminergic activity associated with tic disorders are frequently, but not universally, the result of tic behaviors, is untenable based on the available data.

Cholinergic Mechanisms

The study of dopaminergic mechanisms has led to the assessment of neurochemical systems in close neuroanatomic juxtaposition. Dysfunction of cholinergic systems in TS has been specifically postulated on the basis of the effects of cholinergic and anticholinergic agents on tic symptoms (Stahl & Berger, 1981). However, the evidence supporting a central role of cholinergic mechanisms in the pathophysiology of TS is not convincing. Intravenous physostigmine, a selective and potent inhibitor of acetylcholinesterase, has been reported by some investigators acutely to decrease motor and phonic tics (Stahl & Berger, 1981). In sharp contrast, other investigators have reported that intramuscular physostigmine aggravates motor tics and can block the beneficial effects of scopolamine, a muscarinic blocking agent (Tanner, Goetz, & Klawans, 1982). Clinical trials with choline, lecithin, and deanol have also been disappointing overall (Stahl & Berger, 1982). Although precursor loading with choline and lecithin appears to increase brain acetylcholine levels, evidence does not indicate that the synaptic release of acetylcholine is increased by this maneuver (McIntosh, 1981).

Some peripheral neurochemical data also suggest the involvement of cholinergic systems (Hanin, Merikangas, Merikangas, & Kopp, 1979); however, the report of Singer and coworkers (1984) of normal levels of CSF acetylcholinesterase and butyrylcholinesterase in TS compared to normal controls also argues against a primary defect in brain cholinergic systems.

GABAergic Mechanisms

The benzodiazepine clonazepam has been reported to be effective in the treatment of some patients with TS (Gonce & Barbeau, 1977). Whether this is due to the potentiation of the inhibitory effects of GABA or some other pharmacological effects is unclear since other benzodiazepines, including diazepam (Connell, Corbett, Horne, & Mathews, 1967), have not been reported to diminish tics. In a recent open trial, progabide, a direct GABA agonist, was effective in reducing tics in 2 of 4 patients with TS (Mondrup, Dupont, & Braindgaard, 1985). Taken together, these clinical findings along with the intimate neuro-anatomical relationship between GABA and dopaminergic systems suggest that GABAergic systems warrant further evaluation in TS patients. However, a primary defect in GABAergic mechanisms is not supported by the data of van Woert, Rosenbaum, and Enna (1982), who did not find a significant difference in CSF GABA or whole blood GABA between 15 TS patients and a group of controls.

Serotonergic Mechanisms

Although serotonergic mechanisms have been repeatedly invoked as potentially playing an important role in the pathophysiology of TS, there is very little hard evidence to support this connection. Medications that act by increasing or decreasing serotonergic activity do not consistently alter TS symptoms. Studies of CSF 5-hydroxyindoleacetic acid (5-HIAA), the principal central metabolite of serotonin, have reported a range of low and normal levels in TS patients compared to contrast groups (Butler et al., 1979; Cohen et al., 1978, 1979). Other metabolic data are equally inconclusive (Leckman et al., 1984).

Despite this dearth of evidence, serotonergic hypotheses continue to be attractive. Circumstantial evidence includes the neuroanatomic projections of central serotonergic systems to the substantia nigra and the striatum, reviewed earlier, and their likely involvement in the pathophysiology of obsessive–compulsive disorder and migraine. Both disorders are thought to involve altered serotonergic function and both have been associated with TS (Barabas, Matthews, & Ferrari, 1984; Cummings & Frankel, 1985; Insel, Mueller, Alterman, Linnoila, & Murphy, 1985; Pauls & Leckman, 1986; Rydzewsky, 1976).

Noradrenergic Mechanisms

Despite the prominence of noradrenergic mechanisms in some of the pathophysiological models proposed for TS, evidence of noradrenergic involvement in the pathophysiology of TS is limited and based largely on the reported beneficial effects of clonidine, an imidazoline derivative with specific alpha-2 adrenergic receptor agonist activity (Leckman, Walkup, & Cohen, Chapter 20, this volume). However, the effectiveness of clonidine in TS is controversial, with some investigators reporting positive results that have not been replicated by others.

Biological studies have not generally supported a primary role for noradrenergic mechanisms. In particular, studies of the B_{max} and K_D of ^3H yohimbine binding to alpha-2 receptors on platelets revealed no abnormalities among TS patients versus controls (Silverstein, Smith, &

Johnson, 1984), and subsequent changes in specific binding parameters during clonidine treatment did not parallel the course of clinical improvement. Neurochemical studies of 3-methoxy-4-hydroxyphenylethyleneglycol (MHPG), a major metabolite of brain norepinephrine measured in CSF, plasma, and urine, have not consistently revealed differences between patients and controls (Leckman et al., 1986).

The finding of elevated salivary amylase excretion in TS patients versus a contrast group of ADD children is suggestive of the involvement of beta-adrenergic receptors in the pathophysiology of TS (Selinger, Cohen, Ort, Anderson, & Leckman, 1984). However, a controlled clinical trial found no difference in treatment response to varying doses of propranolol compared to placebo (Sverd, Cohen, & Camp, 1983).

The complex hypotheses involving noradrenergic-dopaminergic and noradrenergic-serotoninergic-dopaminergic interactions have been proposed to account for the effects of clonidine and to establish a connection with the highly stress-sensitive central noradrenergic systems. Although some circumstantial evidence is available to support these hypotheses (Leckman, Walkup, Riddle, Towbin, & Cohen, 1987), there is little direct support. These hypotheses have also been heuristically valuable in leading to a more complete understanding of the functional interrelationship of the noradrenergic locus coeruleus and the nigrostriatal and mesolimbic dopaminergic systems (Deutch et al., 1986).

Endogenous Opioid Mechanisms

Endogenous opioid peptides have been localized in the basal ganglia and the locus coeruleus and appear to play a role in the control of human motor functions and in the pathophysiology of abnormal movement disorders (Buck & Yamamura, 1982). Consequently, endogenous opioid mechanisms have been proposed in TS (Sandyk, 1985) and direct, if limited, neuropathologic evidence has been reported. Specifically, Haber and coworkers (1986) reported that the immunoreactivity of dynorphin in the brain of a single adult TS patient was markedly reduced. If this finding can be substantiated and is determined not to be due to pharmacological effects or technical artifact, this could be a finding of singular importance leading to an array of genetic, neuroimaging, and in vivo pathodynamic studies.

The effects of opioid receptor antagonists have been reported to be dramatic; however, both positive and negative responses have been reported in patients with TS. Additional studies are needed to confirm these provocative single-case studies and anecdotal reports and to delineate the conditions under which the function of endogenous opiates may influence the expression of TS and related disorders.

Gender-Specific Neuroendocrine Mechanisms

Clinical experience confirmed by recent epidemiologic data provides unequivocal evidence that the full expression of TS occurs three to nine times more commonly among males than among females (Zahner, Clubb, Leckman, & Pauls, Chapter 5, this volume). The reasons for this gender difference are poorly understood. The usual prepubertal age of onset of tic disorders suggests that activation of the hypothalamic–pituitary–gonadal axis is not a precondition for onset of tics, although it may affect the course of the disorder and influence the appearance of OCD. In contrast, animal data concerning the effects of sex steroids on the ontogeny of central dopaminergic systems suggest that exposure to androgens early in fetal life may induce enduring changes in dopaminergic receptors in the CNS (Wilson & Agrawal, 1979).

A DEVELOPMENTAL MODEL
OF GENE–ENVIRONMENT INTERACTION

We have previously proposed a stress diathesis model of the pathogenesis of TS and related disorders (Leckman, Walkup, Riddle, Towbin, & Cohen, 1987). A central feature of this model is the transmission through a single major autosomal gene of the vulnerability to develop TS or a related disorder (Pauls & Leckman, 1986). Current analyses suggest that virtually all of the males and half to three-quarters of the females with this susceptibility gene will display at least some features of these disorders. The two major areas of symptomatic expression are tic disorders and OCD. In a majority of instances these manifestations will be time limited and subclinical in character, for example, a chronic motor tic disorder that is noticeable only during periods of stress or fatigue and that improves in adulthood. Or an individual might experience mild OC symptoms that wax and wane and only marginally interfere with his or her school or work performance. The nature of this transmitted vulnerability is unknown but may well involve the neuroanatomic sites and pathophysiological mechanisms already described.

In this model, the genetic vulnerability only accounts for a portion of the range of phenotypic expression. The remainder is determined by the individual's age; gender-specific neuroendocrine factors, perhaps including the effects of androgens on the developing brain; the presence of comorbid conditions such as attention deficit disorder, migraine, and asthma; and a host of pre- and post-natal environmental events (intermittent physical or psychological stresses that are severe enough to overwhelm the individual or the family's coping skills and to activate endogenous stress-responsive neurochemical, neuropeptide, and neuroendocrine systems) and exposures (prenatal exposure to dopaminergic blocking agents, or intermittent exposure to CNS stimulants, sympathomimetics, or antihistamines). In this model, in order for someone to exhibit the most extreme forms of these disorders it is necessary to envision a vicious cycle of adverse events that lead to a progression of the tic and OC symptomatology that is experienced as a major stress and leads, in turn, to even greater exacerbation of symptoms.

If this model is correct, efforts to limit exposures to potential adverse pharmacological agents throughout the life cycle, and to improve the individual's and/or the family's ability to understand this disorder and to cope effectively with its symptoms and sequelae may be more important than prescribing the correct medication to suppress tic or OC behaviors once they are established.

ENDURING CHALLENGES

TS is a complex behavioral disorder that is poised between mind and body, governed by innate vulnerabilities and environmental circumstances. The interaction of these forces within the mediating influences of the individual's personality and interpersonal environment shapes the expression of these disorders and influences the individual's long-term adaptation. The major challenge to the practicing clinician is to treat the individual, not just the symptoms (Cohen, Ort, Leckman, Riddle, & Hardin, Chapter 12; Silver, Chapter 13; Wolff, Chapter 14, this volume).

The challenges for future research are also formidable and include the long-term goals of unraveling the pathobiology of TS from its source through explication of genetic and nongenetic factors.

Explication of the Genetic Mechanisms

The explication of the genetic mechanisms involved in the transmission and expression of this family of disorders is an area of extraordinary promise (Pauls, Chapter 6, this volume). This work will include determination of the chromosomal location of the putative TS gene, identification of the exact DNA sequence of this gene, identification of the gene products responsible for the pathobiology of these disorders, and localization of the regions of the CNS affected by these gene products over the course of development. The clinical consequences that will follow from these anticipated discoveries will be enormous, including vastly improved diagnostic procedures and a rational basis for developing treatment interventions.

Explication of Nongenetic Factors

The explication of the nongenetic factors that influence the range and severity of expression of the putative TS gene is an important area of endeavor. Foremost among these factors is likely to be the role played throughout development by gender-specific neuroendocrine mechanisms. Other important factors to be studied include the impact of specific comorbid conditions and the effects of exposure to specific neuropharmacological agents. Similarly, the role of intermittent stress in exacerbating these syndromes needs to be understood at a biological level. The identification of these nongenetic factors can be anticipated to have a major impact on clinical practice through the development of preventive interventions for individuals known to be at risk. Explication of these factors should also clarify why some individuals develop OCD in the absence of tic behaviors and vice versa.

REFERENCES

Bannon, M.J., Elliot, P.J., Alpert, J.E., Goedert, M., Iversen, S.D., & Iversen, L.L. (1983). Role of endogenous substance P in stress-induced activation of mesocortical dopamine neurons. *Nature, 306,* 791–792.

Barabas, G., Matthews, W.S., & Ferrari, M. (1984). Tourette syndrome and migraine. *Archives of Neurology, 41,* 871–872.

Buck, S.H., & Yamamura, H.I. (1982). Neuropeptides in normal and pathological basal ganglia. In A.J. Friedhoff & T.N. Chase (Eds.), *Gilles de la Tourette syndrome.* New York: Raven.

Bunney, B.S., & DeRiemer, S. (1982). Effect of clonidine on dopaminergic neuron activity in the substantia nigra: Possible indirect mediation by noradrenergic regulation of the serotonergic raphe system. In A.J. Friedhoff & T.N. Chase (Eds.), *Gilles de la Tourette syndrome.* New York: Raven.

Butler, I.J., Koslow, S.H., Seifert, W.E., Jr., Caprioli, R.M., & Singer, H.S. (1979). Biogenic amine metabolism in Tourette syndrome. *Annals of Neurology, 6,* 37–39.

Chase, T.M., Foster, N.L., Fedro, P., Brooks, R., Mansi, L., Kessier, R., & DiChiro, G. (1984). Gilles de la Tourette syndrome: Studies with the fluorine-18-labeled fluorodeoxyglucose positron emission topographic method. *Annals of Neurology, 15,* S175.

Cohen, D.J., Shaywitz, B.A., Caparulo, B.K., Young, J.G., & Bowers, M.B., Jr. (1978). Chronic, multiple tics of Gilles de la Tourette's disease: CSF acid monoamine metabolites after probenecid administration. *Archives of General Psychiatry, 35* (2), 245–250.

Cohen, D.J., Shaywitz, B.A., Young, J.G., Carbonari, C.M., Nathanson, J.A., Lieberman, D., Bowers, M.B., Jr., & Maas, J.W. (1979). Central biogenic amine metabolism in children with the syndrome of chronic multiple tics of Gilles de la Tourette: Norepinephrine, serotonin, and dopamine. *Journal of the American Academy of Child Psychiatry, 18*(2), 320–341.

Connell, P.H., Corbett, J.A., Horne, D.J., & Mathews, A.M. (1967). Drug treatment of adolescent tiqueurs: A double-blind trial of diazepam and haloperidol. *British Journal of Psychiatry, 113,* 375–381.

Cummings, J.L., & Frankel, M. (1985). Gilles de la Tourette syndrome and the neurological basis of obsessions and compulsions. *Biological Psychiatry, 20,* 1117–1126.

Devinsky, O. (1983). Neuroanatomy of Gilles de la Tourette's syndrome: Possible midbrain involvement. *Archives of Neurology, 40,* 508–514.

Deutch, A.Y., Goldstein, M., & Roth, R.H. (1986). Activation of the locus coeruleus induced by stimulation of the ventral segmental area. *Brain Research, 363,* 307–314.

Feinberg, M., & Carroll, B.J. (1979). Effects of dopamine agonists and antagonists on Tourette's disease. *Archives of General Psychiatry, 36,* 979–985.

Friedhoff, A.J. (1982). Receptor maturation in pathogenesis and treatment of Tourette syndrome. In A.J. Friedhoff & T.N. Chase (Eds.). *Gilles de la Tourette syndrome.* New York: Raven Press.

Gonce, M., & Barbeau, A. (1977). Seven cases of Gilles de la Tourette's syndrome: Partial relief with clonazepam: A pilot study. *Canadian Journal of Neurological Sciences, 4,* 279–283.

Haber, S.N., Kowall, N.W., Vonsattel, J.P., Bird, E.D., & Richardson, E.P. (1986). Gilles de la Tourette's syndrome: A postmortem and neurohistochemical study. *Journal of Neurological Sciences, 75,* 225–241.

Hanin, I., Merikangas, J.R., Merikangas, K.R., & Kopp, U. (1979). Red-cell choline and Gilles de la Tourette syndrome. *New England Journal of Medicine, 301,* 661–662.

Hruska, R.E. (1986). Elevation of striatal dopamine receptors by estrogen: Dose and time studies. *Journal of Neurochemistry, 47,* 1908–1915.

Insel, T.R., Mueller, E.A., Alterman, I., Linnoila, M., & Murphy, D.L. (1985). Obsessive–compulsive disorder and serotonin: Is there a connection? *Biological Psychiatry, 20,* 1174–1188.

Iversen, S.D., & Alpert, J.E. (1982). Functional organization of the dopamine system in normal and abnormal behavior. In A.J. Friedhoff & T.N. Chase (Eds.), *Gilles de la Tourette syndrome.* New York: Raven.

Jankovic, J., Glaze, D.G., & Frost, J.D. (1984). Effects of tetrabenazine on tics and sleep of Gilles de la Tourette's syndrome. *Neurology, 34,* 688–692.

Javoy-Agid, F., Ruberg, M., Taquet, H. Studler, J.M., Garbarg, M., Worens, C., Schwartz, D.C., Grovselle, D., Lloyd, K.G., Raisman, R., & Agid, Y. (1982). Biochemical neuroanatomy of the human substantia nigra (pars compacta) in normal and parkinsonian subjects. In A.J. Friedhoff & T.N. Chase (Eds.), *Gilles de la Tourette syndrome.* New York: Raven.

Klawans, H.L., Falk, D.K., Nausieda, P.A., & Weiner, W.J. (1978). Gilles de la Tourette syndrome after long term chlorpromazine therapy. *Neurology, 28,* 1064–1066.

Leckman, J.F., Anderson, G.M., Cohen, D.J., Ort, S., Harcherik, D.F., Hoder, E.L., & Shaywitz, B.A. (1984). Whole blood serotonin and tryptophan levels in Tourette's disorder: Effects of acute and chronic clonidine. *Life Sciences, 35,* 2497–2503.

Leckman, J.F., Cohen, D.J., Price, R.A., Riddle, M.A., Minderaa, R.B., Anderson, G.M., & Pauls, D.L. (1986). The pathogenesis of Tourette syndrome: A review of data and hypothesis. In N. S. Shah & A. G. Donald (Eds.), *Movement Disorders.* New York: Plenum.

Leckman, J.F., Ort, S., Cohen, D.J., Caruso, K.A., Anderson, G.M., & Riddle, M.A. (1986). Rebound phenomena in Tourette's syndrome after abrupt withdrawal of clonidine: Behavioral cardiovascular and neurochemical effects. *Archives of General Psychiatry, 43,* 1168–1176.

Leckman, J.F., Walkup, J.T., Riddle, M.A., Towbin, K.E., & Cohen, D.J. (1987). Tic disorders. In H.Y. Meltzer, W. Bunney, J. Coyle, J. Davis, I. Kopin, C. Schuster, R. Shader, & G. Simpson, (Eds.) *Psychopharmacology: The Third Generation of Progress.* New York: Raven. pp 1239–1246.

McIntosh, F.C. (1981). Acetylcholine. In G.F. Siegel, R.W., Albers, B.W., Agranoff, & R. Katzman (Eds.), *Basic Neurochemistry.* Boston: Little, Brown.

Mondrup, K., Dupont, E., & Braindgaard, H. (1985). Progabide in the treatment of hyperkinetic extrapyramidal movement disorders. *Acta Neurologica Scandanavia, 72,* 341–343.

Pauls, D.L., & Leckman, J.F. (1986). The inheritance of Gilles de la Tourette syndrome and associated behaviors: Evidence for autosomal dominant transmission. *New England Journal of Medicine, 315,* 993–996.

Price, R.A., Pauls, D.L., & Caine, E.D. (1984). Pedigree and segregation analysis of clinically defined subgroups of Tourette syndrome. *American Journal of Human Genetics, 36,* 178S.

Price, R.A., Kidd, K.K., Cohen, D.J., Pauls, D.L., & Leckman, J.F. (1985). A twin study of Tourette syndrome. *Archives of General Psychiatry, 42,* 815–820.

Price, R.A., Leckman, J.F., Pauls, D.L., Cohen, D.J., & Kidd, K.D. (1986). Tics and central nervous stimulants in twins and non-twins with Tourette syndrome. *Neurology, 36,* 232–237.

Quirion, R., Gaudreau, P., Martel, J.-C., St-Pierre, S., & Zamir, N. (1985) Possible interactions between dynorphin and dopaminergic systems in the substantia nigra. *Brain Research, 331,* 358–362.

Rothenberger, A. (1984). Therapie der Tic-Storungen, Z. *Kinder-Jugend Psychiatrie, 12,* 284–301.

Rydzewsky, W. (1976). Serotonin (5HT) in migraine: Levels in whole blood in and between attacks. *Headache, 16,* 16–19.

Sandyk, R. (1985) The endogenous opioid system in neurological disorders of the basal ganglia. *Life Sciences, 37,* 1655–1663.

Seignot, M.J.N. (1961). Un cas de maladie des tics de Gilles de la Tourette guéri par le R1625. *Annual Medical Psychology, 119,* 578–579.

Selinger, D., Cohen, D.J., Ort, S. Anderson, G.M., & Leckman, J.F. (1984). Parotid salivary response to clonidine treatment in Tourette's syndrome: Indicators of noradrenergic responsivity. *Journal of the American Academy of Child Psychiatry, 23,* 392–398.

Silverstein, F., Smith, C.B., & Johnston, M.V. (1984). Effect of clonidine on platelet alpha adrenoreceptors and plasma norepinephrine of children with Tourette syndrome. *Developmental Medicine and Child Neurology, 27,* 793–799.

Singer, H.S., Oshida, L., & Coyle, J.T. (1984). CSF cholinesterase activity in Gilles de la Tourette's syndrome. *Archives of Neurology, 41*(7), 756–757.

Stahl, S.M., & Berger, P.A. (1981). Physostigmine in Tourette syndrome: Evidence for cholinergic underactivity. *American Journal of Psychiatry, 138*(2), 240–241.

Stahl, S.M., & Berger, P.A. (1982). Cholinergic and dopaminergic mechanisms in Tourette syndrome. In A.J. Friedhoff & T.N. Chase (Eds.), *Gilles de la Tourette syndrome.* New York: Raven.

Sweet, R.D., Bruun, R.D., Shapiro, E., & Shapiro, A.K. (1974). Presynaptic catecholamine antagonists as treatment for Tourette syndrome: Effects of alpha methylpara tyrosine and tetrabenazine. *Archives of General Psychiatry, 31,* 857–861.

Sverd, J., Cohen, S., & Camp, J.A. (1983). Brief Report: Effects of propranolol in Tourette syndrome. *Journal of Autism & Developmental Disorder, 13,* 207–213.

Tanner, C.M., Goetz, C.G., & Klawans, H.L. (1982). Cholinergic mechanisms in Tourette syndrome. *Neurology, 32,* 1315–1317.

Uhr, S.B., Berger, P.A., Pruitt, B., & Stahl, S.M. (1985). Treatment of Tourette's syndrome with R022–1319, a D-2-receptor antagonist. *New England Journal of Medicine, 311,* 989.

Van Woert, M.H., Rosenbaum, D., & Enna, S.J. (1982). Overview of pharmacological approaches to therapy for Tourette syndrome. In A.J. Friedhoff & T.N. Chase (Eds.), *Gilles de la Tourette syndrome.* New York: Raven.

Wilson, W.E., & Agrawal, A.K. (1979). Brain regional levels of neurotransmitter amines as neurochemical correlates of sex-specific ontogenesis in the rat. *Developmental Neuroscience, 2*(4), 195–200.

Part II

Clinical Features and Associated Problems

CHAPTER EIGHT

Tourette's Syndrome and Attention Deficit Disorder

David E. Comings
Brenda G. Comings

INTRODUCTION

Tourette's syndrome is a common neurobehavioral disorder of child-hood. Two independent genetic studies both suggest a gene frequency of .006 (Comings, Comings, Devor, & Cloninger, 1984; Pauls & Leckman, 1986). This indicates that approximately 1 in 83 persons carries a TS gene. As such it is one of the most common major gene disorders. Attention deficit disorder with or without hyperactivity (ADDH) is even more common and also shows a strong genetic basis, although the genetic mechanisms are less clear (Cadoret, Cunningham, Loftus, & Edwards, 1975; Cantwell, 1976; Morrison & Stewart, 1971, 1974; Shafer, 1973; Welner, Welner, Stewart, Palkes, & Wish, 1977). If the motor and vocal tics, coprolalia, and compulsive behaviors are excluded, many of the remaining clinical features of TS overlap remarkably with those of ADD/H, and yet we have the ironic situation that the use of stimulants is an accepted treatment of ADDH while some suggest they are absolutely contraindicated in TS (Lowe, Cohen, Dettor, Kremeintzer, & Shaywitz, 1982). Here we discuss the clinical and therapeutic issues concerning these interrelated syndromes.

WHAT PERCENTAGE OF TS PATIENTS HAVE ADDH?

As shown in Table 8.1, reports summarizing 1500 individuals indicate that significant attentional problems and hyperactivity occur in about half of TS patients. In 250 cases of TS, we found ADDH was present in 54 percent (Comings & Comings, 1984, 1985). In a second series (Comings & Comings, 1987), of 246 patients compared to 47 normal controls, 49 percent of TS patients had ADDH, compared to 4.2 percent of controls ($X^2 = 32.5$; $p = <.00001$), and 62 percent of TS patients satisfied the DSM-III criteria of ADD (with or without motor hyperactivity), compared to 6.3 percent of controls ($X^2 = 49.2$; $p = <.00001$). The severity of the TS is an important aspect of examining the relationship between ADDH and TS. To evaluate this, our TS patients were divided into three grades of severity. In grade 1, the tics were too mild to treat. In grade 2, the tics were severe enough to justify treatment. Grade 3 patients differed from grade 2 in that some type of symptom had caused a significant interference in the patient's life. Table 8.2 summarizes the proportion of the three grades of TS in our first and second series and the frequency of ADDH in the three grades. In the second series of consecutive, unselected patients, each new individual had to fill out an extensive 425-item questionnaire modeled on the Diagnostic Interview Schedule (Robins, Helzner, Croughman, & Ratclif, 1981) before his or her first visit to the clinic. This allowed the diagnosis of many DSM-III

Table 8.1. ADDH in Tourette's Syndrome

Reference	Number of Cases	Percentage with ADDH
ADDH		
Fernando, 1966	69	48[a]
Moldofsky et al., 1974	15	67
Erenberg et al., 1978	12	42
Shapiro et al., 1978	250	50
Stefl, 1984	431	48[b]
Comings & Comings, 1984, 1985	250	54[c]
Erenberg et al., 1986	200	35
Pauls et al., 1986	27	63
Comings & Comings, 1987b	246	49
Total and average	1,500	48
ADD		
Comings & Comings, 1987b	246	62

[a]Impulsive and other behavioral problems.
[b]Physician-diagnosed MBD, ADD, or hyperactivity + learning disabled + severe behavioral problem.
[c]Independent of the present 246 cases.

Table 8.2. ADD and ADDH in Two Series of Tourette's Syndrome Patients

	First Series[a]	Second Series[b]	Controls
Number of Cases[c]	250	246	47
ADDH			
Total	54%	49%	4.2%
Grade 1	32%	33%	
Grade 2	51%	46%	
Grade 3	69%	71%	
ADD			
Total	—	62%	6.3
Grade 1	—	47%	
Grade 2	—	58%	
Grade 3	—	83%	

[a]Comings & Comings, 1984, 1985.
[b]Comings & Comings, 1987b.
[c]In the first series 12% were grade 1, 59% grade 2, and 29% grade 3.
In the second series 16% were grade 1, 60% grade 2, and 24% grade 3.

disorders and included detailed questions about all the criteria for ADDH as well as many related questions concerning the age of onset of the symptoms and their relationship to motor and vocal tics. This allowed us to distinguish between ADDH and ADD. A group of 47 random normal controls were also included. It can be seen that the relative proportion of the three grades of TS remained constant throughout the two series (12, 59, and 29 percent in the first series and 16, 60, and 24 percent in the second). There are several important conclusions from this table. First, the frequency of ADDH remained essentially the same in the two series, 54 percent and 49 percent. Second, ADDH was ten times more frequent in TS than in the controls. Third, ADDH was significantly increased in frequency (32 and 33 percent) even in grade 1 TS patients. This is important in relation to the suggestion that ADDH is only present in TS because of selective bias. Forth, ADD was even more common, occurring in 62 percent of the TS patients. This was again ten times more common than in the controls. Finally, ADDH and ADD were extremely common in grade 3 TS patients (ADDH 70 percent and ADD 83 percent). These figures strongly suggest that ADDH is an integral part of TS. Although selection for severe cases can increase the frequency of ADDH, it is still seven to eight times more common in very mild cases than in the general population.

ADDH IS AN EARLY EXPRESSION OF THE TS GENE

In the course of taking a history from TS patients with ADDH we noticed that it was present for several years before the onset of motor or vocal tics. This may suggest ADDH can present as the first manifestation of the putative TS gene. To examine the average duration between the onset of ADDH and the onset of tics, in the first series, we examined 91 TS cases with ADDH where sufficient information was available. The symptoms of ADDH started an average of 3.0 years (SD 2.94) prior to the onset of motor and vocal tics. Recognizing that determining the age of onset of ADDH can be rather inexact, we asked many more detailed questions in the highly structured questionnaire given to the second series of patients. This time adequate information was available on 140 patients. The duration between the onset of ADDH symptoms and TS was 2.4 years (SD 2.85), similar to that in the first series. Thus our experience indicates that when ADDH is present it usually precedes the onset of motor and vocal tics by 2 to 3 years. In some cases the two come on simultaneously. Occasionally the ADDH starts after the onset of tics.

ADDH CAN BE THE ONLY EXPRESSION OF A TS GENE

A more complex question is whether an individual with a TS gene may present as ADDH only and never have tics. The major evidence suggesting that this can occur comes from family studies. An obligate carrier of a TS gene is an individual without motor or vocal tics who has a TS child and a parent or sibling with TS. Many times such an individual has had a history of childhood ADDH. In a recent study in our clinic, a graduate student, Margaret Martin, examined 53 additional new TS patients. ADD was present in 80 percent. The parents of the TS patients, who themselves had no motor or vocal tics, were divided into two groups—obligate carriers ($N = 18$) and noncarriers ($N = 25$). The latter included those where there was insufficient family history to identify who was the carrier and thus included some carrier parents. Among the obligate carriers 33 percent had a childhood or adult history of ADD ($X^2 = 10.2$; $p = .001$). Among the noncarrier group 12 percent had a childhood or adult history of ADD ($X^2 = 1.2$; $p = $ NS). This study provided clear evidence that the TS gene may be expressed as ADD or ADD-residual type (APA, 1980) without motor or vocal tics. In some of these carrier parents their ADDH required medical treatment.

ADDH AND TS SEGREGATE TOGETHER IN FAMILIES

The proposal that ADD and TS are closely related entities has recently been challenged by Pauls and coworkers (1986). This was based on two observations obtained from a small study of 27 families: (1) When the proband had both TS and ADDH, 17.2 percent of the relatives had ADDH, while if the proband did not have ADDH only 2.2 percent of the relatives had ADDH, eight times lower; and (2) in the families where the proband had ADDH, TS and ADDH segregated independently— that is, they occurred in different individuals in the pedigree. It was concluded that the occurrence of ADDH in TS was due to a strong selective bias. Thus if by chance a TS child also had ADDH then that child would be the first one in a family to come to a physician's attention, but the two are really independent entities and are transmitted separately in the family. If the proband does not have ADDH then it is unlikely that the ADDH will also be present in the family and thus the frequency of ADDH in other family members with TS will be no greater than in the general population. Among their 27 probands, 63 percent had ADDH.

   In a reply, we pointed out several problems with this study (Comings & Comings, 1987a).

1. We agree that there is selective bias and that the proband tends to be the most severely affected TS case in a family and the one most likely to have ADDH. However, it is incorrect to generalize to the conclusion that this accounts for all the ADDH in TS. As shown in Table 8.2, ADDH was present in 70 percent of the most severe, grade 3 TS patients. However, it was also present in 32 percent of the grade 1 cases whose tics were so mild they did not require treatment. Thus with selective bias the frequency of ADDH increases from 30 to 70 percent, not 0 to 70 percent.

2. To examine the question of whether ADDH and TS segregate independently, we examined 199 members of the 24 families we are using in linkage studies. All members of these families have been individually interviewed for the presence of TS symptoms and ADDH. These were divided into two groups, those where the proband had ADDH (19 families) and those where the proband did not have ADDH (5 families). When the proband was excluded from the first group, 37 percent of the 91 TS or CMT patients had ADDH, compared to 21 percent in the second group. Thus the frequency of ADDH in other TS patients in the family when the proband did not have ADDH was only 1.5 times lower than when the proband had ADDH, not 8 times lower. By contrast, the frequency of ADDH in members of the family that did not have TS or CMT was only 4.6 percent, no different from the 4.2 percent we found in our random controls. This indicates the TS and ADDH segregated together, not independently.

3. For the families where the TS proband had ADDH, the number of relatives with TS or CMT in Pauls and colleagues' study was very small—16. As a result when their chi-square analysis of segregation of TS and ADD placed individuals in five different cells many of the numbers were quite small. By contrast there were 91 relatives with TS or CMT in our families where the proband had TS and ADDH. The chi-square between the frequency of ADDH in all the TS-CMT relatives (34 percent) and that in family members without TS (4.6 percent) was 20.87 ($p = <.00001$).

4. The claim by Pauls and colleagues (1986) that if the proband does not have ADDH then the frequency of ADDH in other members of the family with TS is no greater than that in the general population does not coincide with another publication of theirs in which a large pedigree was examined (Kurlan et al., 1986). In this pedigree the proband did not have ADDH and 9 of 29 or 31 percent of other members of the family with TS-CMT had ADDH. This is virtually identical to our finding of ADDH in 32 to 33 percent of grade 1 TS patients, and 34 percent in other TS patients in our linkage families.

The sum of all these observations supports the assertion that ADDH is an integral aspect of the expression of the putative TS gene. It is present in approximately one-third of very mild cases and increases to two-thirds in the more severe cases.

Editors' Note: The question of whether or not some forms of ADDH are etiologically related to TS remains controversial. See Pauls & Leckman, Chapter 6, this volume, for another perspective on this issue.

CAN STIMULANT MEDICATION CAUSE TS?

There are numerous reports documenting the onset of motor and vocal tics after the administration of stimulant medication for the treatment of ADDH (Bachman, 1981; Bremness & Sverd, 1979; Golden, 1974, 1982; Lowe et al., 1982; Pollack, Cohen, & Friedhoff, 1977; Sleator, 1980). Lowe and colleagues (1982) felt that "the widespread use of stimulants may be increasing substantially the number of cases (of TS) requiring clinical diagnosis and invervention" (p. 73). They recommended that stimulants not be given to any ADDH child with TS or a family history of TS, and that if tics developed in a child on stimulants the medication should be immediately discontinued. By contrast, based on experience with over 1000 patients, Shapiro and Shapiro (1981) concluded that stimulants did not play a significant role in precipitating TS, and often used these medications to counter some of the side effects of haloperidol. Comings and Comings (1984) concluded the stimulants do not cause TS and that if permanent motor and vocal tics come on during the course of stimulant treatment the ADDH was due to a TS gene. This conclusion is based on the following:

1. ADDH is an integral part of the symptom complex of TS.
2. The natural history of the majority of TS cases is to begin as ADDH and then develop tics and vocal noises.
3. There was no evidence that as a group TS patients receiving stimulant medication before the onset of tics had a shortened duration from onset of ADDH to the onset of tics. This was based on a division of ADDH patients into two groups, those treated with stimulants before the onset of tics, and those treated only after the onset of tics. If stimulants played a significant role in causing TS or precipitating tics, the duration from the onset of ADDH to the onset of tics should be shorter in the group getting the stimulants before the tics than in the group getting stimulants after the tics had already started. In fact this duration was 5.3 years in the stimulants-then-tics group and 1.6 years in the tics-then-stimulants

group. Even when the latter group was corrected for those with an onset of tics within a year of the onset of ADDH (see Comings & Comings, 1984, for rationale), the duration was 4.0 years, still less than the group who had stimulants before the onset of tics. Since the duration was so much longer in the stimulants-then-tics group one might suggest that this group never would have gotten tics if they didn't receive the stimulants. However, the frequency of a positive family history of TS was not significantly different for the two groups (average 75 percent).

We reexamined this question specifically with the second group of 246 patients (Comings & Comings, 1987b). The results were similar. In the stimulants-before-tics group the duration from onset of ADDH to onset of tics was 3.7 years, while in the tics-then-stimulants group it was 2.2 years. When both groups were corrected for those cases with an almost simultaneous onset of ADDH and tics, the duration was 4.25 years for the stimulants-then-tics group and 3.6 years for the tics-then-stimulants group. Thus in two successive studies, each involving about 250 patients, there was no evidence that stimulants hastened the time of onset of tics and vocal noises.

4. A different approach to this question was taken by Price, Leckman, Pauls, Cohen, and Kidd (1986). They reasoned that the question of whether stimulants permanently exacerbate motor and vocal tics could be investigated by studying identical twins. They examined six identical twins, one of each pair receiving stimulant therapy while the other did not. From this and one other case in the literature (Waserman, Lal, & Gautier, 1983), they concluded that "stimulant treatment may not substantially increase the risk for developing or permanently exacerbating tics in many individuals, because the tics also appear in untreated co-twins" (p. 236).

CAN STIMULANT MEDICATION MAKE TS WORSE?

There is no question that stimulant medication can sometimes exacerbate the symptoms of TS. The real questions are how often this happens and whether its occurrence should result in an absolute proscription against the use of such medication in TS. In our second group of patients, 92 were on stimulants during the time they had tics. These patients were about equally divided into those who thought the stimulants had no effect or decreased the tics (31.5 percent) and those who thought the stimulants made them slightly worse or much worse (27.2 percent). (The other 40 percent had no opinion.) In the vast majority of patients in whom the stimulants made the tics worse, the tics were alleviated by the subsequent administration of haloperidol or pimozide. We have only had 7 patients in whom the stimulants had to be discontinued because the tics couldn't be controlled. In our experience, pemoline is more likely to exacerbate tics than methylphenidate, with dextroamphetamine intermediate.

In the study by Price and colleagues (1986), 34 of 170 individuals with TS surveyed by questionnaire were treated with stimulants before age 18. They found that half of the treated individuals reported at least some worsening of the tics. Shapiro and Shapiro (1981) reported that stimulants did not exacerbate the tics of TS individuals who were being treated with haloperidol. In the study by Price and colleagues (1986) there were 11 individuals who received stimulants when they were not on haloperidol. Only 2 of these showed a clear exacerbation of the tics.

As discussed previously (Comings & Comings, 1984), we feel that, if haloperidol or clonidine, alone or in combination, does not control ADDH symptoms that are seriously interfering with the TS child's academic or social development, the judicious use of stimulants, kept at the lowest effective dose, can contribute significantly to the overall treatment. A number of cases are referred to us where a child with ADDH, treated with stimulants, has developed motor and vocal tics. In over 50 percent of these cases, a careful history shows that some tics were present before stimulants were started. The subsequent administration of haloperidol or pimozide almost always results in enough control of the tics that the stimulants can be continued.

Editors' Note: The pharmacological management of individuals with TS is reviewed in detail in Part 4 of this volume. The use of CNS stimulants in the treatment of concurrent ADDH and TS remains controversial. See Golden, Chapter 22, and Shapiro & Shapiro, Chapter 18, for further discussion of this important clinical question.

THE CONCEPT OF ADDH SECONDARY TO A TS GENE

We believe it is useful to divide ADDH into two major categories: pure ADDH and ADDH secondary to a TS gene. The latter we define in the following manner:

1. Meets the DSM-III criteria for ADDH
2. One or both of the following are true:
   a. Has a positive family history of TS or chronic motor tics
   b. Has one or two mild or subtle motor or vocal tics, but not both

This designation is useful for several reasons. It allows us to inform the parents that we believe their child's ADDH is due to the partial or early expression of a TS gene and that he or she may at some future date develop motor or vocal tics. If stimulant medications are prescribed they are told of the possible exacerbation or precipitation of tics by the medication. Depending upon the severity of the particular case either the medication can be discontinued or haloperidol (or other medication) can be added to control the tics. This diagnostic category is also useful in regard to the presence of other symptoms. In our experience such children are likely to manifest other symptoms of TS such as echolalia, palilalia, coprolalia, copropraxia, compulsive behaviors, confrontive personality, and undue interest in sex or overt exhibitionism. Knowledge of the relationship between these behaviors and TS usually helps to avoid treatment modalities that are unlikely to be effective. Let us look at a typical case.

When John was 4 years of age, his mother noticed that he was very aggressive in groups, cried easily, and had a very short attention span. This continued until finally at age 7 the parents began therapy in a behavior modification program with positive rewards for good behavior. This worked for awhile but he soon began to manipulate them to get bigger and better rewards for less and less good behavior. At age 9 he was treated with methylphenidate, and this resulted in real improvement for the next 2 years. The summer before coming to the clinic the parents stopped the methylphenidate and placed him in a summer camp. However, he was thrown out after 1 month because he was lying, stealing, and pulling girls' pants down. When his mother locked him out of the house for several hours in the afternoon because of his aggressive behavior, he would break the windows to get back in. When school started he didn't want to go and frequently smashed things in fits of anger. When seen in the clinic he fit all the criteria for ADDH and was treated with imipramine, which resulted in a striking improvement in his attention span and decrease in his short temper and aggressive behavior. He never had motor and vocal tics and would normally have been diagnosed simply as ADDH. However, the family was riddled with other members with Tourette's syndrome (mother, uncle, two cousins, and grand-uncle) (see Fig. 8.1). His grandmother had severe obsessive–compulsive behaviors, another cousin antisocial behavior (juvenile delinquency and drug abuse), and a second cousin ADDH and severe behavioral problems. Thus the diagnosis became ADD secondary to a TS gene.

Our clinical impression is that ADD secondary to a TS gene is associated with more severe behavior problems than occur in pure ADD. In our study of the second series of 246 TS patients, we also had 17 patients with pure ADDH and 15 with ADD secondary to a TS gene. This pro-

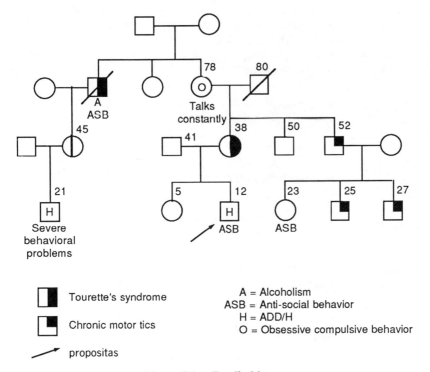

Figure 8.1. Family history.

vided us with the opportunity to ask whether indeed there were any personality characteristics that were more common in ADD 2° to TS compared to pure ADD. Figure 8.2 compares the frequency of various behavioral features of controls, TS patients, and these two types of ADD. It was surprising that obsessive–compulsive behaviors were present in a significant number of patients with both ADD and ADD secondary to a TS gene (26 to 35 percent). The presence of conduct disorder in 26 and 32 percent of the ADD groups was not too surprising, given the clear relationship between the two (Stewart, Cummings, Singer, & DuBlois, 1981). Based on our experience with TS patients and conduct problems (Comings & Comings, 1985; 1987c) we thought conduct disorder would be more frequent in ADD secondary to a TS gene than in pure ADD, but this was not the case. However, a larger number of cases will have to be studied to verify this either way. We were also surprised by the relatively high frequency of occasional or frequent exhibitionism in both types of ADD. Stuttering and panic attacks were more common in ADD secondary to a TS gene than ADD. However, of all the behaviors, depression was the most striking, being present in 20 percent of ADD secondary to a TS gene versus 0 percent of the ADD patients.

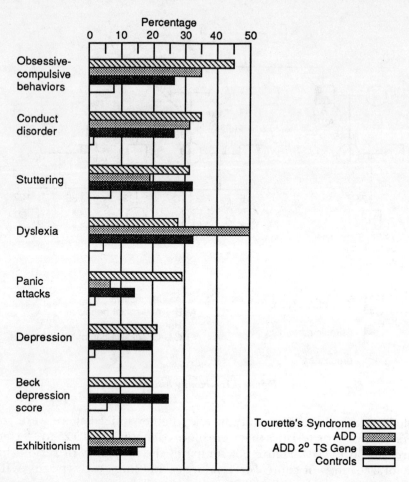

Figure 8.2.   Comparison of behaviors in Tourette's syndrome, ADD, and ADD 2° TS.

The other major feature that distinguishes ADD from ADD secondary to a TS gene is the age of onset. While both may begin very early in life, in our experience the ADD associated with TS not infrequently begins after 7 years of age, the cutoff time for the DSM-III criteria of regular ADD. This is consistent with the fact that the onset of TS itself is some-times delayed until 15 years of age. If it is associated with ADD, which comes on at the same time or a few years earlier, the age of onset of the ADD can be as late as 13 to 15 years of age. We have yet to see a case of ADDH with an age of onset of later than 7 years that was not ADD secondary to a TS gene.

These findings further illustrate the many interweaving similarities between TS and ADD and the role that ADDH plays in the symptomatology of TS. In a similar manner, we are impressed with the role that the TS gene plays in ADDH. We find a positive family history of TS or CMT in approximately 50 percent of the ADDH cases we evaluate.

TREATMENT OF ADDH SECONDARY TO A TS GENE

We feel that children with a diagnosis of ADD secondary to a TS gene do not need to be treated any differently than children with pure ADDH, with the following possible exceptions. (1) We are likely to push harder for a more extensive trial of alternative treatments, such as special structured classes, special diets (Egger, Carter, Graham, Gamley, & Soothill, 1985), and/or first trying clonidine or imipramine (or desipramine). (2) If these fail it is imperative that the parents be given a thorough understanding of the fact that their child's ADDH appears to be due to a TS gene, and because of this tics and vocal noises are very likely to develop at some future date, and these may require the additional use of haloperidol.

THE NEUROPATHOLOGY OF ADD AND TS

One of the major conceptual problems with treating ADDH in Tourette's syndrome with stimulants is that methylphenidate and dextroamphetamine promote the release of dopamine while haloperidol and pimozide are dopamine antagonists. How can we justify treating the same patient with both medications? A detailed analysis of the possible pathophysiology of ADD and TS has been presented elsewhere (Comings, 1987). This analysis suggests that the initial lesion in TS is a defect in dopaminergic neurons from the mesencephalic limbic system to the prefrontal lobe, resulting in ADDH (Shaywitz, Yager, & Klopper, 1976) and resembling symptoms of a frontal lobe syndrome (Mattes, 1980; Pontius, 1973). With time there is a compensatory hyperactivity of subcortical dopamine neurons leading to motor and vocal tics. The combined picture is that of a disinhibition of the limbic system. In this conceptual framework, where there are some areas of dopaminergic hypoactivity and other areas of dopaminergic hyperactivity, the simultaneous administration of dopamine agonists and antagonists is not so unusual. There are, in fact, some reports of the beneficial effect of dopamine agonists, such as L-dopa, on ameliorating the symptoms of TS (Friedhoff, 1982; Nomura & Segawa, 1982). A similar approach using dopamine agonists and antagonists has been suggested for the treatment of both the negative and positive symptoms of schizophrenia (Chouinard & Jones, 1978).

SUMMARY

TS may present with a wide range of symptoms, from a few isolated tics and vocal noises too mild to treat to a crippling disorder with severe ADDH, learning disabilities, coprolalia, compulsive behaviors, conduct disorder, panic attacks, phobias, depression, mania, and schizoid behaviors (Comings & Comings, 1987b, 1987c, 1987d, 1987e, 1987f, 1987g). Many patients require multiple modes of treatment, and the use of stimulants in conjunction with haloperidol or other medications can sometimes make the difference between a functioning and a nonfunctioning child.

REFERENCES

American Psychiatric Association. (1980). *Diagnostic and statistical manual of mental disorders* (3rd ed.). Washington, DC.

Bachman, D.S. (1981). Pemoline-induced Tourette's disorder: A case report. *American Journal of Psychiatry, 138,* 1116–1117.

Bremness, A.B., & Sverd, J. (1979). Methylphenidate-induced Tourette syndrome: A case report. *American Journal of Psychiatry, 136,* 1334–1335.

Cadoret, R.J., Cunningham, L., Loftus, R., & Edwards, J. (1975). Studies of adoptees from psychiatrically disturbed biological parents. II. Temperament, hyperactive, antisocial, and developmental variables. *Journal of Pediatrics, 87,* 301–306.

Cantwell, D.P. (1976). Genetic factors in hyperkinetic syndrome. *Journal of the American Academy of Child Psychiatry, 15,* 214–223.

Chouinard, G., & Jones, B.D. (1978). Schizophrenia as a dopamine-deficiency disease. *Lancet, 2,* 99–100.

Comings, D.E. (1987). A controlled study of Tourette syndrome: VII. Summary: A common genetic disorder causing disinhibition of the limbic system. *Amer. J. Hum. Genet.* 41, 839–866.

Comings, D.E., & Comings, B.G. (1984). Tourette's syndrome and attention deficit disorder with hyperactivity: Are they genetically related? *Journal of the American Academy of Child Psychiatry, 23,* 138–146.

Comings, D.E., & Comings, B.G. (1985). Tourette syndrome: Clinical and psychological aspects of 250 cases. *American Journal of Human Genetics, 37,* 435–450.

Comings, D.E., & Comings, B.G. (1987a). Tourette syndrome and ADDH [Letter to the editor]. *Archives of General Psychiatry, 44,* 1023–1024.

Comings, D.E., & Comings, B.G. (1987b). A controlled study of Tourette syndrome: I. Attention deficit disorder, learning disorders and school problems. *American Journal of Human Genetics, 41,* 701–741.

Comings, D.E., & Comings, B.G. (1987c). A controlled study of Tourette syndrome: II. Conduct. *American Journal of Human Genetics, 41,* 742–760.

Comings, D.E., & Comings, B.G. (1987d). A controlled study of Tourette syndrome: III. Phobias and panic attacks. *American Journal of Human Genetics, 41,* 761–781.

Comings, D.E., & Comings, B.G. (1987e). A controlled study of Tourette syndrome: IV. Obsessions compulsions and schizoid behaviors. *American Journal of Human Genetics, 41,* 782–803.

Comings, B.G., & Comings, D.E. (1987f). A controlled study of Tourette syndrome: V. Depression and mania. *American Journal of Human Genetics, 41,* 804–821.

Comings, D.E. and Comings, B.G. (1978g). A controlled study of Tourette Syndrome. VI. Early development, sleep problems, allergies and handedness. *American Journal of Human Genetics, 41,* 822–838.

Comings, D.E., & Comings, B.G., Devor, E.J., & Cloninger, C.R. (1984). Detection of major gene for Gilles de la Tourette syndrome. *American Journal of Human Genetics, 36,* 586–600.

Egger, J., Carter, C.M., Graham, P.J., Gumley, D., & Soothill, J.F. (1985). Controlled trial of oligoantigenic treatment in the hyperkinetic syndrome. *Lancet, 1,* 540–54.

Erenberg, G., & Rothner, A.D. (1978). Tourette syndrome: A childhood disorder. *Cleveland Clinic Quarterly, 45,* 207–212.

Erenberg, G., Cruse, R.P., & Rothner, A.D. (1986). Tourette syndrome: An analysis of 200 pediatric and adolescent cases. *Cleveland Clinic Quarterly, 53,* 127–131.

Fernando, S.J.M. (1966). Gilles de la Tourette's syndrome. *British Journal of Psychiatry, 113,* 607–617.

Friedhoff, A.J. (1982). Receptor maturation in pathogenesis and treatment of Tourette syndrome. In A.J. Friedhoff & T.N. Chase (Eds.), *Gilles de la Tourette syndrome.* New York: Raven.

Golden, G.S. (1974). Gilles de la Tourette's syndrome following methylphenidate administration. *Developmental Medicine & Child Neurology, 16,* 76–78.

Golden, G.S. (1982). [Letter to the editor]. *Journal of the American Medical Association, 248,* 1063.

Kurlan, R., Behr, J., Medved, L., Shoulson, I., Pauls, D., Kidd, J.R., & Kidd, K.K. (1986). Familial Tourette's syndrome: Report of a large pedigree and potential for linkage analysis. *Neurology, 36,* 772–776.

Lowe, T.L., Cohen, D.J., Detlor, J., Kremenitzer, M.W., & Shaywitz, B.A. (1982) Stimulant medications precipitate Tourette's syndrome. *Journal of the American Medical Association, 247,* 1729–1731.

Mattes, J.A. (1980). The role of frontal lobe dysfunction in childhood hyperkinesis. *Comprehensive Psychiatry, 21,* 358–369.

Moldofsky, H., Tullis, C., & Lamon, R. (1974). Multiple tic syndrome (Gilles de la Tourette's syndrome). Clinical, biological and psychological variables and their influence with haloperidol. *Journal of Nervous & Mental Disease, 159,* 282–292.

Morrison, J.R., & Stewart, M.A. (1971). A family study of the hyperkinetic child syndrome. *Biological Psychiatry, 3,* 189–195.

Morrison, J.R., & Stewart, M.A. (1974). Bilateral inheritance as evidence for polygenicity in the hyperactive child syndrome. *Journal of Nervous & Mental Disease, 158,* 226–228.

Nomura, Y., & Segawa, M. (1982). Tourette syndrome in oriental children: Clinical and pathophysiological considerations. In A.J. Friedhoff & T.N. Chase (Eds.), *Gilles de la Tourette syndrome.* New York: Raven.

Pauls, D.L., & Leckman, J.F. (1986). The inheritance of Gilles de la Tourette syndrome and associated behaviors. *New England Journal of Medicine, 315,* 993–997.

Pauls, D.L., Hurst, C.R., Kruger, S.D., Leckman, J.F., Kidd, K.K., & Cohen, D.J. (1986). Gilles de la Tourette's syndrome and attention deficit disorder with hyperactivity. *Archives of General Psychiatry, 43,* 1177–1179.

Pollack, M.A., Cohen, N.L., & Friedhoff, A.J. (1977). Gilles de la Tourette's syndrome. Familial occurrence and precipitation by methyphenidate therapy. *Archives of Neurology, 34,* 630–632.

Pontius, A.A. (1973). Dysfunction patterns analogous to frontal lobe system and caudate nucleus syndromes in some groups of minimal brain dysfunction. *Journal of the American Medical Association, 26,* 285–292.

Price, R.A., Leckman, J.F., Pauls, D.L., Cohen, D.J., & Kidd, K.K. (1986). Gilles de la Tourette's syndrome: Tics and central nervous system stimulants in twins and nontwins. *Neurology, 36,* 232–237.

Robins, L.N., Helzer, J.E., Croughman, J., & Ratclif, K.S. (1981). National Institute of Mental Health Diagnostic Interview Schedule. *Archives of General Psychiatry, 38,* 381–389.

Shaywitz, B.A., Yager, R.D., & Klopper, J.H. (1976). Selective brain dopamine depletion in developing rats: An experimental model of minimal brain dysfunction. *Science, 191,* 305–307.

Shafer, D. (1973). A familial factor in minimal brain dysfunction. *Behavioral Genetics, 3,* 175–186.

Shapiro, A.K., Shapiro, E., Bruun, R.D., & Sweet, R.D. (1978). Gilles de la Tourette syndrome. New York: Raven.

Shapiro, A.K., & Shapiro, E.S. (1981). Do stimulants provoke, cause, or exacerbate tics and Tourette syndrome? *Comprehensive Psychiatry, 22,* 265–273.

Sleator, E.K. (1980). Deleterious effects of drugs used for hyperactivity on patients with Gilles de la Tourette syndrome. *Clinical Pediatrics, 19,* 452–454.

Stefl, M.E. (1984). Mental health needs associated with Tourette syndrome. *American Journal of Public Health, 74,* 1310–1313.

Stewart, M.A., Cummings, C., Singer, S., & DuBlois, C.S. (1981). The overlap between hyperactive and unsocialized aggressive children. *Journal of Child Psychology & Psychiatry, 22,* 35–45.

Waserman, J., Lal, S., & Gauthier, S. (1983). Gilles de la Tourette's syndrome in monozygotic twins. *Journal of Neurology, Neurosurgery & Psychiatry, 46,* 75–77.

Welner, Z., Welner, A. Stewart, M. Palkes, H., & Wish, E. (1977). A controlled study of siblings of hyperactive children. *Journal of Nervous & Mental Disease, 165,* 110–117.

CHAPTER NINE

Obsessive–Compulsive Symptoms in Tourette's Syndrome

Kenneth E. Towbin

In the 100 years since Gilles de la Tourette's original publication, a consensus has emerged about cardinal tic features of the disorder he described. There is continued uncertainty, however, about whether other associated features such as impulsivity and inattention, self-injurious acts, violence, and obsessive-compulsive symptoms (OCS) are intrinsic manifestations or epiphenomena of Tourette's syndrome (TS). Research has only begun to clarify the significance of the association between TS and OCS and to describe the features of OCS in TS patients. These obsessional symptoms are highly variable in presentation, often appearing late in the course of illness. They manifest the same general form as "classic" obsessional phenomena, which are involuntary in onset, disturbing, cannot be suppressed (often despite efforts of resistance), disrupt social or occupational function, and are accompanied by recognition that the origin is psychological or lies within the sufferer, as opposed to being a product of an external reality. The purpose of this chapter is to address the current understanding of the association of OCS and TS and identify its broader implications.

FUNDAMENTAL PROBLEMS

Clinically, both TS and obsessive–compulsive disorder (OCD) are conventionally defined. Each is a syndromic collection of signs and symptoms that occur together that may not be due to the same cause. Such syndromes have no external validity, no biological test that can independently identify the disorder without invoking its initial clinical definition. Despite the apparent, remarkable congruence of clinical descriptions of OCS, from Esquirole in 1838 through the DSM-III (APA, 1980), major problems confront those attempting to clarify the relationship between TS and OCS. Where is the boundary between obsessive–compulsive disorder (OCD) and obsessive–compulsive personality disorder (OCP), or between normal behavior and OCD? How can we distinguish OCD reliably from other disorders (e.g., schizophrenia, phobic anxiety disorders, depression) where obsessions and compulsions are present? When viewed from the perspective of a clinician who has experience with TS, the clinical uncertainty regarding OCS bears a striking resemblance to efforts using clinical observations alone to draw distinctions between everyday "nervous habits" and mild, nondisturbing tics, or between tics and tardive dyskinesia in patients treated for TS with neuroleptic medication for many years. Thus OCS are frequently confused

The author acknowledges the collaboration of Eric D. Caine, M.D., University of Rochester School of Medicine, in the conceptualization of this area.

with OCP and, when they are features associated with other disorders, the diagnosis of OCD may be made to the exclusion or neglected in favor of the coincident disorder.

In the efforts to understand differences between TS and OCD itself, three additional sources contribute to the confusion. Both TS and OCS are capable of involving virtually any function or movement from the repertoire of human activity; there are no pathognomic features. Both may have an aura associated with the behaviors, and both may involve an internal struggle or resistance that precedes manifest actions. Lastly, the content of the behaviors often is associated with, or in reaction to, sexual or scatological concerns. It can be readily seen that a complex motor tic that involves a repeated set of typical movements, such as tapping a specified number of times until the sufferer "feels right," and a compulsion may be indistinguishable.

Although it had been hoped that a distinction between OCS and tics might be based on whether there was an internal experience in anticipation of a movement, it is clear now that the relationship between these is ontogenically complex. For some individuals, the anticipatory experience develops *after* the movement, but is nevertheless invariably associated with it as they struggle to find some rationalization for their symptoms. The internal experience actually precedes or prompts the behaviors for others. One usually sees patients long after the cycle has established itself, when the question becomes unanswerable.

Even if the distinctions could be made clear, other problems would present themselves. Foremost is the measurement of severity. The dilemmas of quantification and symptom comparison facing those who attempt to develop assessment methods for tics present themselves to those evaluating OCS. To date, no valid scales have been developed for the monitoring of symptom severity and frequency in OCS. As pointed out in the chapter on assessment methods, the ability to suppress symptoms for periods of time and the variability of symptoms over time pose serious challenges to quantifying the overall direction of illness (Leckman, Towbin, Ort, & Cohen, Chapter 4, this volume). If compulsions or obsessions increase when tics diminish, one cannot speak of improvement.

An additional hurdle confronts those attempting to evaluate obsessional ideas: A subject's internal state of mind is a critical variable that cannot be observed "objectively." Since the degrees of felt distress, resistance, and interference figure so prominently in the definition of the disorder, subtle changes in these mental experiences should form a cornerstone of measurement. Unlike the overt manifestations of tics, obsessions and the patient's mental response to compulsions are beyond the rater's view, a subjective experience exclusively. The validity of measurements thus can become a reflection of a respondent's motivation or ability to perceive and understand differences in these inner experiences.

To summarize, the fundamental problems in understanding the association of TS and OCS stem from a substantial ignorance about the course and phenomenology of OCS itself, the ambiguity about the differences between similar features of the disorders, difficulties in measurement that are shared, and the additional burden of needing to quantify an internal state.

A REVIEW OF FINDINGS

Gilles de la Tourette originally identified OCS as features present in one of his cases (1885). Meige and Feindel (1907) also indicated that OCS were more prevalent in persons with tics than in the general population, although they offered no figures. Anecdotal case descriptions, (e.g., Samuel Johnson) have suggested that obsessional phenomena were quite common among TS sufferers and that they often appeared to develop late in the disease course, perhaps 10 to 15 years following the emergence of simple motor tics. Some investigators have gone so far as to propose that TS was actually a specific subtype of OCS (Singer, 1963; Yaryura-Tobias, 1981).

Drawing on published reports and personal experience making a total of 69 cases, Fernando (1967) was the first to make an effort to describe the prevalence of OCS in TS patients. While the method of relying on published reports might result in an underestimation, he argued, he discovered that less than 30 percent had OCS. Morphew and Sim (1969) gave a figure of 35 percent of patients while Kelman (1965) reported a prevalence of 11 percent among the subjects in their reviews of case reports. The criteria used to arrive at the diagnosis of the OCS were not specified in either of these studies and they appear to have combined OCP and OCS. Yaryura-Tobias (1981) reached a similar conclusion, stating that 35 percent of his TS patients had OCD, although he too failed to define his diagnostic criteria. In a larger study, Jagger and coworkers (1982) surveyed 75 anonymous TS patients who were members of the Tourette Syndrome Association (TSA) and found 55 percent reported some OCS during their illness. Finally, in the largest community epidemiologic investigation to date, the Ohio TSA commissioned a needs assessment study and found that among 431 patients reportedly diagnosed with TS a point prevalence of 74 percent suffered from OCS "sometimes" or "often" during their illness (Stefl, 1983).

Figures relying on direct interviews and specified criteria for detection are also available. Nee, Caine, Polinsky, Eldridge, and Ebert (1980) found that 34 of 50 (68 percent) TS patients had OCS using the equivalent of DSM-III criteria. Subsequently, Nee, Polinsky, & Ebert (1982) described an older population of 30 TS patients and found 90 percent had some form of OCS using DSM-III criteria. A family study (Montgomery, Clayton, & Friedhoff, 1982) of 15 TS patients revealed that 10 probands (67 percent) had "definite" obsessive–compulsive illness according to Feighner criteria. A more recent, larger family study (Pauls, Towbin, Leckman, Zahner, & Cohen, 1986) found 14 of 27 TS probands (51 percent) had associated OCS and in fact met DSM-III criteria for OCD (without the exclusionary criterion) when the interviews were subjected to a "best estimate" method of diagnosis (Leckman, Sholomskas, Thompson, Belanger, Weissman, 1982).

Recently, there have been attempts to employ more reliable assessments for OCS, such as the Leyton Obsessional Inventory (Cooper, 1970), to the TS population. Traditionally, though equivocally, this instrument has been considered a valid tool for differentiating normal persons from patients with OCD. Frankel and coworkers (1986) modified the Leyton inventory and administered it to a sample of 33 United Kingdom and 30 United States adult TS patients, 11 OCD outpatients, and 41 normals. They reported that 51 percent of the sample of combined U.K. and U.S. TS patients suffered from OCD based on Leyton scores greater than 70, compared to 82 percent of OCD patients and 12 percent of normal controls. It also appeared that a greater portion of the younger, American TS sample (13 of 31 or 58 percent) reported high Leyton scores, compared to the British TS group where 15 of 33 (45.5 percent) scored high. Using a younger population, Grad, Pelcovitz, Olson, Mathews, and Grad (1987) discovered 7 of 25 TS outpatients (28 percent), average age 11.1 years, met criteria for OCD based on results of the child version of the Leyton Obsessional Inventory (Berg, Rapoport, & Flament, 1986) and teacher and parent checklists. This study also employed a control population of normal volunteers who were matched for age, socioeconomic status, race, and sex. The prevalence of OCD in the control population using this method was 2 of 25 (8 percent).

These figures are to be compared to the community surveys of Rudin (1953) and the Epidemiologic Catchment Area (ECA) program (Robins et al., 1984), which found lifetime prevalences of 0.05 and 2 to 3 percent, respectively, for OCD. Clearly the prevalences mentioned earlier suggest a significant increase of OCD among TS sufferers, although the caveat that OCS and OCD are not identical must be added. Features of the ECA methodology suggest that comparing the Ohio, Jagger, and family study figures with the ECA figure may give a rough indication of differences in prevalence between the general population and those with TS in spite of the diagnostic difficulties.

Although the studies cited above offer useful information about the prevalence of OCS among TS probands, their greatest value derives from what can be learned about the inheritance of these disorders. In Montgomery and coworkers' study (1982), 5 of the 30 first-degree relatives (17 percent) met Feighner criteria for OCD. In a study of 30 monozygotic twin pairs in which at least one cotwin had TS, Price, Kidd, Cohen, Pauls, and Leckman (1985) surveyed for concordance of TS and OCS using a telephone/mail questionnaire. Fifty-three percent of the pairs were fully concordant for TS and another 23 percent were partially concordant. While the diagnoses of OCS were not definitive and the degree of impairment was not assessed, it appeared that 83 percent of the individuals had OCS and that concordance for OCS was roughly equal to that for TS (52 percent).

In the more extensive family study of Pauls and coworkers (Pauls, Cohen, Heimbuch, Detlor, & Kidd, 1981; Pauls, Kruger, Leckman, Cohen & Kidd, 1984), 103 relatives of 27 probands were interviewed directly using a semistructured instrument validated for the diagnosis of all major psychiatric disorders and expanded for the examination of tics and OCS. In addition, each relative was asked to report on symptoms in each of his or her first-degree relatives. A "best estimate" method was used in which experts, blind to proband diagnoses, reviewed all available data, including specialized self-reports and relatives' reports on one another, in order to make diagnostic estimates. Twenty-three of 103 of first-degree relatives (22 percent) met DSM III criteria for OCD (minus the exclusionary criterion). Moreover, when the data were stratified according to whether probands had OCD or not, the prevalence of OCD in relatives was equivalent in each proband group. These findings indicate that the inheritance of OCD in first-degree relatives of TS patients is independent of whether the proband had OCD. They imply that OCD may be an alternative expression of TS. This conclusion is bolstered further by the finding that 13 relatives (13 percent) had OCD in the absence of any history of tics.

A different approach to this question was taken by Green and Pittman (1986), who compared results of a structured interview for tics and other disorders in 16 adult patients with TS, average age 31, 16 adult patients diagnosed with primary OCD, average age 40, and 16 normal adults. In their study, 11 of 16 OCD adults (69 percent) had tics at some time in their lives or a family history of tics. This was compared with 1 of 16 normal controls. Eight of 16 (50 percent) OCD adults and 12 of 16 (75 percent) TS adults had a family history of tics. Similarly, 6 of 16 OCD adults had a lifetime history of tics.

Taken together, these data suggest that OCS are considerably more prevalent among TS sufferers and their first-degree relatives than in the general population. Also, it may be that some patients considered to have OCD are manifesting the expression of a TS etiology. The data raise the possibility that OCD in some patients may be an alternative expression of the etiology that is responsible for TS (Pauls & Leckman, 1986; Pauls, Towbin, Leckman, Zahner & Cohen, 1986).

TREATMENT

Since the treatments for the pure forms of OCD and TS remain problematic, it is not surprising that there is a special complexity in the treatment of serious OCS in TS patients. Few studies have looked carefully at the response of associated behaviors such as OCS to pharmacologic treatment. Recommendations for intervention are further hampered by an incomplete understanding of their natural history and phenomenology. To date, no studies have been designed to examine specifically the effects of behavioral or pharmacologic treatment for OCS in a TS population. Nevertheless, as long as patients continue to present with disabling OCS in combination with TS or CMT, some treatment guidelines will be necessary. Currently, the standard considerations for pharmacologic treatment of TS are haloperidol, clonidine, and pimozide. Although anecdotal reports indicate that OCS in TS may respond to haloperidol (Shapiro, Shapiro, Bruun, & Sweet, 1978), as may some patients with OCD (O'Regan, 1970), many patients find little relief or that side effects outweigh the benefits. No reports on effects of pimozide on OCS are available now. Indications that OCS in TS patients may respond to clonidine (Cohen, Detlor, Young, & Shaywitz, 1980; Cohen, Leckman, & Shaywitz, 1985; Leckman et al., 1982) are complemented by a report of a positive response in one patient with pure OCD (Knesevitch, 1982).

OCD drug treatment studies would suggest, despite serious methodologic shortcomings, that tricyclic antidepressants (especially clorimipramine), monoamine oxidase inhibitors, and other agents may be useful in TS patients with severe OCS (Towbin, Leckman and Cohen, 1987). Unfortunately, little has been published on the effects of these agents in TS patients, and the general view from clinical experience is that TCAs and MAOIs may exacerbate tics. The literature on the use of these medications to treat tics makes no mention of the effects on associated behaviors. Abuzzahab and Anderson (1973) reviewed the International Registry in 1973 and found 13 of 17 TS patients treated with antidepressants failed to respond. Only three reports of systematic trials using TCAs were discovered and revealed 1 of 6 patients worsened significantly in response to 150 mg of clorimipramine (Caine, Polinsky, Ebert, Rapoport, & Mikkelsen, 1979), another worsened on 25 mg/per day of imipramine (Fras & Karlavage, 1977), while 2 adult patients treated with combinations of imipramine plus haloperidol or amitriptyline plus haloperidol appeared to improve (Fras, 1978). Five patients receiving clorimipramine crossing over to desipramine, 150 mg each, demonstrated no changes in symptoms on either medication (Caine, et al., 1979). Anecdotal experience suggests that, during withdrawal from these agents, tics may become worse. Faced with a paucity of studies, it is impossible to extend any treatment recommendations confidently. Nevertheless, for TS patients with *severe* OCS, or for whom OCS may be the most disturbing or disabling feature of their malady, it may be necessary to consider implementation of TCAs such as imipramine or clorimipramine, or other potentially valuable agents such as fluoxetine (Fontaine and Chouinard, 1986) or fluvoxamine (Price, Goodman, Charney, Rasmussen & Heninger, 1987) alone or in combination with standard treatments when there is failure to respond to standard treatments alone.

Current neurochemical theory would predict that TCAs would worsen TS since increases in noradrenergic activity from their (or their metabolites') action opposes the putative effects of drugs like clonidine, haloperidol, and pimozide (Leckman et al., 1985; Leckman, Walkup, Riddle, Towbin, & Cohen, 1987; Shapiro et al., 1978; Shapiro, Shapiro, & Eisenkraft, 1983a, 1983b). It should be remembered, however, that all these agents have diffuse effects, each having impacts at noradrenergic, serotonergic, and dopaminergic sites (Charney, Menkes, & Heninger, 1981; Halaris, Belendiuk, & Freedman, 1975; Nose & Takamoto, 1975; Seeman & Lee, 1975; Serra, Argiolas, Klimek, Fadd & Gessa, 1979; Svensson, Bunney, & Aghajanian, 1975). It has been thought that serotonin plays a key role in OCD (Kahn, Westenberg, & Jolles, 1984; Prasad, 1984; Rassmussen, 1984; Yaryura-Tobias; 1977, Zohar, Mueller, Insel, Zohar-Kadouch, & Murphy, 1987), although it is likely that alterations in many neuro-physiologic functions are necessary to yield a syndrome as complex as OCD (Insel, Mueller, Alterman Linnoila and Murphy, 1985; Zohar and Insel, 1987). Further work using pharmacologic probes in patients with TS and OCS might clarify central mechanisms and illuminate distinctions between these disorders.

IMPLICATIONS FOR THE FUTURE

A review of our current understanding of the relationship between OCS and TS shows that we are at the earliest stages of investigation. Having identified the increased prevalence of OCS in TS patients, the task is to describe better the phenomenology, course, treatment response, and pathophysiology of these complex obsessional symptoms. It will be necessary, in future TS research, to pay close attention to the occurrence and treatment response of OCS in patients as well as to recognize the presence of these symptoms in first-degree family members. In order to do this effectively, we will need clearer definitions of the boundaries between OCS and tics and valid, reliable instruments for measurements of severity and improvement.

Data suggesting that the etiology underlying TS also gives rise to OCD are provocative. Such findings imply that clinically homogeneous groups of OCD patients may have etiologically distinct disorders. Findings from studies of heredity, phenomenology, and treatment response among OCD patients that have failed to consider the presence of etiologically distinct populations will need reevaluation. Future investigations will need to consider comorbid conditions in a direct, systematic fashion. Investigations should take note of tics in the proband and his or her family members just as they must now give a careful accounting of depression, phobic anxiety, and psychosis. Consideration of comorbidity opens the way toward a clearer understanding of the relationship between basic neurobiological disease mechanisms and the variety of clinical expressions that may result.

Clinically, those responsible for the treatment of TS patients need to inquire about and evaluate the severity of OCS in their routine interviews. For many patients these are often unrecognized yet deeply troubling and closely guarded features of their illness. In clinical research, it will be important to begin focusing specifically on patients with disabling OCS and TS in pharmacologic and metabolic studies, in order to offer some relief from the dilemma of current therapies that can either antagonize or fail to alleviate one or the other manifestation of their syndrome.

REFERENCES

Abuzzahab, S.R., & Anderson, F.O. (1973). Gilles de la Tourette's syndrome: International registry. *Minnesota Medicine, 56,* 492–496.

American Psychiatric Association. (1980). *Diagnostic and Statistical Manual of Mental Disorders.* (3rd ed.). Washington, DC: Author.

Berg, C.J., Rapoport, J.L., & Flament, M.F. (1986). The Leyton Obsessional Inventory—Child Version. *Journal of the American Academy of Child Psychiatry, 25*(1), 84–92.

Caine, E.D., Polinsky, R.J., Ebert, M.H., Rapoport, J.L., & Mikkelsen, E.J. (1979). Trial of chlorimipramine and desipramine for Gilles de la Tourette syndrome. *Annals of Neurology, 6,* 305–306.

Charney, D.S., Menkes, D.B., & Heninger, G.R. (1981). Receptor sensitivity and the mechanisms of action of antidepressant treatment: Implications for the etiology and therapy of depression. *Archives of General Psychiatry, 38,* 1160–1180.

Cohen, D.J., Detlor, J., Young, J.G., & Shaywitz, B.A. (1980). Clonidine ameliorates Gilles de la Tourette's syndrome. *Archives of General Psychiatry, 37*, 1350–
1357.

Cohen, D.J., Leckman, J.F., & Shaywitz, B.A. (1985). The Tourette syndrome and
other tics. In D. Shaffer, A.A. Ehrhardt, & L. Greenhill (Eds.), *The Clinical Guide
to Child Psychiatry.* New York: Free Press.

Cooper J. (1970). The Leyton Obsessional Inventory. *Psychological Medicine, 1,*
48–64.

Fernando, S.J.M. (1967). Gilles de la Tourette's syndrome: A report on four cases
and a review of published case reports. *British Journal of Psychiatry, 113*, 607–
617.

Frankel, M., Cummings, J.L., Robertson, M.M., Trimble, M.R., Hill, M.A., & Ben-
son, D.F. (1986). Obsessions and compulsions in Gilles de la Tourette's syndrome. *Neurology, 36*, 378–382.

Fras, I. (1978). Gilles de la Tourette syndrome: Effects of tricyclic antidepressants. *New York State Journal of Medicine, 78*, 1230–1232.

Fras, I., & Karlavage, J. (1977). The use of methylphenidate and imipramine in
Gilles de la Tourette's disease in children. *American Journal of Psychiatry, 134*(2),
195–197.

Fountaine, R. and Chouinard, G. (1986). An open trial of fluoxetine in the treatment of obsessive-compulsive disorder. *Journal of Clinical Psychopharmacology,*
6(2), 98–101.

Gilles de la Tourette, G. (1982). Study of a neurologic condition characterized
by motor incoordination accompanied by echolalia and coprolalia. (C. G.,
Goetz, & H. L. Klawans, Trans.). In A. J. Friedhoff & T. N. Chase (Eds.), *Gilles
de la Tourette Syndrome.* New York: Raven.

Grad, L.R., Pelcovitz, D., Olson, M., Matthews, M., & Grad, G. (1987). Obsessive-
compulsive symptomatology in children with Tourette's syndrome. *Journal of
the American Academy of Child Psychiatry, 26*(1), 69–74.

Green, R.C., & Pittman, R.K. (1986). Tourette syndrome and obsessive compulsive disorder. In M. A., Jenike, L. Baer, & W.E. Minicheillo (Eds.), *Obsessive
Compulsive Disorders: Theory and Management.* Littleton, MA: PSG.

Halaris, A.E., Belendiuk, K.T., & Freedman, D.X. (1975). Antidepressant drugs
affect dopamine turnover. *Biochemistry & Pharmacology, 24*, 1896–1898.

Insel, T.R., Mueller, E.A., Alterman, I., Linnoila, M., & Murphy, D.L. (1985). Obsessive–compulsive disorder and serotonin: Is there a connection? *Biological
Psychiatry, 20*, 1174–1181.

Jagger, J., Prusoff, B.A., Cohen, D.J., Kidd, K.K., Carbonari, C.M., & John, K. The
epidemiology of Tourette's syndrome. *Schizophrenia Bulletin, 8*(2), 267–278.

Kahn, R.S., Westenberg, H.G., & Jolles, J. (1984). Zimelidine treatment of obsessive–compulsive disorder: Biological and neurophysiological aspects. *Acta
Psychiatrica Scandinavica, 69*, 259–261.

Kelman, D.H. (1965). Gilles de la Tourette's disease in children: A review of the
literature. *Journal of Child Psychology & Psychiatry, 6*, 219–226.

Knesevitch, J.M. (1982). Successful treatment of obsessive–compulsive disorder with clonidine hydrochloride. *American Journal of Psychiatry, 139,* 364–365.

Leckman, J.F., Sholomskas, D., Thompson, W.D., Belanger, A, & Weissman, M.M. (1982). Best estimate of lifetime psychiatric diagnoses: A methodological study. *Archives of General Psychiatry, 39,* 879–883.

Leckman, J.F., Cohen, D.J., Detlor, J., Young, J.G., Harcherik, D., & Shaywitz, B.A. (1982). Clonidine in the treatment of Tourette syndrome: A review of data. In A.J., Friedhoff, & T.N. Chase (Eds.), *Gilles de la Tourette Syndrome.* New York: Raven.

Leckman, J.F., Detlor, J., Harcherick, D., Ort, S.I., & Cohen, D.J. (1985). Short-and long-term treatment of Tourette's disorder with clonidine: A clinical perspective. *Neurology, 35,* 343–351.

Leckman, J.F., Walkup, J.T., Riddle, M.A., Towbin, K.E., & Cohen, D.J. (1987). Psychopharmacology of Tourette's syndrome: An update. In R.Y. Meltzer, W. Bunney, J. Coyle, J. Davis, I. Kopin, R. Schuster, R. Shader, G. Simpson, *Psychopharmacology, the Third Generation of Progress.* New York: Raven.

Meige, H., & Feindel, F. (1907). *Tics and Their Treatment.* London: Appleton.

Montgomery, M.A., Clayton, P.C., & Friedhoff, A.J. (1982). Psychiatric illness in Tourette syndrome patients and first-degree relatives. In A.J. Friedhoff, & T.N. Chase (Eds.), *Gilles de la Tourette Syndrome.* New York: Raven.

Morphew, J.A., & Sim, M. (1969). Gilles de la Tourette's syndrome: A clinical and psychopathological study. *British Journal of Medical Psychology, 42,* 293–301.

Nee, L.E., Caine, E.D., Polinsky, R.J., Eldridge, R., & Ebert, M.H. (1980). Gilles de la Tourette syndrome: Clinical and family study of 50 cases. *Annals of Neurology, 7*(1), 41–49.

Nee, L.E., Polinsky, R.J., & Ebert, M.H. (1982). Tourette syndrome: Clinical and family studies. In A.J. Friedhoff, T.N. Chase (Eds.), *Gilles de la Tourette Syndrome.* New York: Raven.

Nose, T., & Takamoto, H. (1975). The effect of penfluridol and some psychotropic drugs on monoamine metabolism in central nervous system. *European Journal of Pharmacology, 31,* 351–359.

O'Regan, J.B. (1970). Treatment of obsessive–compulsive neurosis with haloperidol. *Canadian Medical Association Journal, 103*(2), 167–168.

Pauls, D.L., Cohen, D.J., Heimbuch, R.C., Detlor, J., & Kidd, K.K. (1981). The familial transmission of Tourette's syndrome. *Archives of General Psychiatry, 38,* 1091–1093.

Pauls D.L., Kruger, S.D., Leckman, J.F., Cohen, D.J., & Kidd, K.K. (1984). The risk of Tourette's syndrome and chronic multiple tics among relatives of Tourette's syndrome patients obtained by direct interview. *Journal of the American Academy of Child Psychiatry, 23*(2), 134–137.

Pauls, D.L., & Leckman, J.F. (1986). The inheritance of Gilles de la Tourette's syndrome and associated behaviors: Evidence for an autosomal dominant transmission. *New England Journal of Medicine, 315,* 993–997.

Pauls, D.L., Towbin, K.E., Leckman, J.F., Zahner, G.E.P., & Cohen, D.J. (1986)

Gilles de la Tourette syndrome and obsessive–compulsive disorder: Evidence supporting a genetic relationship. *Archives of General Psychiatry, 43*(12), 1180–1183.

Prasad, A. (1984). A double blind study of imipramine versus zimelidine in the treatment of obsessive–compulsive neurosis. *Pharmacopsychiatry, 17*(2), 61–62.

Price, L.H., Goodman, W.K., Charney, D.S., Rasmussen, S.A. and Heninger, G. R. (1987). Treatment of severe obsessive-compulsive disorder with fluvoxamine. *American Journal of Psychiatry* 144(8), 1059–1061.

Price, R.A., Kidd, K.K., Cohen, D.J., Pauls, D.L., & Leckman, J.F. (1985). A twin study of Tourette syndrome. *Archives of General Psychiatry, 42*(8), 815–820.

Rasmussen, S. (1984). Lithium and l-tryptophan augmentation in clomipramine resistant obsessive–compulsive disorder. *American Journal of Psychiatry, 141,* 1283–1285.

Robins, L.N., Helzer, J.E., Weissman, M.M., Orvashel, H., Gruenberg, E., Burke, J.D., & Regier, D.A. (1984). Lifetime prevalence of specific psychiatric disorders in 3 sites. *Archives of General Psychiatry, 41*(10), 949–959.

Rudin, E. (1953). Ein Beitrag zur Frage der Zwangskrankheit, inbesondere ihre hederitaren Beziehungen. *Archiv für Psychiatrie und Nervenkrankheiten. 191,* 14–54.

Seeman, P., & Lee, T. (1975). Antipsychotic drugs: Direct correlation between clinical potency and presynaptic action on dopamine neurons. *Science, 188,* 1217–1219.

Serra, G., Argiolas, A., Klimek V., Fadd, F., and Gessa, G.L. (1979). Chronic treatment with antidepressants prevents the inhibitor effect of small doses of apomorphine on dopamine synthesis and motor activity. *Life Sciences, 25,* 415–424.

Shapiro, A.K., Shapiro, E.S., Bruun, R.D., & Sweet, R.D. (1978). *Gilles de la Tourette Syndrome.* New York: Raven.

Shapiro, A.K., Shapiro, E.S., & Eisenkraft, G.J. (1983). Treatment of Gilles de la Tourette syndrome with pimozide. *American Journal of Psychiatry, 140,* 1183–1186.

Shapiro, A.K., Shapiro, E., & Eisenkraft, G.J. (1983). Treatment of Tourette syndrome with clonidine and neuroleptics. *Archives of General Psychiatry, 40,* 1235–1240.

Singer, K. (1963). Gilles de la Tourette disease. *American Journal of Psychiatry, 120,* 80–81.

Stefl, M.E. (1983). *The Ohio Tourette Study.* University of Cincinnati, School of Planning.

Svensson, T.H., Bunney, B.S., & Aghajanian, G.K. (1975). Inhibition of both noradrenergic and serotonergic neurons in brain by the alpha-adrenergic agonist clonidine. *Brain Research, 92,* 291–306.

Towbin, K.E., Leckman, J.F., & Cohen, D.J. (1987). Drug treatment of obsessive–compulsive disorder: A review of findings in the light of diagnostic and metric limitations. *Psychiatric Developments, 5*(1), 25–50.

Yaryura-Tobias, J.A., Neziroglu, F., Howard S., & Fuller, B. (1981). Clinical aspects of Gilles de la Tourette syndrome. *Journal of Orthomolecular Psychiatry*, *10*(4), 263–268.

Yaryura-Tobias, J.A. (1977) L-tryptophan in obsessive-compulsive disorders. *American Journal of Psychiatry* 134(11):1298–1299.

Zohar, J., Mueller, E.A., Insel, T.R., Zohar-Kadouch, R.C., and Murphy, D.L. (1987). Serotonergic responsivity in obsessive-compulsive disorder. *Archives of General Psychiatry* 44(11): 946–951.

Zohar, J. and Insel, T.R. (1987) Obsessive-compulsive disorder: Psychobiological approaches to diagnosis, treatment and pathophysiology. *Biological Psychiatry* 22: 667–687.

CHAPTER TEN

Behavioral Symptoms in Tourette's Syndrome

Mark A. Riddle
Maureen T. Hardin
Sharon I. Ort
James F. Leckman
Donald J. Cohen

Various psychiatric and behavioral disturbances have been associated with Tourette's syndrome (TS) since Tourette's original description (Cohen, 1980; Comings & Comings, 1985; Gilles de la Tourette, 1885; Leckman, Detlor, & Cohen, 1983; Mahler & Rangell, 1943). A review of the literature indicates that patients, especially children, with TS have a greater incidence of behavioral problems than other populations (Comings & Comings, 1985). The most common associated behavioral symptoms—obsessions and compulsions, hyperactivity, distractibility, and impulsivity—are discussed in separate chapters in this volume (Comings & Comings, Chapter 8; Towbin, Chapter 9). This chapter will focus primarily on the behavioral problem—failure of inhibition of aggression—that is a major source of intrapsychic pain and social impairment for many patients with TS. In addition, the relationship of TS to other major psychiatric disorders will be discussed. Finally, several behavioral problems, such as school refusal and social isolation, that are thought to develop in response to having TS will be described.

LITERATURE REVIEW

Various authors have described behavioral symptoms in patients with TS and have attempted to understand their significance or explain their etiology. Table 10.1 reviews the literature.

FAILURE OF INHIBITION OF AGGRESSION

For a substantial subgroup of patients with TS, associated behavioral symptoms, particularly aggression directed toward others, can be the most disabling and confusing clinical problems. The recent Ohio survey suggests that as many as 25 to 30 percent of TS patients may often experience extreme temper or aggressive behavior (Stefl, 1983). Aggression may be expressed in numerous ways, such as yelling and screaming; throwing objects, hitting, biting, scratching, kicking, or spitting at a parent or sibling; destroying favorite toys or objects; punching holes in walls; or breaking windows. Failure of inhibition of aggression generally is manifested in a predictable pattern over time. Tics commonly have an onset between the ages of 4 and 12 years. A careful history, however, may reveal preexisting difficulties with regulation of activity, temper tantrums, and aggressive behavior, often starting in the toddler years. During their early school years, these children frequently are identified as having difficulties with distractibility, hyperactivity, impulsivity, as well as unpredictability in their regulation and expression of anger. Frequently a diagnosis of attention deficit disorder is made. Peer relation-

Table 10.1. Behavioral Symptoms in Tourette's Syndrome: A Literature Review

Author	Date	Explanation
Gilles de la Tourette	1885	Psychological features cause expression of tics
Mahler & Rangell	1943	Term "incontinence of the emotions" used to describe individuals with TS
Ascher	1948	Hostile reaction to authority figures seen more commonly in TS
Torup	1962	Restlessness, sensitivity, and anxiety are common features in TS
Shapiro et al.	1972	Psychopathology and behavioral difficulties occur only in response to having a chronic illness (e.g., TS)
Cohen	1980	Some patients with TS exhibit "failure of inhibition of aggression," impaired cognitive development, and delayed social and emotional development
Wilson et al.	1982	Behavior problems seen in TS patients are similar to those seen in children with learning disorders and behavior problems

ships commonly are lacking or highly charged with bursts of anger. With the development of motor and phonic tics the child and family are confronted with yet another problem. The child, who often is acutely aware of his or her behavioral difficulties and tics, makes conscious efforts to control them voluntarily. At the same time, he or she may receive repeated messages from parents, teachers, siblings, and peers that these behaviors and tics are negative and should be stopped. Parents may have difficulty identifying what sets the child off. Some children are able to suppress the tics and behavioral difficulties while in school but explode into a surge of symptoms on returning home with parents or siblings. They often appear irritable and anger easily. Cohen describes such children as frightened and pained by what they feel they cannot control or as possessed by a force that makes them place into action the most dreaded sexual and aggressive ideas that suddenly come into their minds (1980).

The following clinical vignette illustrates some of the features of the failure of inhibition of aggression seen in many patients with TS.

Max, now a 13-year-old boy, first came to our attention at age 7, when he was evaluated for multiple motor and phonic tics. The history revealed a child who was more active than average from birth and by age 3 had significant difficulty adjusting to nursery school. At an early age he was described as "always in motion," with peer problems, including difficulty sharing and frequent fighting. At age 6, Max developed his first motor tic. Within 6 months his tics increased in number and frequency and eventually progressed to phonic tics. During this time his behavior also deteriorated. In school the problems included overactivity, distractibility, and difficulty reacting to peers. He was the object of teasing about his tics. Despite these difficulties, he was seen by his teachers as bright, submissive, and eager to please.

At home the situation was very different. By the time he was 7 his behavioral difficulties were escalating. The slightest situation would cause a temper outburst of yelling, banging things, and retreating to his room. By age 10 Max was argumentative with his parents, especially his mother. When asked why he talked back to his parents, Max would respond, "I don't want to do it, it just seems to come out. I feel real bad afterwards. I wish I never said those things." Max started swearing around his mother and siblings but less so around his father. The swearing occasionally involved a combination of sexual and aggressive overtones, such as writing "fuck off." His parents were bewildered and at first attempted to explain his aggressive behavior as preadolescent rebellion. As his behavior gradually began to increase in severity, his parents' concerns increased. His mother felt that she no longer was able to set boundaries with him. A new behavior developed—hitting his mother during times of temper outbursts. It was at this point that the parents agreed to seek professional help. Max's physical aggression toward his mother and siblings never was as painful as it was frightening. There never was physical harm, but everyone was tense and felt abused.

Max was bewildered by his own behavior. He complained of being out of control. He acknowledged the wish to hurt his mother. Yet he said that he felt bad after he yelled at her or punched her. He acknowledged some ability to control his behavior. He couldn't stop himself completely from punching at his mother, but he could "pull the punches" so that he avoided hurting her seriously. When asked, "Why do you hit your mother?" Max replied, "I don't know. There's something about her that makes me mad—I'm not sure what it is. I know she loves me and cares about me. But sometimes she makes me mad, and I just feel the urge to hit her. I wish I didn't do it. But I can't stop. Sometimes I feel like something is inside me, making me do these things."

At age 13, after Max entered eighth grade, school stresses intensified, and his motor and phonic tics increased. At the same time his aggressive behavior at home became worse. His mother began to fear his acting out, saying, "He takes pleasure in hurting my feelings and frequently describes the wish to kill someone." He also started punching walls, destroying furniture, and on one occasion impulsively pulled a knife on his mother. His anxiety level increased to the degree that he was overeating, had difficulty falling asleep at night, and described feelings of being totally out of control.

The particular manner in which aggressive symptoms are manifested varies from patient to patient. In the case of Max, the failure of inhibition of aggression was expressed to an extreme. Neither he nor his parents were able to create order or boundaries for his inappropriate, frightening behavior. Initially, patients with TS may express aggression passively, for example, refusing to carry out simple tasks such as picking up clothes or carrying out the trash. The first direct expressions of aggressive behavior usually are verbal and include "talking back" to parents and siblings. This often is followed by abusive verbalizations that may include swearing. Some parents describe "Jekyll and Hyde" behavior in their children, for example: "Most of the time he's sweet, and he behaves well, but occasionally he changes dramatically—it's as though there's this monster inside. It's very confusing, and I never know when he's going to explode." Yelling back and forth between child and parent may escalate into physical abuse. Usually the Tourette's patient does not hurt seriously the object of the physical aggression. The behavior typically is more threatening and scary than directly harmful. Shadowboxing or "pulled" punches are common. As these verbal and physical behaviors continue, the whole family can develop a sense of being out of control. Parents may be confused by the combination of predominantly "good" behavior combined with occasional, seemingly unpredictable, "bad" behavior. Parents often wonder whether or not they should hold their child responsible for these aggressive behaviors.

Because society expects adults to have more control over their behavior than children, failure of inhibition of aggression is an especially disabling problem for adult TS patients.

Mr. W, a 23-year-old patient with severe motor and phonic tics, punches holes in his car's dashboard, yells out obscenities in social situations, and is quick to lose his temper and throw things. Despite above-average intelligence and a college degree, he is unable to obtain steady employment. His aggressive outbursts, not tics, have led to the loss of numerous jobs.

Mrs. T, a 26-year-old mother of two young children, talks about her frightening, aggressive thoughts, which include the following images: "When I'm walking with my 2-year-old son and holding his hand, I have this overwhelming urge to squeeze him until he cries. When I'm changing my baby, I have this desire to push in on the soft spot on top of his head."

Examples are numerous of adults who appear to have a "good" and "bad" self. Their unpredictable outbursts and preoccupation with suppressing aggressive thoughts can create marital and parenting problems that, in turn, may lead to chaos in the family, divorce, and emotional responses in their children.

Mr. A is a 31-year-old married father of two children who first came to us because he had developed significant side effects while taking haloperidol. When he was off this medication, not only were his tics more severe, but his aggressive outbursts were intolerable. He constantly yelled at his wife and children and would punish his children physically for minor offenses. He also developed two self-abusive behaviors—digging at his gums and biting his lips until they were sore and painful.

The specific etiology of failure of inhibition of aggression in patients with TS is not known. Patients, parents, and teachers often ask whether the behavioral symptoms are involuntary or whether they can be controlled voluntarily. Framing the question in this way, although useful in legal or philosophical discussions, fails to capture the patients' experience in a clinically meaningful way. We have found it more helpful to describe the patient as having a "thin barrier" between aggressive thoughts or feelings and the expression of aggressive acts. Some patients prefer the term "short fuse." Thus, these patients with TS are similar to others in that they experience aggressive thoughts and express aggressive behaviors; they are different in that the aggression is expressed more frequently and more "easily." In addition, the patient's environment, particularly the family, as well as his or her psychological makeup, play an important role in determining the specificity and intensity of the aggressive behaviors. Adolescents and adults talk about either a lack of control or a feeling of being out of control. The lack of control usually is described in the following terms: "I don't know what happens, I get so mad that I hit my brother ... I feel so bad afterwards." A feeling of being out of control stirs up not only guilt but anxiety at not having the ability to control frightening behavior. For some, the feeling of being out of control can exceed the expression of the behavioral symptoms and the tics. An example of this feeling of being out of control is the adolescent who states: "Once it starts, I can't seem to stop. It's like the feelings have all taken over. I get so mad it scares me."

The patient's perception of what causes this lack of control or feeling of being out of control also varies. Some blame external events and deny their own involvement in causing the behavior. Others may view the events as random and spontaneous. An example of the former is the patient who explains: "My brother made me so mad, he's always messing up my things." An example of the latter is the patient who states: "I don't understand what sets me off. Sometimes it could just be my mother walking in front of me."

Whatever the description or perception of the behavior, the individual's internal controls of angry and aggressive feelings are lacking. Whether this poor impulse control differs in degree or description from that of other children with similar difficulties but without TS is not known.

Motor and phonic tics are more severe during times of excitement or stress. They usually are seen most frequently at home, where the patient feels most comfortable and least afraid of embarrassment or retaliation. Acts of aggression also occur most commonly in the home. Perhaps the most difficult aspect of the aggressive behaviors for parents and spouses to understand and accept is the observation that they most commonly are directed at the most loved and important people in the patient's life. From an analytic perspective, those people with whom we are involved most intimately are the ones toward whom we experience the most intense thoughts and feelings, not only of love and caring, but also of anger and aggression. While other individuals may experience similar thoughts and feelings, it is the intensity of the verbal and physical response that may be different in the individual with TS.

Patients often channel their aggressive behavior along specific lines. Our observations suggest that the targets of aggression are "selected" to minimize the possibility of retaliation. For example, if other children in the neighborhood or at school become the targets of aggression, it usually is younger, smaller children who are selected. Patients usually are not consciously aware of having selected a particular target, beyond occasional awareness that someone has annoyed or irritated them. Pets also are a common target for aggressive behavior. Initially, aggressive behavior commonly is directed toward parents, sibling, or pets in the home—patients seem to have sufficient ability to control aggressive behaviors with peers and schoolmates. However, if the intensity of the aggressivity escalates, the behaviors may spill over into the neighborhood or classroom.

Careful clinical evaluation will reveal some failure of inhibition of aggression in many patients with Tourette's syndrome. The intensity of the failure to control aggression often parallels the severity of the motor and phonic tic symptoms, but this is not always true. Whether certain subgroups of patients with Tourette's syndrome have more difficulties with aggression than with, for example, associated attention deficit disorder with hyperactivity or obsessive-compulsive features is not known. Empirical studies are needed to clarify this issue.

Occasionally a patient may develop psychotic symptoms related to his difficulty controlling aggressive thoughts and behaviors. These symptoms usually are described as indistinct voices or other environmental cues (e.g., the television telling the patient to commit a violent act). The patient also may describe delusional fears of retaliation. The psychotic symptoms usually are connected to aggressive themes and a pervasive sense of being out of control. Generally, they are not accompanied by other psychotic symptoms.

ASSOCIATED PSYCHIATRIC DISORDERS

Previous and current studies have found that obsessive–compulsive symptoms frequently are associated with TS, but other types of psycho-pathology are not related directly (Jagger et al., 1982; Nee, Caine, Polin-sky, Eldridge, & Ebert, 1980; Pauls, Cohen, Heimbuch, Detlor, & Kidd, 1981; Pauls & Leckman, 1986; Pauls, Towbin, Leckman, Zahner, & Co-hen, 1986). In the past, various psychopathological states, such as schizo-phrenia and schizoid personality, were thought to be associated with TS. Shapiro, in a study involving 34 patients, found that the incidence of general psychiatric disturbance, including schizoid personality traits, was higher in patients with TS than the general population but that the incidence of schizophrenia and other underlying psychoses was not significantly higher (Shapiro, Shapiro, Wayne, & Clarkin, 1972).

Comings and Comings (1985), in a large study concerning the psycho-logical aspects of TS, found that no major psychiatric disturbance was commonly seen except obsessions in many patients, but the frequency of clearly diagnosable major affective disorder was not determined. Corbett and coworkers found that parents of children with tics showed a higher proportion of affective illness as compared to a psychiatric population (Corbett, Mathews, Connell, & Shapiro, 1969). Whether or not the affec-tive illness resulted from living with a child with a chronic disorder is not known.

Unfortunately, there have been no reports of well-designed studies of the frequency of carefully diagnosed, major psychiatric disorders in patients with TS. In the near future, the Yale Tourette Syndrome Family Genetic Study under the direction of Dr. David Pauls should provide important information regarding this question.

SECONDARY BEHAVIORAL PROBLEMS

Two other behavioral problems—school refusal and social isolation—seen in patients with TS appear to develop in response to living with a chronic neuropsychiatric disorder. Frequently, parents of children with TS complain about the difficulties they have getting their children to attend school willingly. Usually, this complaint is heard only after the child has become the object of teasing or punishment about the tics. Some children are direct in expressing their wish not to attend school. Others may complain of aches and pains in the morning before leaving for school. Obviously, the wish not to attend school is fairly common among school-age children in general. What is striking about children with TS is the relationship between teasing by schoolmates or reproachment by teachers and the wish to stay home.

Another common problem seen in patients with TS is social isolation. Many patients, both children and adults, will acknowledge a wish to have more friends and to be more involved socially. Although there appears to be an obvious connection between the patient's embarrassment about his or her tics and social isolation, it is our impression that many patients are not consciously aware of such a connection. Other symptoms that can contribute to social isolation include aggressive and impulsive behaviors.

Frequently, social maturation is delayed or, as in some of our adult patients, never achieved. For example, Max was described by his parents and teachers as never being able to take the right steps in making a friend or relating to peers. One very bright male patient made the following comment: "I never had many friends and never played sports because it was always too painful to have to deal with their curiosity and questions about my tics."

ASSESSMENT AND MANAGEMENT

Assessment and management of behavioral difficulties in TS depend on several factors: (1) the severity of the behavioral symptoms; (2) the patient's experience of these symptoms; (3) the family's abilities to recognize and respond to the patient's needs; and (4) the strength of the support system outside the family.

Behavioral symptoms are assessed by the amount of interference or disruption the behavior causes the patient and family. For many, the degree of difficulty caused by aggressive symptoms is greater than that caused by tics. Behavior causing disruption in the family and/or the classroom commonly is the initial reason for bringing a child to a physician for help. Parents describe their own feelings of frustration and despair at the constancy of their child's outbursts, the inability to predict these outbursts, and finally the difficulty they have in establishing external controls. The outbursts, as mentioned previously, can be either yelling and screaming or a combination of verbal attacks and hitting, kicking, or throwing things. Success in management, in our experience, seems related proportionately to severity. Thus not only the description of the behavior but also the frequency and degree of resulting disruption are important.

Success in management also depends on the ability of the individual to gain insight into what causes his or her difficulties and thus to learn to use alternate ways of responding to troublesome situations. The patient who is able to use insight may benefit from individual psychotherapy. Otherwise, a behavioral approach to therapy may be useful.

The ability of the parents to provide an accepting and therapeutic environment for the child depends largely on their own emotional health. TS can be a chronic illness; that alone can be wearing and damaging to the emotional strength of a family. The clinician frequently is asked to provide education, support, and, as necessary, referral for therapy. This therapy may take various directions. It may be aimed at helping parents channel their own feelings of frustration, anger, and guilt or may be directed at teaching them appropriate patterns of responses or how to construct appropriate controls for their children.

For many children the behavioral difficulties extend to the classroom, causing problems in social adjustment and learning. For adult patients, these difficulties may cause chronic employment problems or, in severe situations, frequent loss of employment. Education by the clinician concerning TS, in conjunction with individual therapy and family support, may be all that is needed. In situations where the behavior is more disruptive, special class placement for the child may be necessary. For adults, vocational counseling often is helpful.

Pharmacological intervention may be necessary when behavioral symptoms become severe. It is our impression that the common agents used to treat the core symptoms (tics) also are helpful in decreasing behavioral difficulties. Thus the behavioral components of TS become an important consideration when medication is being considered (i.e., clonidine, haloperidol, or pimozide). This also is the case in assessing the efficacy of the medication. It is important to assess not only the decrease in tics but the decrease in behavioral difficulties. The use of medication without some form of individual and family support generally is unproductive. A combination of pharmacotherapy, individual and family counseling, and special school or vocational intervention usually is the most successful approach.

Specific treatment recommendations are difficult to discuss because of the variation in symptoms and the variation in needs of each patient. The following interventions are ones that we find most successful. Individual or group psychotherapy focusing on the difficult behavior is the most common treatment recommendation. The therapist's understanding of the nature and course of the tic disorder is most important because of the relationship this has with the aggressive behavior. For children and adolescents, the school can be an important area for management. When the behavioral difficulties overflow into the school and learning is impaired, a program that is highly structured, small in class size, and involves special attention to learning needs generally is most successful. Likewise, for children and adolescents, the use of behavioral techniques by the individual therapist or special education professional also can be productive for both the patient and the family. When the aggressive symptoms become severe, such as violent outbursts or an overwhelming sense of being out of control, pharmacological intervention or evaluation and treatment on an inpatient unit may be necessary.

CONCLUSION

The associated behavioral symptoms seen in patients with TS—failure of inhibition of aggression and secondary behavioral problems of social isolation and delayed maturation—are observed frequently and often are socially disabling. The evaluation of a patient with TS should include a thorough review of these associated behaviors. Effective treatment of these symptoms often requires involvement of the patient, family, and school. The goal of research in this area is to understand the pathogenesis of aggressive behavior, to define more clearly the clinical features of this aspect of TS, and to identify more effective means of intervention.

(*Editors' Note:* Parts 3, 4, and 5 of this volume also address various aspects of evaluation and treatment of TS. Cohen, Ort, Leckman, Riddle, & Hardin, Chapter 12; Hagin, Chapter 15; Wolff, Chapter 14; and Azrin & Peterson, Chapter 16, are particularly germane to the issues raised in this chapter.)

REFERENCES

Ascher, E. (1948). Psychodynamic considerations in Gilles de la Tourette's disease (Maladie des tics). *American Journal of Psychiatry, 105,* 267–276.

Cohen, D.J. (1980). The pathology of the self in primary childhood autism and Gilles de la Tourette syndrome. *Psychiatric Clinics of North America, 3*(3), 383–402.

Comings, D.E., & Comings, B.G. (1985). Tourette syndrome: Clinical and psychological aspects of 250 cases. *American Journal of Human Genetics, 37,* 435–450.

Corbett, J.A., Mathews, A.M., Connell, P.H., & Shapiro, D.A. (1969). Tics and Gilles de la Tourette's syndrome: A pilot study. *Schizophrenic Bulletin, 8,* 269–278.

Gilles de la Tourette, G. (1885). Étude sur une affection nerveuse caractérisée par de l'incoordination motrice accompagnée d'echolalie et de coprolalie. *Archives de Neurologie, 9,* 19–42.

Jagger, J., Prusoff, B.A., Cohen, D.J., Kidd, K.K., Carbonari, C.M., & John, K. (1982). The epidemiology of Tourette's syndrome: A pilot study. *Schizophrenia Bulletin, 8,* 269–278.

Leckman, J.F., Detlor, J., & Cohen, D.J. (1983). Gilles de la Tourette syndrome: Emerging areas of clinical research. In S.B. Guze, F.J. Earls, & J.E. Barrett (Eds.), *Childhood Psychopathology and Development.* New York: Raven.

Mahler, M.S., & Rangell, L. (1943). A psychosomatic study of maladie des tics (Gilles de la Tourette's disease). *Psychiatric Quarterly, 17,* 519–605.

Nee, L.E., Caine, E.D., Polinsky, R.J., Eldridge, R., & Ebert, M.H. (1980). Gilles de la Tourette syndrome: Clinical and family study of 50 cases. *Annuals of Neurology, 7,* 41–49.

Pauls, D.L., Cohen, D.J., Heimbuch, R., Detlor, J., & Kidd, K.K. (1981). Familial pattern and transmission of Gilles de la Tourette syndrome and multiple tics. *Archives of General Psychiatry, 38,* 1091–1093.

Pauls, D.L., & Leckman, J.F. The inheritance of Gilles de la Tourette syndrome and associated behaviors: Evidence for autosomal dominant transmission. *New England Journal of Medicine, 315,* 993–997.

Pauls, D.L., Towbin, K.E., Leckman, J.F., Zahner, G.E.P., & Cohen, D.J. (1986). Gilles de la Tourette's syndrome and obsessive compulsive disorder. *Archives of General Psychiatry, 43,* 1180–1182.

Shapiro, A.K., Shapiro, E., Wayne, H., & Clarkin, J. (1972). The psychopathology of Gilles de la Tourette's syndrome. *American Journal of Psychiatry, 192, 129*(4), 87–94.

Stefl, M.E. (1983). The Ohio Tourette study: An investigation of the special service needs of Tourette syndrome patients. Ohio Tourette Syndrome Association.

Torup, E. (1962). A follow-up study of children with tics. *Acta Paediatrica, 51,* 261–268.

Wilson, R.S., Garron, D.C., Tanner, C.M., & Klawans, H.L. (1982). Behavior disturbance in children with Tourette syndrome. In A.J. Friedhoff & T.N. Chase (Eds.), *Gilles de la Tourette syndrome.* New York: Raven.

CHAPTER ELEVEN

Stereotyped and Self-Injurious Behaviors in Disorders Other Than Tourette's Syndrome

Fred R. Volkmar
Joel D. Bregman

OVERVIEW

Repetitive behaviors, or stereotypies, and self-injurious behaviors (SIB) are observed in a variety of neuropsychiatric disorders and, occasionally, in otherwise normally developing children. Disorders in which such behaviors are common include mental retardation, infantile autism, Tourette's syndrome, and certain heritable metabolic syndromes, for example, Lesch-Nyhan syndrome. These behaviors can be viewed from a variety of theoretical perspectives and may, depending on their intensity or severity, be appropriate targets of intervention. This chapter presents a brief overview of research findings, theoretical models, and potential interventions related to these behaviors. Clinicians attempting to evaluate an individual case or to design specific intervention programs are encouraged to consult primary sources.

Stereotyped behaviors are defined, most simply, as rhythmic, purposeless, repetitive behaviors ranging from the thumb sucking of a normal infant to the profound engagement in a variety of self-stimulatory behaviors common in autistic individuals (Baumesiter & Forehand, 1973; Hoder & Cohen, 1983; Thelen, 1981). Repetitive behaviors that have obvious purpose or adaptive function are not encompassed within this definition, nor are other abnormal movement patterns such as those associated with tic disorders, epilepsy, chorea, and so on (Hoder & Cohen, 1983). Similarly, self-injurious behaviors may be defined as behaviors that are potentially or actually harmful to the subject. These behaviors may range in complexity from the head banging of an infant to more complex self-injurious behaviors observed in severely impaired and retarded individuals. Though self-injurious behaviors are less commonly observed than stereotypies and may be apparent only in quite specific situations (Bachman, 1972), observational studies suggest important relationships between these two classes of behavior (Volkmar, Hoder, & Cohen, 1985). Some investigators suggest that these two classes of behavior should be regarded as distinctive (see Barron & Sandman, 1983). Repetitive movements and episodes of self-injurious behavior may be observed in individuals with Tourette's syndrome; the primary focus of this chapter will be on these behaviors as they relate to other disorders, most notably mental retardation and pervasive developmental disorders. However, being retarded or manifesting symptoms of pervasive developmental disorders does not preclude the appearance of tic behaviors in combination with stereotypic movement disorders as reviewed by Fahn and Erenberg (Chapter 3, this volume).

DEVELOPMENTAL PERSPECTIVES

Self-stimulatory behaviors are commonly observed early in life and are not necessarily pathologic. Repetitive movements in utero and in early childhood may serve an important function as the developing child gains increased motor differentiation and mastery (Brazelton, 1973). Such movements are, however, typically transient and, in the absence of other factors, such as environmental or sensory deprivation, they do not commonly become preferential modes of activity. These behaviors, in the otherwise normally developing infant, tend to follow a characteristic developmental course and cephalocaudal progression (Gesell & Ilg, 1937). For example, nonnutritive sucking of the hand can be observed in utero and in normal babies within hours after birth and reaches a peak in the later half of the first year of life (Kravitz & Boehm, 1971). Similar patterns are observed for movements of the lower extremities.

Body rocking, head banging, and head rolling differ from other stereotyped behaviors in the degree to which they involve significant vestibular stimulation. Although differences in the definitions of these behaviors make comparisons between reports difficult, such behaviors may be observed in a significant number of normal children and are most common when the child is alone or at the onset or cessation of sleep and again follow a predictable developmental course in most cases (Hoder & Cohen, 1983). Body rocking and head rolling and nodding are relatively commonly observed (Kravitz & Boehm, 1971). Body rocking is usually a transient, self-limited behavior occurring within the first year of life. Head rolling has a somewhat later onset and may result in significant hair loss. Head banging is the most dramatic of these behaviors and is observed in 5 to 15 percent of normal children (Hoder & Cohen, 1983). It may occur in association with otitis media or teething, and may be associated with significant injury. This behavior is particularly distressing to parents; high rates (up to 80 times per minute) may be observed. Although usually self-limited, head banging is sometimes so persistent or severe as to require intervention.

Other behaviors with a strong repetitive component include bruxism, nail biting, trichotillomania, and so forth. Bruxism, the habit of grinding the teeth together, is observed after the eruption of teeth and may be seen in as many as 56 percent of normal infants (Kravitz & Boehm, 1971), particularly during sleep. Bruxism can be associated with various disorders. Nail biting is a particularly common habit in childhood and adulthood. Nail biting usually develops after 4 or 5 years of age and becomes most common in later childhood before decreasing. Although usually not associated with serious injury, this behavior can be of concern to parents and can be effectively treated with various behavioral interventions.

Trichotillomania, hair pulling, is relatively uncommon in childhood. Hair can be removed from any body area and is plucked, twisted, or rubbed off. Trichotillomania must be differentiated from other disorders resulting in hair loss, for example, alopecia areata, tinea capitis, and so forth. It may be highly resistant to treatment. Skin diseases can predispose to self-injurious behaviors such as biting, scratching, and so on.

In autistic and mentally retarded children stereotyped behaviors may fail to disappear over the course of development and instead become preferential modes of activity. The autistic child may be content to spend hours on end engaged in hand flapping or other stereotyped behaviors (Ritvo, Ornitz, & La Franchi, 1968). Self-injurious behaviors may also become common, particularly in lower-functioning individuals (Schroeder, Mulick, & Rojahn, 1980).

Stereotyped movement disorders, as outlined in DSM-III, are also characterized by repetitive motor (and sometimes phonic) movements that are variably expressed and can be voluntarily suppressed for brief periods. Movements in these disorders typically are a cause of distress and are not preferred modes of activity, as they are with autism or mental retardation. Additionally, they have a spasmodic nature. Transient tic disorder is characterized by motor tics of varying intensity most commonly involving the face and lasting for more than a month but less than a year. As defined in DSM-III, chronic motor tic disorder is characterized by invariant intensity of the tics with duration of over a year. Tourette's disorder is characterized by both motor and phonic tics that vary in intensity and last for more than a year. The atypical stereotyped movement disorder category in DSM-III is reserved for conditions, such as head banging, involving nonspasmodic, voluntary movements. The relationship of the stereotyped movement disorders, that is, the possibility that they represent a continuum of severity, is not well established, though a progression of the disorder is apparent in many cases. Self-injurious behaviors are also commonly observed in patients with certain inborn errors of metabolism, most notably in Lesch-Nyhan syndrome, and in children with sensory defects and those suffering from environmental deprivation (Edelson, 1984).

THEORETICAL PERSPECTIVES

Various attempts have been made to understand the etiology and pathogenesis of stereotyped and self-injurious behaviors within the context
of various psychological or biological theories. At present, the available
evidence does not appear to support either perspective exclusively. Psychological models and research reports concerned with these behaviors
have been based on a variety of theoretical orientations ranging from
psychodynamic to learning theory. These theories differ in their emphasis on environmental versus intrinsic factors and the nature of factors that act to sustain these behaviors. Some investigators suggest that
these behaviors are manifestations of neuromuscular development
(Thelen, 1979), serve important practice functions (Sallustro & Atwell,
1978), reflect inherent drives to activity and self-stimulation (Baumeister & Forehand, 1973), or are manifestations of high levels of arousal
or anxiety perhaps related to CNS factors. Learning theorists view these
behaviors as acquired by inadvertent reinforcement and maintained by
environmental contingencies. As described subsequently, many of the
most sophisticated behavioral interventions have been conducted with
this framework. Given the degree to which such behaviors may interfere
with remedial efforts, it is not surprising that they are commonly viewed
as targets for intervention. The degree to which such efforts are successful, though gratifying, does not necessarily establish a particular pathogenic mechanism; for example, behavior modification procedures may
be helpful in reducing such behaviors but do not account for their initial presence.

The importance of neurobiological factors in the pathogenesis of
stereotyped and self-injurious behaviors is suggested by several lines
of evidence. Such behaviors may be elicited in animals by the administration of dopamine or the dopamine agonist amphetamine and by ablation
of specific cortical regions and inhibited by administration of dopamine
antagonistics, for example, the neuroleptics. Similar behaviors can
sometimes be observed in humans following administration of amphet-
amines and other stimulants or after cortical damage; stimulant administration typically exacerbates stereotyped behaviors that are commonly
diminished by neuroleptics (Young, Kavanagh, Anderson, Shaywitz, &
Cohen, 1982). A variety of experimental manipulations, for example,
sensory isolation, maternal deprivation, and stress, may potentiate
stereotyped behaviors. The importance of dopaminergic systems in the

production of these behaviors seems relatively clear although other neurotransmitter systems may significantly modify their expression (Young et al., 1982). A variety of technical and practical problems have complicated research studies of children in this area.

ASSESSMENT AND TREATMENT

Stereotyped and self-injurious behaviors may be observed in individuals with various psychiatric and medical conditions and with varying degrees of intellectual impairment. Accordingly, the first obligation of the clinician, after ensuring the patient's safety, is to conduct a thorough assessment. Generally, this would include a psychiatric assessment, physical examination, developmental or intellectual testing, and an assessment of adaptive functioning. Additional laboratory studies, for example, urine for genetic screening, blood for chromosome analysis, and so forth, and specialized consultation, pediatric or neurologic, may be indicated. The patient's psychosocial environment may also be an important aspect of assessment and intervention efforts. Treatments should be based on such comprehensive assessments. Interventions should, to the extent possible, be minimally intrusive. Assessment and treatment methods for stereotyped and self-injurious behaviors in otherwise normally developing children have been reviewed by others (Hoder & Cohen, 1983); the assessment and treatment of tic disorders are discussed elsewhere in this volume. Although the discussion of treatment studies here will largely focus on individuals with mental retardation and pervasive developmental disorders (PDD) and will exclude discussion of patients with Tourette's disorder, it is important to recognize that there are many individuals who display both disorders.

Stereotypic and self-injurious behaviors are appropriate targets for clinical intervention when they pose the potential for injury or significantly interfere with learning and rehabilitation. However, the treatment of these behaviors poses a formidable clinical challenge since their etiology may be multifaceted and they may be observed in association with a variety of conditions. For treatment to succeed, interventions must be individualized and directed toward the various factors underlying or maintaining these behaviors.

During the past 20 years, a number of treatment approaches have been investigated. These have included surgery, ECT, psychoactive medications, psychotherapy, and various behavioral procedures (primarily of an operant, instrumental nature). Psychopharmacologic and behavioral interventions are currently the most popular. Ideally, the choice of treatments should be based upon etiological as well as ethical and legal considerations. Treatment should generally employ the least restrictive procedure possible (Dorsey, Iwata, Ong, & McSween, 1980; Rapoff, Altman, & Christophersen, 1980), with positive reinforcement techniques used in preference to aversive procedures (Durand, 1982).

Although hundreds of studies have been conducted in an attempt to determine the safest and most effective treatments for SIB and stereotypy among those with pervasive developmental disorders and mental retardation (for reviews see LaGrow & Repp, 1984; Singh, 1981, 1985), few definitive conclusions can be drawn since much of the available literature suffers from serious methodological problems. These problems include issues concerning appropriate experimental design, reliability of data, generalization of behavioral change, and maintenance of treatment effects over time. This chapter will focus on the two treatment approaches, behavioral and psychopharmacologic, that appear to offer the greatest benefit. While other approaches, for example, psychotherapy and surgery, have been employed, ethical, legal, or experimental problems complicate the interpretation of such studies. For example, a number of studies, some well designed, suggest the effectiveness of electric shock as an aversive deterrent to SIB (Singh, 1981), but ethical and legal constraints argue for extremely judicious use of such procedures. Similarly, electroconvulsive therapy appeared to be very effective in curtailing head banging in a severely retarded man with a pervasive developmental disorder (Bates & Smeltzer, 1982) after various pharmacologic and behavioral interventions had failed. However, the dramatic response may well have reflected an underlying affective disorder. Conversely, no studies suggest that such treatments are either effective or desirable approaches for Tourette's syndrome.

Pharmacologic Treatments

Various psychoactive agents, including the neuroleptics, stimulants, sedative–hypnotics, antimanics, and others (such as opiate antagonists, GABA analogues, and 1-5-hydroxytryptophan), have been employed, though few studies have been well designed or adequately controlled (see Singh, 1985, for a review). The neuroleptics are the most commonly used agents prescribed for control of stereotypies and SIB; they may be used in as many as 50 percent of institutionalized and community based mentally retarded individuals. These agents may provide some measure of behavioral control and sedation in appropriately selected patients.

Singh (1985) reviewed nine studies evaluating the effects of several commonly used neuroleptics on SIB in mentally retarded individuals. Eight of these studies reported clinical benefits, though all suffered from various methodological problems, for example, lack of appropriate experimental design, placebo controls, reliable assessments, and so on. In one single case report, Kinnell (1984) noted that fluphenazine, in daily doses of 36 to 48 mg, dramatically eliminated the incessant head punching and banging of a 17-year-old mentally retarded adolescent after physical restraint and various behavioral procedures had been unsuccessful. Similarly, in a placebo-controlled, crossover study, Aman, White, and Field (1984) found that relatively low doses of chlorpromazine (2–3 mg/kg/day) produced a 35 percent suppression of stereotyped body rocking in four profoundly retarded adolescents and young adults; however, administration of this agent significantly decreased performance on a learning task and the study's methodological problems (lack of a true "blind," relatively low dose of medication, brief treatment and drug wash-out periods) complicate its interpretation.

In a series of well-designed double-blind, placebo-controlled studies, Campbell and her associates have found haloperidol to be of significant benefit in reducing the stereotypic behaviors of autistic children without impairment of cognitive functioning. Campbell and colleagues (1978) noted that haloperidol, in doses of 0.5 to 4.0 mg per day, significantly reduced stereotypies and social withdrawal in hospitalized, young, autistic subjects. Cohen and colleagues (1980) found dramatic reductions in stereotypy and increased orienting responses in a similar group of subjects receiving equivalent doses of haloperidol. Subsequently, Campbell and colleagues (1982) found haloperidol, in doses of 0.5 mg to 3.0 mg per day, superior to placebo in reducing stereotyped behaviors, social withdrawal, and hyperactivity. These studies suggest that, in relatively low doses, haloperidol can induce behavioral improvement in young autistic individuals without adversely affecting cognitive function.

The utility of sedative–hypnotics in reducing stereotypy and SIB remains essentially untested. Singh (1985) in his recent review reported only one study assessing the efficacy of these agents; although diazepam was reported to be of benefit in reducing SIB in moderately and severely retarded adults, methodological problems make this report suspect. Primrose (1979) noted a significant decrease in SIB in 28 institutionalized mentally retarded young adults during treatment with baclofen (a GABA analogue), though again methodological problems complicate the interpretation of this result. In another case-control study of 100 mentally retarded adolescents (Barron & Sandman, 1983), various paradoxical responses to the agents, for example, excitation, restlessness, aggression, and so forth, were noted.

A few studies have assessed the potential benefit of lithium carbonate on SIB in mentally retarded patients (Singh, 1985). Though occasionally patients appeared to respond, methodological problems complicate the interpretation of these studies, and the utility of lithium remains to be established. Several investigators have suggested that SIB might repre-

sent a disturbance of the endogenous opiate system (related to a toni-
cally elevated pain threshold and/or addictive phenomena). In a well-
designed study, Sandman and colleagues (1983) found that the opiate
antagonist naloxone significantly attenuated SIB in one profoundly retarded young adult and eliminated it in another; "low frequency" SIB
appeared to be most sensitive, particularly at the lowest dose employed.
Similar results have been noted by other investigators; for example,
Davidson, Kleene, Carroll, and Rockowitz (1983) noted a decrease in intensity, though not frequency, of head banging in an 8-year-old severely
retarded boy. Though studies of the endogenous opiate system offer interesting possibilities for our understanding of some forms of SIB, the
usefulness of naloxone is limited by its short duration of action and par-
enteral administration. Studies of the effects of 5-hydroxytryptophan, a
serotonin precursor, have been contradictory (Singh, 1985).

Behavioral Interventions

Behavioral techniques have been the best researched and have generally
yielded encouraging results for the treatment of SIB and stereotypy associated with PDD and mental retardation (see: Azrin and Peterson,
Chapter 16, this volume). These techniques generally are derived from
learning theory that views such behaviors as maintained either by association with a reinforcement (e.g., attention) or by subsequent avoidance or termination of unpleasant situations (e.g., avoidance of social
interaction or educational tasks). Positive reward (reinforcement) techniques include differential reinforcement, via praise, attention, food,
tokens, and so forth, of other more adaptive behaviors (differential reinforcement of other behaviors or DRO) and differential reinforcement of behavior incompatible with the targeted maladaptive behavior
(DRI). Punishment procedures have included electric shock, aromatic
ammonia capsules, bitter tastes, the spraying of mist into the face, requirements for restitution and positive practice (overcorrection), and
withdrawal of positive reinforcement (e.g., timeout or response cost).
Associated techniques prevent the pleasurable feedback accompanying
a particular behavior (e.g., sensory extinction). Another approach focuses on the manipulation of antecedent events rather than subsequent
responses, for example, physical exercise. Behavioral interventions
generally are well designed; however, the small numbers of subjects
studied and questions regarding the generalizability of results to other
subjects or situations are potential problems in their interpretation.

The reinforcement of socially adaptive behaviors as a means of reducing stereotypy and SIB has significant appeal for both practical and
theoretical reasons. Such behaviors may be maintained by a lack of

ample environmental stimulation (Donnellan, Anderson & Mesaros, 1984; Volkmar, Hoder & Cohen, 1985). Situations that provide high degrees of environmental stimulation may reduce stereotypic responses (Frankel, Freeman, Ritvom, & Pardo, 1978). A general strategy has been the reinforcement of any adaptive behavior (DRO) and/or reinforcement of any behavior incompatible to the maladaptive one (DRI). Several studies (see Singh, 1985) suggest that DRO techniques may dramatically reduce SIB, though other studies are less encouraging. Tarpley and Schroeder (1979) compared the efficacy of DRO and DIR in reducing SIB in three profoundly retarded individuals. DRI was appreciably more rapid and effective; however, no information on the generalizability of the findings or their temporal maintenance was provided.

Time-out procedures involve the temporary removal (time-out) of an individual from a positively reinforcing environment contingent upon engagement in the maladaptive behavior. Overcorrection procedures represent mild degrees of punishment, most commonly consisting of repetitive practice of alternative forms of adaptive behaviors. Several studies suggest the potential utility of such procedures (Denny, 1980; Luiselli, Pemberton, & Helfen, 1978; Matson, Stephens, & Smith, 1978). Sensory extinction procedures, for example, the use of protective equipment such as padded gloves or helmets, have also been reported significantly to reduce SIB (Aiken & Salzberg, 1984; Dorsey, Iwata, Reid, & Davis, 1982). Visual screening, using the hand to block vision, has been reported to be effective in eliminating stereotypy and SIB (McGonigle, Duncan, Cordisco, & Barrett, 1982). Therapeutic effects of sensory extinction procedures may also, conceivably, be accounted for by the mildly aversive situations they present. Aversive procedures have also been employed for the PDD and mentally retarded populations, and they often appear to be effective. However, problems in research design may complicate their interpretation, and, given their potential for abuse, determination of the least restrictive treatment alternative suggests that they should be used only after other approaches have been unsuccessful.

Other studies have focused on antecedent behavioral manipulations. Kern et al., (1982a,b) reported that jogging reduced self-stimulatory behaviors in intellectually impaired autistic children while simultaneously improving task behavior, classroom motivation, and compliance. Behavioral changes were reliably documented and generalized across settings. Effects were sustained for 1 ½ to 2 hours following exercise. The authors postulated that effects might be related to exercise-induced stimulation of the endogenous opiate system, although this notion is at variance with the studies of Davidson and colleagues (1983) and Sandman and colleagues (1983) reviewed earlier. Subsequently, Kern (1984) demonstrated that only vigorous exercise (jogging vs. ball play) consistently reduced stereotypies in three autistic children. Similar findings have been reported in mentally retarded individuals (Baumeister & MacLean, 1984; Lancioni, Smeets, Ceccarani, Capodaglio, & Campanari, 1984). Finally, the interaction between pharmacologic and behavioral treatments is an important area of research. When used together such treatments may be more effective than when used separately (Campbell et al., 1978; Durand, 1982; McConahey, Thompson, & Zimmerman, 1977).

Treatment planning for patients with stereotypic and self-injurious behaviors associated with mental retardation or PDD must be based upon a careful psychiatric–behavioral assessment that identifies specific underlying disorders and contributory environmental factors. A search for contributing medical problems is always warranted. In those situations in which etiology remains obscure, treatment should begin with positive behavioral approaches, for example, differential reinforcement of other or incompatible behaviors, and then proceed to mildly aversive procedures, for example, time-out, overcorrection, and so on. Unfortunately, it is not possible to predict which behavioral approaches will be most useful for a given patient; differential treatment responses do not appear to be related to such factors as diagnosis, degree of intellectual impairment, or demographic variables. Should behavioral interventions prove unsuccessful, a trial of psychoactive medication is indicated. For those patients without other contributing disorders, a trial of neuroleptics, for example, haloperidol, appears to offer the greatest likelihood of success; the potential for adverse effects of these agents, particularly in relation to sedation, must always be weighed against the potential benefits. Other agents, such as lithium, may be helpful on occasion. The sedative–hypnotics and stimulants appear typically to worsen such behaviors. Because of their restrictiveness and potential for abuse, aversive procedures, such as electric shock, should be reserved for those cases that prove resistant to other approaches.

REFERENCES

Aiken, J.M., & Salzberg, C.L. (1984). The effects of a sensory extinction procedure on stereotypic sounds of two autistic children. *Journal of Autism & Developmental Disorders, 14,* 291–299.

Aman, M.G., White, A.J., & Field, C. (1984). Chlorpromazine effects on stereotypic and conditioned behavior of severely retarded patients: A pilot study. *Journal of Mental Deficiency Research, 28,* 253–260.

Bachman, J.A. (1972). Self-injurious behavior: A behavioral analysis. *Journal of Abnormal Psychology, 80,* 211–224.

Barron, J., & Sandman, C.A. (1983). Relationship of sedative-hypnotic response to self-injurious behavior and stereotypy by mentally retarded clients. *American Journal of Mental Deficiency, 88,* 177–186.

Bates, W.J., & Smeltzer, D.J. (1982). Electroconvulsive treatment of psychotic self-injurious behavior in a patient with severe mental retardation. *American Journal of Psychiatry, 139,* 1355–1356.

Baumesiter, A.A., & Forehand, R. (1973). Stereotyped acts. In N.R. Ellis (Ed.), *International Review of Research in Mental Retardation.* New York: Academic Press.

Baumeister, A.A., & MacLean, W.E., Jr. (1984). Deceleration of self-injurious and stereotypic responding by exercise. *Applied Research in Mental Retardation, 5,* 385–393.

Brazelton, T.B. (1973). *Neonatal Behavioral Assessment Scale.* Philadelphia; Lippincott.

Campbell, M., Anderson, L.T., Cohen, I.L., Perry, R., Small, A.M., Green, W.H., Anderson, L., & McCandless, W.H. (1982). Haloperidol in autistic children: Effects on learning, behavior, and abnormal involuntary movements. *Psychopharmacology Bulletin, 18,* 110–111.

Campbell, M., Anderson, L.T., Meier, M., Cohen, I.L., Small, A.M., Samit, C., & Schar, E.J. (1978). A comparison of haloperidol and behavior therapy and their interaction in autistic children. *Journal of the American Academy of Child Psychiatry, 17,* 640–655.

Cohen, I.L., Campbell, M., Posner, D., Small, A.M., Tribel, D., & Anderson, L.T. (1980). Behavioral effects of haloperidol in young autistic children—An objective analysis using a within-subjects reversal design. *Journal of American Academy of Child Psychiatry, 19,* 665–677.

Davidson, P.W., Kleene, B.M., Carroll, M., & Rockowitz, R.J. (1983). Effects of naloxone of self-injurious behavior: A case study. *Applied Research in Mental Retardation, 4,* 1–4.

Denny, M. (1980). Reducing self-stimulatory behavior of mentally retarded persons by alternative positive practice. *American Journal of Mental Deficiency, 84,* 610–615.

Donnellan, A.M., Anderson, J.L., & Mesaros, R.A. (1984). An observational study of stereotypic behavior and proximity related to the occurrence of autistic child–family member interactions. *Journal of Autism & Developmental Disorders, 14,* 205–210.

Dorsey, M.F., Iwata, B.A., Ong, P., & McSween, T.E. (1980). Treatment of self-injurious behavior using a water mist: Initial response suppression and generalization. *Journal of Applied Behavioral Analysis, 13,* 343–353.

Dorsey, M.F., Iwata, B.A., Reid, D.H., & Davis, P.A. (1982). Protective equipment: Continuous and contingent application in the treatment of self-injurious behavior. *Journal of Applied Behavioral Analysis, 15,* 217–230.

Durand, M.V. (1982). A behavioral/pharmacological intervention for the treatment of severe self-injurious behavior. *Journal of Autism Development & Disorders, 12,* 243–251.

Edelson, S.M. (1984). Implications of sensory stimulation in self-destructive behavior. *American Journal of Mental Deficiency, 89,* 140–145.

Frankel, F., Freeman, B.J., Ritvom, E., & Pardo, R. (1978). The effect of environmental stimulation upon the stereotyped behavior of autistic children. *Journal of Autism & Developmental Disorders, 8,* 389–394.

Gesel, A.L., & Ilg, F.L. (1937). *Feeding behavior of infants.* Philadelphia: Lippincott.

Hoder, E.L., & Cohen, D.J. (1983). Repetitive behaviors of childhood. In M. Levine & W. Carey (Eds.), *Developmental-behavioral Pediatrics.* Philadelphia: Saunders.

Kern, L., Koegel, R.L., & Dunlap, G. (1982a). The influence of vigorous versus mild exercise on autistic stereotyped behaviors. *Journal of Autism & Developmental Disorders, 14,* 57–67.

Kern, L., Koegel, R.L., Dyer, K., Blew, P.A., & Fenton, L.R. (1982b). The effects of physical exercise on self-stimulation and appropriate reasoning in autistic children. *Journal of Autism & Developmental Disorders, 12,* 399–419.

Kinnell, H.G. (1984). 'Addiction' to strait jacket: A case report of treatment of self-injurious behavior in an autistic child. *Journal of Mental Deficiency Research, 28,* 77–79.

Kravitz, H., & Boehm, J.J. (1971). Rhythmic habit patterns of infancy: Their sequence, age of onset, and frequency. *Child Development, 42,* 399–413.

LaGrow, S.J., & Repp, A.C. (1984). Stereotypic responding: A review of intervention research. *American Journal of Mental Deficiency, 88,* 595–609.

Lancioni, G.E., Smeets, P.M., Ceccarani, P.S., Capodaglio, L., & Campanari, G. (1984). Effects of gross motor activities on the severe self-injurious tantrums of multi-handicapped individuals. *Applied Research in Mental Retardation, 5,* 471–482.

Luiselli, J.K., Pemberton, B.W., & Helfen, C.S. (1978). Effects and side-effects of a brief overcorrection procedure in reducing multiple self-stimulatory behavior: A single case analysis. *Journal of Mental Deficiency Research, 22,* 287–293.

Matson, J.L., Stephens, R.M., & Smith, C. (1978). Treatment of self-injurious behavior with overcorrection. *Journal of Mental Deficiency Research, 22,* 175–178.

McConahey, O.L., Thompson, T., & Zimmerman, R.L. (1977). A token system for retarded women: Behavior therapy, drug administration and their combination. In T. Thompson & J. Grabowski (Eds.), *Behaviour modification of the mentally retarded.* New York: Oxford University Press.

McGonigle, J.J., Duncan, D., Cordisco, L., & Barrett, R.P. (1982). Visual screening: An alternative method for reducing stereotypic behaviors. *Journal of Applied Behavioral Analysis, 15,* 461–467.

Primrose, D.A. (1979). Treatment of self-injurious behavior with a GABA (gamma-aminobutyric acid) analogue. *Journal of Mental Deficiency Research, 23,* 163–173.

Rapoff, M.A., Altman, K., & Christophersen, E.R. (1980). Suppression of self-injurious behavior: Determining the least restrictive alternative. *Journal of Mental Deficiency Research, 24,* 37–46.

Ritvo, E.R., Ornitz, E.M., & LaFranchi, S. (1968). Frequency of repetitive behaviors in early infantile autism and its variants. *Archives of General Psychiatry, 19,* 341–347.

Sallustro, F., & Atwell, C.W. (1978). Body rocking, head banging and head rolling in normal children. *Journal of Pediatrics, 93,* 704–708.

Sandman, C.A., Datta, P.C., Barron, J., Hoehler, F.K., Williams, C., & Swanson, J.M. (1983). Naloxone attenuates self-abusive behavior in developmentally disabled clients. *Applied Research in Mental Retardation, 4,* 5–11.

Schroeder, S.R., Mulick, J.A., & Rojahn, J. (1980). The definition, taxonomy, epidemiology, and ecology of self-injurious behavior. *Journal of Autism & Developmental Disorders, 10,* 417–432.

Singh, N.N. (1981). Current trends in the treatment of self-injurious behavior. *Advances in Pediatrics, 38,* 340–377.

Singh, N.N., & Millichamp, C.J. (1985). Pharmacological treatment of self-injurious behavior in mentally retarded persons. *Journal of Autism & Developmental Disorders, 15,* 257–267.

Tarpley, H.D., & Schroeder, S.J. (1979). comparison of DRO and DRI on rate of suppression of self-injurious behavior. *American Journal of Mental Deficiency, 84,* 188–194.

Thelen, E. (1979). Rhythmical stereotypies in normal human infants. *Animal Behavior, 27,* 699–715.

Thelen, E. (1981). Kicking, rocking, and waving: Contextual analysis of rhythmical stereotypies in normal human infants. *Animal Behavior, 29,* 3–11.

Volkmar, F.R., Hoder, E.L., & Cohen, D.J. (1985). Compliance, "negativism," and the effect of treatment structure on behavior in autism: A naturalistic study. *Journal of Child Psychology & Psychiatry, 26,* 865–877.

Young, G.J., Kavanagh, M.E., Anderson, G.M., Shaywitz, B.A., & Cohen, D.J. (1982). Clinical neurochemistry of autism and associated disorders. *Journal of Autism & Developmental Disorders, 12,* 147–165.

Part III

Psychosocial and Behavioral Perspectives

CHAPTER TWELVE

Family Functioning and Tourette's Syndrome

Donald J. Cohen
Sharon I. Ort
James F. Leckman
Mark A. Riddle
Maureen T. Hardin

OVERVIEW

The daily experiences and long-term course of an individual with a persistent illness of any type influence and, in turn, are shaped by the life of a family. Life within a family is a particularly potent force in buffering the impact of chronic illness on overall social and emotional development during childhood or increasing the degree of functional handicap that may result from a disability (Feinstein & Berger, 1987). A child's world is in very large part charted by his or her internalization of relations with parents and siblings; the child's internal world of self-worth and self-perception is shaped by their view of him or her and how they help him or her in understanding relations with others. For most adults, as well, the world of the family provides the experiences, gratifying or painful, that most deeply affect mood and self-esteem. To be a successful and effective spouse and a parent, to be an adult offspring who can provide for parents and justify their years of support—these are the ingredients of which adult self-esteem are created, and for most people the ways in which competence can best be displayed.

For a child or adult with Tourette's Syndrome (TS), life within the family will deviate in very important ways from what normally can be anticipated. Individuals with TS generally will provide ambivalent pleasure for their parents, pose special challenges for their siblings, and experience different, indeed, unique, problems in their roles as offspring, brother or sister, husband and wife, father or mother. That an individual with TS will pose such challenges to families, and experience difficulties in trying to be a rewarding and beloved member and creator of a family, is almost self-evident. As a serious, chronic illness, TS presents realistic strains on family functioning. Yet, over and above such nonspecific factors, TS disrupts family life in ways that often are more difficult to overcome. These stresses relate to the natural history of the disorder; its symptoms; the familial nature of the condition; the possibility of suppressibility; inadequate public information; and the types of treatment offered (Cohen, Detlor, Shaywitz, & Leckman, 1982).

NATURAL HISTORY

After many years of perfectly normal development, children who will eventually have TS slowly develop symptoms that grow upon parental awareness as worthy of note. Their simple childhood tics fail to disappear. At dinnertime, a father will reprimand a child for making a noise; a mother will scold the boy for making funny faces. Tension mounts: Soon, there is hardly a time when the family assembles that the child is not scolded for his noises, gestures, or facial expressions. Parents generally are more sensitive to their children's shortcomings as well as assets than are others; thus parents may experience the child's tics as more disruptive, odd appearing, or louder than do others. Each tic may be felt as painful by the parents, who may try to look away or ignore its occurrence for some period of time but then lose their temper and reprimand the child. In spite of parental response, tics worsen, with one type of tic leaving and others taking its place. Some of these may be very odd, such as bending down to touch the floor, making faces, sticking out the tongue, hawking, spitting, coughing, and the like. Their peculiarity makes the family increasingly uncomfortable, edgy, and worried. As they progress from the appearance of the first "childhood" tic to the reassuring pronouncement by family doctor or pediatrician that this is just a "nervous habit" to the ultimate realization that the child is suffering from TS, the child and family may feel very much alone and confused. Children may experience the onset of TS as so bewildering that they may feel they are going crazy; parents may have the same worries. Occasionally, parents will resort to physical aggression, such as spanking or striking their children, or to bribes and threats, as described by Wolff (Chapter 14, this volume). The years that transpire between onset and diagnosis may shape patterns of interaction that are long-lived, as well as bitter memories of abuse and guilt. In front of their very eyes, parents see their lovely children dissolve into anxious, preoccupied ticquers and they feel impotent, angry, and hurt.

For those children whose tics are preceded by attentional and behavioral problems—whose problems may later be the most severe—the onset of the tics may follow upon several years of tension between parents and children. The hyperactive, disruptive, inattentive, and naughty 4-year-old child can wreak havoc on a family. Parents may feel the child is willfully or intentionally mean, and the child may be excluded from nursery school, day care, and play groups, and ostracized by other children and families. Exhausted mothers naturally will feel furious and are likely to have scolded and disciplined the child. Thus the onset of tics is within a matrix, in such cases, of already existing negative interactions. Such children are likely to feel that they are "bad" and "mean" or "unloving"; it is at a suprisingly early age that children are able to take in and make a part of themselves the reactions that they have elicited in others. The unfolding of tics may be seen by both child and parent as an expression of the child's anger.

Whether the child has had, or concurrently develops, attentional and behavioral difficulties along with the tics, or whether the tics appear in a child who was a "perfect angel," the tics are often quickly related to issues surrounding anger and aggression. Parents will feel angry with their children; they will feel that they are doing what they are doing out of spite, and children will feel anger with themselves and with others.

They may try to cover the anger by being super-nice, just as parents may be able to deal with their own hurt and angry feelings by being very loving. Many years ago, these secondarily emergent, angry feelings were seen as a primary cause of the tics and TS. We now recognize their reactive nature, but this does not minimize their clinical importance in understanding the experience of a family.

Because of their deep concern, parents will often seek help from several physicians before they finally receive a diagnosis of TS. Even at this point, the search may not cease, and parents may travel considerable distances in hope of finding something more optimistic to hold on to. Early misdiagnoses may lead to prolonged skepticism about physicians; these doubts are placed alongside their sense of needing and searching for a competent one.

SYMPTOMS AND THE FAMILY

Unlike the symptoms of most organic disorders, those of TS are bewildering in their variety and are often socially distressing. While most physical disorders are clearly "organic" in appearance and elicit sympathy, if they are also distancing, those associated with TS are more likely to elicit criticism as well as annoyance. There are obvious reasons for this. The symptoms seem, at times, to be under control. Children may be without symptoms or with few apparent tics when in school or when friends are nearby, and then demonstrate nonstop tics when alone with their families. Their ability to hold tics back then makes them seem willful when they are exhibited. Sometimes, symptoms are reserved for those whom children feel closest to. For example, children may use their most abusive language or actually strike out physically in relation to their parents. The mother's sense that she has suffered more than anyone on behalf of her child—and her knowledge of how much he or she needs her—makes her pain all the more poignant when the child calls her a "fat ass" in the supermarket or can't seem to stop pinching her "tits."

The community may pull back from children in wheelchairs or with cerebral palsy. Retarded children who drool may upset storekeepers. Classmates may wonder about the child with cystic fibrosis who coughs. But these reactions are counterbalanced by sympathy and concern. The children are seen as brave, if not as ones who are easily invited to play. This is not so for children with TS, whose symptoms are experienced by others as signs that they are badly disciplined or neglected or intentionally malicious. Thus parents are approached in public with advice, just as they are given advice by relatives, about how they should handle the child's movements or sounds. In school, teachers complain that the child's noises prevent others from concentrating. Parents and siblings do not receive communal support for their efforts as the family of a child with an illness, nor are they able cognitively to understand or conceptualize the nature and cause of the problems as "organic" and not under the child's control; they do not feel like the parents of a handicapped child who, in spite of their pain, may also feel special pride in their devotion and achievements (Jagger, Prusoff, Cohen, Kidd, Carbonari, & John, 1982; Stefl, 1983).

Among the greatest symptomatic problems for parents and siblings are the obsessive and compulsive features seen in up to 50 percent of the more severely impaired TS patients, as well as the behavioral problems that may stem from the TS either directly or indirectly. "We just don't know what is the TS and what isn't. How do we know what to discipline and what to ignore?" Nor can the child answer the question of how to define the boundaries. The obsessive and compulsive symptoms may become the center of the patient's problems during adolescence, while the tics fade into a subsidiary, hardly noticeable role. At such a time, there are further challenges to the family and patient in conceptualizing and dealing with the illness (Comings & Comings, 1985; Nee, Caine, Polinsky, Eldridge, & Ebert, 1980).

PHARMACOLOGICAL TREATMENT

During the past decades, medication has emerged as the mainstay of treatment of TS. Early years of medication management, with haloperidol primarily, led to increased optimism about TS as well as newly associated problems (Shapiro, Shapiro, & Wayne, 1972). In particular, large doses of haloperidol often led to weight gain, dysphoria, parkinsonian side effects, cognitive and memory blunting, phobias, and loss of ebullience. Under the influence of haloperidol, bright and engaging children were converted into lethargic "zombies," and parenting became focused on doses and side effects, symptoms and their regulation. Parents were often in a dilemma, wishing to rid themselves and their children of the TS while at the same time dreading what they were doing to the children. Children were compliant with the treatment, more often than not, although frequently miserable. The distortions in family relations from these earlier periods remain as residual problems in some of the more severely impaired TS adults. The problems have not fully disappeared with the recognition, over the past years, that smaller doses of haloperidol or other neuroleptics such as pimozide are sufficient for the medication to be useful.

Normal parent–child relations may be influenced in profound ways by the impact of deciding upon and then dealing with medication. The decision to "medicate" a child for symptoms that are neither painful nor dangerous and that may in fact seem to the child to be not so very important is a difficult one for a family. No medication available today can cure TS. The goal of medication management, thus, is to help children move along with their development by making normal experiences more open to them—primarily to enable them to participate more fully in school and recreational activities and to feel more comfortable with themselves. Parents must weigh the potential gains against the short and long-term potential dangers. This is a burden on parents, who may feel considerable anxiety.

When medications are less than fully satisfactory, or when there are changes in medications, the use and effects of drugs may become a major focus of child-family relations. Children are not just played with or talked with; they are observed. They themselves may feel not "normal," but somewhat intoxicated or odd. These subtle and not-so-subtle alterations in parental perception and self-perception affect the basic quality of social development.

In addition to medication and the effects of initiation, maintenance, and withdrawal, there are other effects of the medicalization of TS on family functioning. These include the nature of having a diagnosis, the family's knowledge and fantasies about the course of illness, and the child's sense of suffering from something affecting the brain (most often described in terms such as "chemical imbalance," whatever this might imply for a child).

One cannot take lightly the meaning of carrying a diagnosis. A sweet child with tics one moment leaves the doctor's office with a disease bearing a strange name the next. What does this mean to the child? To the family? As parents read about TS, see TV shows, attend meetings, and the like, they will learn about the most extreme possibilities. That the vast majority of patients with TS get through life reasonably well or very well, and that only a small minority have severely incapacitating symptoms, is not the impression they are likely to gather from first encounters with public information. Instead, they will feel dread about the emergence of coprolalia, and they will wonder whether their child's tics will be as incessant and pronounced as the worst they have ever seen. This worry, too, must have its impact on the quality of family life, leading parents to overprotect or feel terrible anxiety when their child develops a new tic. Parents may be too worried to ask for clarification about course and prognosis.

When coprolalia or copropraxia does emerge, the family may feel an increase in humiliation, as does the patient. Parents may feel ashamed to go out with the child, and the child may feel the need to apologize.

The very seeking out of diagnosis and treatment is time-consuming, frustrating, and expensive. By the time parents and family have learned what is available, found a physician with whom they can work, and come to a balance about medication, years may have gone by and large amounts of money may have been spent.

Dealing with teachers, special educators, school boards, social security, and other institutions also pits the child and family against society. Instead of feeling the support of educational professionals, parents will often feel their antipathy; they will have to become their children's advocates to keep them in the correct classroom or find a suitable alternative program. This may lead to multiple meetings and then formal hearings and ultimately legal battles. The anger and pain generated by these processes—let alone their cost and the time taken from work and life—are not without impact on the loving and caring nature of family life. Parents are people, and when they are exhausted and in the midst of battle, they cannot help but feel annoyed with the person in whose behalf they are struggling. Without a doubt, children will hear, see, and experience what is going on. Instead of having the sense that parents and school are on the same team—which generally is the case for children, including TS patients—many TS patients will hear their parents' criticisms of teachers and school, and hear of their parents being in battles or experience the rebound from these in school.

ADULTHOOD

As TS patients leave the family for college and adult life, the transition often cannot be accomplished with the same sense of security that it can for other children, even those with chronic medical illnesses. The diabetic or asthmatic college student will have troubles, but he or she has also learned coping skills and ways of explaining problems to peers. Teachers will never recognize the difficulties of the college senior with colitis, and will marvel at the achievements of a law student in a wheelchair. There are no provisions equivalent to the ramps and handicapped parking offered to the TS patient who barks in the middle of lectures or scribbles on exams. The college student and young adult will have to explain his or her problems to individuals who may be well educated in math and humanities but have never heard the name of the disorder and cannot begin to understand the anguish of the sufferer. Nervous, odd, weird, crazy: classmates and coworkers are likely to have these and other thoughts until they can meet the TS patient and see through his or her symptoms to the underlying person.

Many TS patients, in spite of their difficulties, will become spouses and parents. Then they are back into the family as the primary social unit. As spouses and parents, TS patients experience a range of difficulties. If a spouse married a TS patient when the symptoms were mild, there may be considerable anger as the symptoms exacerbate. A woman may overlook her future husband's compulsions, and even become his champion with her own critical family; after marriage, the continuation of symptoms, his need to be rougher than she might like during fore-play or sex, his getting up to check and count, and the like may become more and more annoying. Particularly problematic may be those associ-ated behavioral features such as inattentiveness and poor frustration tolerance. Living with a TS patient day in and day out may be far differ-ent than courtship, particularly as the excitement and ebullience of the TS patient fade during the years of marriage while the obsessive perfec-tionism persists.

The decision to parent is particularly worrisome in light of newer knowledge about the genetics of TS (Pauls, Kruger, Leckman, Cohen, & Kidd, 1984; Price, Kidd, Cohen, Pauls, & Leckman, 1985). Young couples are confronted with the knowledge that the vulnerability to TS is likely to occur in up to half of their offspring. At the same time, they cannot yet be reassured about the severity (from very mild to quite troubling) of the symptoms any child who does develop TS is likely to have, or whether any particular fetus is the bearer of the gene. Should they go ahead with a family or adopt? However they decide, the decision is among the most difficult for any couple to face. If they move ahead with parenthood, as many are choosing to do, there is a twinge of concern with each of the child's actions and movements. The earliest signs of tics and TS are screened, and each puckered lip or blink is felt as possi-bly the first signs of what is uppermost in their minds.

Mothers and fathers with TS may be fine parents, of course, of both normal children and those with TS. Yet, at times, parenting is doubly burdened for TS patients by having an offspring whose symptoms mimic their own. Their children's tics bring to TS parents the feeling, shared by many parents of children with physical or other problems, even when the facts do not support it, that they are guilty of having brought this fate upon their children. TS parents know they have been the transmitter of a painful burden and that they have handed this in-heritance on to the individual they love the most. Further, the short attention and easy frustration experienced by parents with TS may be exacerbated by children who are overactive, inattentive, and the like. The apple, not falling far from the tree, serves as a chronic irritant in just the spot the parent can least tolerate. Parents with short fuses often have children who are easily ignited, and the cycle may lead to frequent episodes of spontaneous combustion.

The situation is further complicated when the TS parent has promi-nent obsessive or compulsive symptoms and the child has tics or atten-tional problems. In all cases of TS parent–child transmission, there may be increased parental sensitivity to the child's difficulties. But often, this is functionally overwhelmed by the increased guilt, anxiety, and negative reverberations. An added force in this is the sense of the non-TS parent (and his or her family) that the TS patient is "to blame" for the child's problems. Outright or more subtly, grandparents will accuse their sons- or daughters-in law, of transmitting their problems to their grandchildren.

Throughout their lives, patients with TS and obsessive and compulsive problems may have troubles in work and family. As they do, they will have an impact on their spouses and children. For example, children will have to explain to other children why their mother or father grimaces and calls out funny names and makes sounds. Sometimes, the parent will be so embarrassed that he or she will avoid going out with the children; the children may feel less worried about the tics than the parent. At other times, the children try to keep others from seeing the afflicted parent, or in other ways cover over ("he's got a cold," etc.). It is very painful indeed for a child to have a parent who is different from the parents of other children; for example, children may tell their foreign-born parents not to talk when their friends are over, so that their accent will not mark them out as different. Children may be very protective of their parents and will not mention to them why they are ashamed. Yet children wish their parents to be perfect, and parents with TS fall short of the ideal in obvious ways. The offspring of parents with TS may take on a parental, protective role. But nice as this may be in some ways, it is a deviation from the normal parent–child relationship with considerable impact on adult patients' sense of themselves and on the family they wish to create.

From the very earliest phases of the emergence of tics and TS and throughout the life span, anxiety and stress seem to be intimately related to the etiology and severity of the problems (Leckman, Cohen, Price, Minderaa, Anderson & Pauls, 1986). Initially, there may be a triggering of TS by acute or chronic stress; later, symptoms are worsened by changes, excitement, and upsetting situations. Thus the family's reactions surrounding the young child's early symptoms may catalyze further difficulties, just as their calm and secure response may buffer the child's problems. The tensions in "TS families" may be extreme when there are two or more sibs with TS or when a parent and offspring have TS. In such situations, the stress may be contagious, and symptom severity may spread.

FAMILY DIAGNOSIS AND DYNAMICS

The assessment and treatment of children (and adults) with TS require a thoughtful understanding of them in relation to the important people in their world. This type of assessment involves understanding the way in which TS patients relate to their parents, the patients' internal pictures of their role and the parents' responses to them, the parents' portraits of their children and their symptoms, and the parents' understanding of the causes of their children's basic troubles and associated problems. By "family dynamics" we mean the ways in which each person in a family has a powerful impact on others, the balance between love and hatred, the ways in which needs are satisfied or frustrated, the recognition of the individuality of each family member, the modes for expression of irritations and sharing of fondness. Dynamics include the channels and efficacy of communication (who talks to whom, when, about what, and with what effect), and how thoughts and feelings are expressed in addition to talking (thoughtfulness, caring, forgetting, doing favors, sabotaging the other's plans, etc.). To what degree do family members feel that their basic needs are satisfied, that they are being as effective as they would like to be, that they find it fulfilling to be at home? When things become too much to bear, what escape valves exist for each member, and at what cost are they used? Is family life a haven of security or a jungle with beasts lurking here and there? Does the child feel he or she can retreat into the family to be protected or is this where the most sharply felt wounds are inflicted? Does the father come home or go to a bar to unwind? Where is the child sent when the noises become too much, or are they never felt as too much? Where does the child go to do his or her tics? Does the child feel most comfort when unleashing the pent-up symptoms alone? Are there other relatives who can buffer the nuclear family's strongest feelings—grandparents who can step in, aunts who can be visited for meals—or others in the community who can be counted upon? Is the family isolated or part of a larger network? Can they trust or are they a combat unit against the larger world? What takes place between the siblings that is fun, and what happens when they get out of hand? How do brothers and sisters explain the TS patient's symptoms to their friends, or do they avoid bringing them into the house? Do they worry that they will develop TS, or even fear that the TS symptoms are contagious?

Understanding the workings of a family does not result from a single interview, however long and sensitive. Most often, it is based upon reports of various family members, observations of how they actually relate in front of the clinician, and months of involvement. The physician becomes entrained in the family dynamics and experiences, along with the family, the ways in which they treat each other (and the physician as a transference figure) and outsiders (and how this makes the physician feel, in the countertransference). The clinician will recognize how parents keep secrets and reveal them, even at the first meeting. "You know, dear, that you sometimes do clench your eyes and throw back your shoulders when you're tired," the wife may say, gently raising the subject that she noted her husband's tics long before bringing their son for evaluation. "Do I? I didn't really notice," he may initially claim, only months later to reveal how he had "loads of tics as a child." The clinician may experience the parents' anxiety in the form of verbal attacks on him or her (or other professionals the family has seen), or through the parents not "listening" to the clinician's explanations. Through such observations, one can learn about the family's modes of dealing with the stress of the illness. The clinician may find himself or herself in the midst of a full-blown argument between child and parents and hear directly how parents won't let the child speak or how they accuse the child of disrupting their family.

To define information concerning family dynamics, the clinician needs to allow opportunities for the family to be seen together, to talk as a family, as well as individually, and to express their strongest feelings and concerns. This process of family diagnosis must be done tactfully and out of a sense of concern, without conveying or perpetuating a family's sense of self-blame; the parents may feel that they have brought the child and not themselves for treatment and evaluation, and may need, implicitly or explicitly, some explanation for the clinician's interest in the broader field of the child's life. Dealing with these issues of the close interconnections between child and family comes most easily for child psychiatrists and others who work naturally with family units, and who can convey their sense of the importance of the family. Any clinician will wish to have a detailed knowledge about the family's history of medical and psychiatric problems, and, of course, about the presence of tics, obsessions, compulsions, and other problems within the family. In the process, parents may make themselves the explicit focus of concern, for example, by asking for help for depressive or anxiety disorders or other problems.

Almost without exception, families feel a sense of relief in telling their story. This family story—the childhood and family experiences of the parents, the continuing involvement with their parents and siblings, and how the children fit into their dreams and now their agonies—is also, almost without exception, richer and more varied than one would predict from the "social surface." As the story is spun, the child takes on a history that precedes birth, stretching back to the childhood of the parents and their sense of what sort of a life they wished for themselves, and moving forward to their vision of the child's future. Often, this story is very poignant, with sadness, illness, loss, and disappointment that may still be sharply felt even though "objectively" in the historical past.

The child's TS symptoms are thus not isolated medical phenomena, but meaningful: They take on their meaning in relation to the specifics of how the family is constituted and the fantasies and aspirations of the parents and others.

Special problems arise in defining the "family" in situations of divorce, particularly when there is remarriage of one or both partners. In such situations, the child may sometimes be seen as one of the precipitants of the dissolution of the marriage; in fact, the presence of a child with a handicap is often the last straw on a relationship, or leads to a cycle of estrangement. When this occurs, questions of identifying where the child inherited TS may take on a more acute form. One parent may overidentify with the child, overgratifying and taking too good care of the child in an attempt to be the super-parent; or a parent may take off completely out of pain and hurt feelings, leaving the child to the other parent as her or his sole responsibility. Bringing divorced parents together for parental discussions, with the child present and in the child's absence, may be essential for trying to understand the child's life and the forces he or she is dealing with. Such meetings can easily become tense and difficult and require an expertise and interest, but they should not be avoided because of the heat they generate. The very difficulty suggests the experiences of the child, perhaps moving from household to household or finding himself or herself a proxy for the expression of anger and disappointment, a vector for communicating complaints, or a spy. The child too may wonder—or actually have heard—about being the "cause" of the divorce.

TREATMENT OF FAMILIES

All authentic therapy for a patient with TS is, in some sense, treatment of the patient's family. To a greater or lesser degree, families are involved in and benefit from the treatment, or suffer from ill-conceived or badly executed treatment programs. This being so, the fundamental question is the degree to which the clinician engages in systematically thinking about the family as an object of concern and plans interventions with the family in mind. Families will need more or less specific, targeted intervention, depending on the results of the clinician's assessment and the family's interest in and/or capacity for extracting benefits from a therapy that involves them. Not every family wishes to be engaged, and some will resist even direct offers; other families are very much in need of help, reach out for it, and fail to have therapeutic opportunities offered to them.

From the very first encounters with a knowledgeable person, the family benefits from a reduction in anxiety and an increased sense of security. Most physicians are aware of the therapeutic nature of their very presence, and use their positions of authority to assert control and convey a sense of hope. For TS patients and their families, in particular, the clinician's technical knowledge, ability to diagnose, capacity to educate, and understanding may end a quest of many years' duration. They have genuinely been perplexed and alone. They now feel they have a handle on the problem and are engaged with someone who can guide them.

By allowing a family to tell its story, over one or several sessions, the clinician provides opportunities for ventilation, sharing of information, and clarification of feelings. In this context, the child may reveal to the parents worries that they did not suspect, as well as symptoms (especially obsessive thoughts or habits involving areas such as bathroom behavior) or fantasies (such as being possessed by a devil or being afraid the parents would send the child away forever) of which they were unaware. Parents are helped with the process of "mourning" for their idealized child—the child they dreamed of having and may actually have had before the onset of the tics. And they may for the first time share and put into perspective their feelings about in-laws, parents, and siblings. For the first time, as well, they can share their rage—at teachers, relatives, people in the street, other physicians who misdiagnosed or misprescribed or did not deal with side effects. In the course of this early treatment, clinicians may also deal with emergent misperceptions of themselves, for example, the family's wish to idealize them (often disguised in their criticism of other physicians) or place them in the role of someone who will do more than a clinician possibly can for the child.

Over the course of the diagnostic involvement with a family, the clinician can also assess ways in which the family can cope and what assistance may be needed to help with coping. The process of providing supports and resources includes both allowing the family to become aware of needs and how they themselves can address them and providing the family with specific suggestions. This aspect of the treatment of the family may include guidance in relation to how to explain the symptoms of TS to others (including meetings with grandparents and others with whom the family is involved), working with schools, providing information to other professionals and agencies, securing residential or other special educational and treatment facilities, and so forth. In many of these activities, the clinician shares his or her power and authority with the family, for example, in working with schools. The clinician provides opportunities for them to see new ways of relating to each other, based on his or her own ways of listening and relating and their new experiences of open discussion.

All of these processes may go on through periodic visits and in the context of providing "medical" care to the patient with TS. For the majority of families, specific family therapy is not required nor desired.

On the other hand, therapy that has the family in mind—which is seen as being framed by the family—is part of the comprehensive care of a patient with TS, just as much as monitoring symptoms and medication.

In general, clinicians will have only episodic engagement with TS patients and their families, once the initial evaluation is over. The episodic visits may be more frequent where medication is part of the treatment or where there are serious learning and behavioral difficulties. Visits may become much more frequent at times of exacerbation of symptoms or other crises. More important than the precise frequency of such encounters is the clinician's ability to create a situation in which the family feels that they are being "held" —that they are heard, that their problems are appreciated, and that they can trust—and that authentic clinical knowledge is available to them. Since TS is a persistent illness, the temporal dimensions for intervention can be quite long. The clinician should not feel the need to act quickly in altering long-standing patterns within a family, even if these are seen as having serious consequences for a child's development. Most often, such gangbuster clinical tactics are met with an equal and opposite reaction that vividly demonstrates the powers of familial inertia. Instead, the clinician needs to respect a family's homeostasis and individuality and display readiness to be available on demand, as the needs arise.

In this long-term relationship, clinicians must also prepare themselves for inevitable crises. These crises will occur when there are exacerbations of symptoms; when the young child becomes a rebellious adolescent and begins to cause grief through unruliness and drinking; when a side effect develops; when the marriage collapses; when a parent becomes ill; or when the doctor makes a mistake. To be a physician at such times means to be exposed to the rage of those who have trusted in him or her and who feel let down. It is to be sitting on the hot seat. Clinicians can use their own sense of disappointment and the anger they may experience (e.g., in reaction to a sharp comment from a family that makes the clinician feel unappreciated) to understand how the family is feeling. Rather than acting on their feelings ("Well, if you want to see another doctor, go ahead. Just don't call me up next week when you need another refill."), clinicians can use them sensitively to guide treatment. Serious work with a family means that one becomes, in fantasy and in some ways in reality, a member of the family. And no member of the family is immune to the most deep feelings, not always loving, that we reserve for those closest to us.

The overriding goal of all treatment of TS is to help patients to move forward. It is to help children feel good about themselves and succeed in the tasks of life—learning, working, making friends, falling in love, dealing with losses; it is to help adults succeed as workers, lovers, and parents. The clinician working with families in which there is TS thus must help parents keep their eyes on the basic target: to help their off-spring move ahead. To achieve this, the parents must be able to balance realistic concern for their children and their special needs with realistic assessment of what they can accomplish in spite of their problems. By and large, this means that parents must be helped to see through the tics—to see their children with tics as children, and not as patients or as burdens. Adults must be helped to recognize what they can achieve, in spite of their lifelong troubles. These are not easy clinical tasks. Sometimes parents must be helped to be not too worried or concerned, and to encourage their children into entering social and other situations where they might be embarrassed, just as adults must be willing to expose themselves. Through work with the family, the child's symptoms can become less encrusted with the feelings, fantasies, dashed hopes, and angers that have grown up over many years or decades. In some deep way, this often means that the mysterious symptoms of TS are again made into "nervous habits" that the child is allowed to have rather than horrible evidence of some basic defect in the child, the parents, or the entire family.

THE FAMILIAL NATURE AND IMPACT OF TS

TS is a familial illness in several senses. First, it aggregates within families, and one can see the transmission over generations of tics, obsessions, and compulsions. Second, the symptoms of TS are first discovered by the family, and quickly evoke strong feelings in parents. Third, the child learns what it is to have tics by seeing the reactions they cause in others in his or her family. Just as with other persistent illnesses, the degree of handicap experienced by a child with TS is not only a function of the severity of the underlying illness and the resultant behavioral disability. It is a function, at least as much, of the ways in which the family can cope with the problems of social stigma, personal guilt, and the like, and the coherence they present to the child in the face of the crisis of the illness. For a child with TS, perhaps more than for sufferers of many other illnesses, the outside world will be critical, rather than supportive; only in the child's home can he or she hope for a buffer against being teased, mocked, nicknamed, and isolated. Willy-nilly, parents will either provide this domain of respite or contribute to the child's tensions (Stefl, 1984).

The child's first mirror is the mother's eyes; the power of those eyes to behold the child's successes and failures, how he or she shines and shames, never is dimmed. Children see themselves through the eyes of their parents, and they will feel as much confidence in their value as they feel valued. Children with TS disappoint the deepest aspirations of their parents to be perfect. If the parents have TS themselves, they disappoint the hopes of the parents to undo their own problems and do better for their children than their parents did for them.

Clinical work with children and adults with TS forces the appreciation of the role of the family in mediating the impact of the disorder on the patient—as a support for the patient or as contributing to his or her anxieties and self-hate. Through such work, one recognizes how powerful the family experiences of a child are in shaping the ultimate impact on development of having TS. The spunky family who can stick with the child, in spite of their pain, and force the child to do what he or she can, in spite of the tics, is far more important than any medication we now have in ensuring that the child has the best chance of growing into competent adulthood. And nothing can be more important than a caring spouse when an adult suffers from an exacerbation of tics or is facing a difficult oral presentation at the office.

Caring for the family, then, is essential to caring for the child or adult with TS. In doing so, clinicians can be guided by their knowledge of family dynamics and the impact of illness on families, as well as by sensitivity to the special challenges to family and personal development posed by TS: its unknown etiology; public visibility and audible symptoms that may seem provocative, intentional, and weird; the lack of social acceptance and sympathy and the criticisms that may be evoked from teachers and strangers, as well as those close to the patient; not knowing what symptoms will come next, and why they get better and worse; and the lack of any respite.

Many years ago, clinicians sometimes believed that TS was "caused" by families or, in some simple sense of the term, that it was an emotional disorder related to internal dynamics whose origin was familial. These concepts are now no longer sustained by informed clinicians. As they were discarded, so was an interest in the more subtle and pervasive ways in which familial factors are involved in the development of individuals with TS and how such individuals affect their families. We are now in a position to understand such interrelationships without increasing the burdens on families or blocking other types of treatment and research.

Future genetic knowledge will elucidate the basis of TS for many individuals. This may bring new stresses to family life by providing a means of defining the transmission of the disorder, by posing issues of family planning, and by leading families to await the expression of the disorder in children who bear the genetic vulnerability. Since the expression of a genetic diathesis is often modified by environmental factors, it is possible that the clarification of genetics will help guide better understanding of the relations between family experiences and the emergence and severity of TS symptoms. At the same time, better understanding of the pathobiology of TS may help improve its treatment and lead toward the achievement of full amelioration.

Over the next years, with increasing knowledge, understanding the role of the family in relation to TS and trying to care for families with TS are likely to remain of central importance. In the past, an emphasis on psychological factors may have inhibited research on biological issues; in the more recent past, an emphasis on medications in the treatment of TS may have obscured the importance of thinking about patients with TS as whole people. Today, we can attempt a balance, appreciating the biological underpinnings of TS as well as the fundamental fact that patients with TS grow and live in families, and create families of their own. Sensitive awareness of how life is lived in the matrix of a family—and the special meaning of this process for an individual with an illness—should help improve the care of TS patients and increase clinical knowledge of how best to be of help.

REFERENCES

Cohen, D.J., Detlor, J., Shaywitz, B.A., & Leckman, J.F. (1982). Interaction of biological and psychological factors in the natural history of Tourette syndrome: A paradigm for childhood neuropsychiatric disorders. In A.J. Friedhoff & T.N. Chase (Eds.), *Gilles de la Tourette Syndrome*. New York: Raven Press.

Comings, D.E., & Comings, B.G. (1985). Tourette syndrome: Clinical and psychological aspects of 250 cases. *American Journal of Human Genetics, 37*, 435–450.

Feinstein, C., & Berger, K. (1987). The chronically ill or disabled child. In J. Nosphitz (Ed.), *Basic Handbook of child psychiatry*. New York: Basic.

Jagger, J., Prusoff, B.A., Cohen, D.J., Kidd, K.K., Carbonari, C.M., & John, K. (1982). The epidemiology of Tourette's syndrome: A pilot study, *Schizophrenia Bulletin, 8*, 267–277.

Leckman, J.F., Cohen, D.J., Price, R.A., Minderaa, R.B., Anderson, G.M., & Pauls, D.L. (1986). The pathogenesis of Gilles de la Tourette's syndrome: A review of data and hypotheses. In N.B. Shah & N.S. Shah (Eds.), *Movement disorders*. New York: Plenum.

Nee, L.E., Caine, E.D., Polinsky, R.J., Eldridge, R., & Ebert, M.H. (1980). Gilles de la Tourette's syndrome: Clinical and family study of 50 cases. *Annals of Neurology, 7*, 41–49.

Pauls, D.L., Kruger, S.D., Leckman, J.F., Cohen, D.J., & Kidd, K.K. (1984). The risk of Tourette's syndrome and chronic multiple tics among relatives of Tourette's syndrome patients obtained by direct interview. *Journal of the American Academy of Child Psychiatry, 23*, 134–137.

Price, R.A., Kidd, K.K., Cohen, D.J., Pauls, D.L. & Leckman, J.F., (1985). A twin study of Tourette syndrome. *Archives of General Psychiatry, 42*, 815–820.

Shapiro, A.K., Shapiro, E., & Wayne, H. (1972). Birth, developmental, and family histories and demographic information in Tourette's syndrome. *Journal of Nervous & Mental Disease, 155,* 335–344.

Stefl, M.E. (1983). *The Ohio Tourette study: An investigation of the special service needs of Tourette syndrome patients.* Ohio Tourette Syndrome Association.

Stefl, M.E. (1984). Mental health needs associated with Tourette syndrome. *American Journal of Public Health, 74,* 1311–1313.

CHAPTER THIRTEEN

Intrapsychic Processes and Adjustment in Tourette's Syndrome

Archie A. Silver

RECIPROCAL INTERACTION BETWEEN ENVIRONMENT AND INTRAPSYCHIC PROCESSES

A fundamental characteristic of the individual with Tourette's syndrome is the impulse to movement, to motor discharge that manifests itself in motor tics and phonic utterance. The persistent and dystonic quality of the motor tics and the nature of the vocal noises from throat clearing to coprolalia and palilalia mark these people as "different" and evoke responses from peers, family, teachers, and employers varying from quiet acceptance and understanding support to rejection and impossible demands. Just how the world reacts, however, is in part determined by the behavior, the attitudes, the psychological defenses of the Tourette's patient. Thus the social adjustment of the patient with Tourette's syndrome depends not only upon the environment but also upon the forces from within the patient that drive him or her. This chapter will focus on these forces, identify a communality in intrapsychic responses and in visual–motor function, illustrate how they affect social adjustment, and consider problems in management. The data upon which this chapter is based were gathered from the study and management of 25 successive children ages 5 years to 17 years with Tourette's syndrome, 21 boys, 4 girls, referred in the past 18 months to the Child Study Center at the University of South Florida Medical School. Twenty of the 25 earned Full Scale IQ on the Wechsler Intelligence Scale for Children in the normal range, 2 were borderline, and 3 were in the bright normal range.

COMMUNALITY OF INTRAPSYCHIC PROCESSES

Awareness of the Impulse to Action

We have said that the impulse to action is characteristic of Tourette's syndrome. The action is largely involuntary but the *impulse* to action is reflected in an *awareness* that the particular action will occur, a conscious sensation of specific tension building within oneself (Bliss, 1980). The discharge of the tension in motor action may, for a time, relieve that tension only to have it build up again. One child says, "I can feel it when I have to say these [bad] words. They keep coming into my mind. I say them to myself over and over again. I try to stop it but it has to come out."

Clarence, age 16, was referred because he is disruptive in a special class for severely emotionally disturbed children. He says, "Tourette's disease just maddens me. Sometimes I would like to holler out loud. I try to hold myself back but it comes out." The impulse to shouting is in his awareness; he feels all the sound and movement repeating in his mind, but finally he loses control and is sent to the principal because of his behavior. His teacher does not understand him and even in a special class, he is considered crazy. His anger at himself is projected to his teacher.

Brian, age 10 1/2, has a compulsion to tap his pencil against his math paper so hard that he occasionally breaks the pencil point. The tapping must be done in patterns of three and is sometimes accompanied by stamping his foot on the floor. Brian says, "I know it's coming. I can feel it in my hand. It is urging me to put a dot there." In spite of his awareness of this impulse and his attempt to control it, he cannot do so.

Even at age 5 the struggle between the impulse and the action may be seen. Laura, a verbal, bright 5-year-old, has a grunting vocalization accompanied by spitting. She says, "I know I'm spitting but I can't help it. I feel like yelling. I think about it and I do it."

The obsession may involve not only repetition of words, but also obsessive iteration of the mental representation of a motor pattern. A ritualistic act is imagined in the child's mind, felt in the muscles, repetitively before it actually occurs. Whether the obsessive repetition is an attempt of the ego to contain the impulse or whether the obsession is somehow linked to the underlying pathological physiology in the striato–limbic–cortical pathways is not known. Whatever the cause, the obsession is a disturbing phenomenon, not only because it causes anxiety in itself, but also because, as an attempt at control, it is only minimally successful. As tension builds, the motor act or the vocal tic escapes from control into impulsive movement. Thus in school as the child attempts to conform to the teacher's instruction to sit in his or her seat, the short periods of quiet the child manages to sustain are broken by sudden dystonic movement, an impulsive jumping from the chair, a torrent of grunts or words. At times, the uncontrolled movements are channeled into a bizarre clowning that only serves to disrupt class and teacher. William, age 15, is typical of this group. At times he feels helpless to fight against it and he "acts crazy" in class. "I feel my arms wanting to move. I just stand up, do my arms all around. Sometimes my arms tighten up." At such times, William gets angry; he says, "I just want someone to shoot me."

Thus the motor and phonic tics and the ritualistic behavior of the child with Tourette's syndrome may be preceded by an obsessive awareness of the action, with attempts at control over the action but final escape of the action into involuntary behavior.

Reaction to Loss of Control

Important as the actual impulsive movement or vocalization is in marking the child as different and affecting acceptance by peers, teachers, and even parents, the inability to control thoughts and impulses is equally important to the child's own ego. The child feels that his or her body or thoughts are not in control. Charles, age 9, puts it succinctly. "I do not have a mind over matter." Two types of response, frequently blurred together in the same child, may appear. In the first the impulse and the action are projected onto some sinister force that is controlling the child. William, age 15, says, "It is an affliction of Satan who is trying to take over my life, telling me to do these things." William looks in the mirror and sometimes he sees not his own image but Satan looking back at him. "I looked red and I had a knife. I thought Satan was going to stab me." When Kenny, age 11, looks in the mirror he sometimes thinks that his image is really someone else forcing him to think and say the things he considers bad. Robert, age 10, is afraid that "an insane guy" will come into his house. He says, "I convince myself that if I hide under the blanket with my dog, I can't be shot by some insane guy." (As he told of this fear, Robert stopped and said that *he* sometimes does crazy things that he cannot help doing and that he is afraid of the crazy thoughts he has. He was able to identify with the "insane guy" whom he fears.) The projections of Patsy, age 12, have become hallucinations of "some evil person telling me to make these faces" (her facial tics).

At the other extreme are children whose impulses are ego-syntonic. They blame themselves for the behavior they cannot control. The explosive outburst, the tic, becomes a part of themselves and they are in consistent conflict over the "bad" or evil things, the uncontrolled things they do, and the good things the world expects them to do. Guilt and its consequence, depression, arise from the conflict. Kenny, age 11, talks to God "a lot." He says, "I pray to be forgiven for all the bad things I do especially when I curse my mother." He constantly needs God's assurance that he will be forgiven. Michael, age 13, fights a constant battle between good and evil, between God who tells him what to do and what not to do and the devil who argues with God, telling Michael to steal.

Andy, age 17 years, feels his thoughts are so bad that he is afraid to say anything or bad thoughts will emerge. He sits rigidly in the chair, struggling to talk, wanting very much to communicate, yet only capable of looking to the examiner for understanding. Andy's paralyzing obsessions were preceded by a hypomanic episode lasting for about 6 months, characterized by denial of his gross peri-oral tics, occasional sniffing sounds, and choreform movements of the arms and shoulders. The denial was abetted by his mother, who refused to accept the diagnosis.

Even where the child has adapted an outgoing friendly and apparently relaxed adjustment, the undercurrent of self-blame and depression may be seen. Jennifer, age 17, is a physically mature young lady whose Tourette's syndrome manifests itself in an occasional explosive echolalic repetition of her own affect-charged verbal responses and in an occasional jerky movement of her head. Her outgoing demeanor changes, however, when she says how bad she is, when in spite of her efforts to prevent it, an explosive, expletive outburst is directed to her mother. Jennifer also has been placed in a class for physically handicapped children. She says that is where she belongs and is most comfortable.

Attenuation of the Stimulus Barrier

The lack of balance between impulse and restraint, the difficulty in control of motor tics and vocalization, the constant battle between good and evil, the undercurrent of guilt and depression evoke additional problems that make socialization difficult. All of the children seen by us were driven by anxiety. The cause of the anxiety, however, may not be clear. Just as the obsessions and compulsions may be multidetermined, the anxiety in these children may also be multidetermined. Anxiety may indeed spring from the conflicts created by the specific consequences of poor impulse control, the guilt, and the depression. In addition, however, the very biological substrate of Tourette's disease may predispose to anxiety, attenuate the stimulus barrier so that it is inadequate to deal with forces from within the organism or with those impinging upon it. Physiological as well as psychological homeostasis is precariously balanced, and the child becomes a labile organism, quick to react to any stimulus viewed as threatening, demanding immediate, sometimes irrational, gratification of needs as he or she perceives them. When these needs cannot be met, as sooner or later they cannot be, the child easily erupts into a tantrum. Robert, age 11, is such a child, tyrannizing his parents, who try to give in to his every whim. Robert has become a tyrant, controlling his parents and trying to get everyone else in the world to do just as he wishes.

This anxiety may emerge as specific fear. How this occurs may be seen in Kenneth, age 11 years. He is afraid to be in his room alone. Even when his grandmother sleeps with him he cannot fall asleep. He is afraid of ghosts and burglars, so afraid that he has a knife and access to his father's gun. He has terrifying dreams of being attacked and overwhelmed. He dreams he was "in a trailer or a house, and a big thing came through the door, a wolf. I gave him something to eat but he attacked me"; and "I was living in a trailer on the beach. A big storm came and pushed me into the water." His anxiety as well as possible ambivalence toward his mother is seen in another dream: "Some person came and hit my mother and threw her down. They slapped her in the face. I shot this guy, but plenty others kept coming." These dreams are most disturbing to Kenny, especially since he thinks the dreams will come true. While the resurgence of anxiety and the emergence of unresolved developmental issues are not unusual in early adolescence, in Kenneth and other children we have seen, symptoms of anxiety are often severe enough to be considered an anxiety disorder. All have difficulty falling asleep and all have similar dreams. Robert, age 9, says, "I just can't fall asleep. I just sit there and look at the moon." He dreams, "A monster is about to eat me. I took a sword and stabbed him in the side but he ran after me." Charles, a bright 10-year-old, says, "I have a wooden sword. If a monster came in I would cut him in half." Patsy, age 12, says, "I'm afraid of being in a room by myself. A killer could bust my window with a rock." She describes a dream: "White puppy dogs are biting me. I eat them for dinner." Robert, age 14, hears "noises in the ceiling." This dream evoked panic. All children we have seen attempt to protect themselves by bedtime rituals, checking doors, windows, closets, under the bed, sometimes, as 13-year-old James felt compelled to do, for 15 minutes at a time. James is so afraid of burglars coming into his room that he sleeps in the linen closet at the foot of his mother's bed.

Even compulsions, of course, cannot defend against the recurring anxiety, the feelings of being overwhelmed and hurt. Illusions of a face coming out of the closet or of a person emerging from clothing or from the shadows of furniture are not infrequent. Thus their anxiety alone tends to make these children prisoners of themselves; they are afraid to sleep overnight with other children and many resist any change in their own routines. According to some of our children, (Robert A., age 10, Robert D., age 9, Kenny, age 11, Michael, age 12, James, age 13, William, age 15, Clarence, age 17) their main problem is that they cannot get to sleep. As a result, they ask, how can they be expected to wake up in time for school? This becomes an excuse for refusing to go to school. It also becomes a focal point of tension between mother and child as she tries with increasing frustration to get him or her out of bed and on the school bus.

COMMUNALITY IN VISUAL–MOTOR DEFECT

Each of the 25 children we have seen has some form of school difficulty. Ten of our 25 patients were suffering from a specific learning disability with perceptual functioning, in one or more areas, significantly below their intelligence as measured by the Wechsler Intelligence Scale for

Children. Most (21 of the 25) of our children however have significant difficulty with visual–motor function. As expected the 40 percent with specific learning disabilities had problems with angulation and the persistence of verticalization in their visual–motor function. In *all* children we have seen, however, writing was slow and perseverative, with difficulty in the physical effort of writing. Clarence, for example, in doing the Bender Gestalt test, drew figure 1 stretched across the page from one side to the other with no concern for the number of dots. Similarly figure 2 was drawn from one side of the page to the other and even continued onto the desk top. Tasks demanding writing, therefore, require more than the time allotted in school, and written homework is endlessly protracted. These findings are consistent with those of Hagin, Beecher, Pagano, and Kreeger (1982).

COMMUNALITY IN PATIENT'S CONCEPT OF THE DISEASE

The universal presence of visual–motor difficulty in children with Tourette's syndrome becomes an additional burden for them, contributing to their difficulty with school adjustment. Their lack of success adds to their already low opinion of themselves. They are bewildered by their disease and are generally pessimistic about their future. Michael, for example, with a Full Scale IQ of 109 on the Wechsler Intelligence Scale for Children—Revised, feels that his brain is worthless and all he can ever hope to become is a garbageman. Kenneth feels he is ugly and other kids hate him. He has many physical complaints; headaches and chest pain "like a sword going through me." Robert says, "If my Tourette's gets worse, I would do something." Clarence is concerned about what his disease "will do to my brain in the future." Charles says, "Why do I have to be me? Why is my soul put in this body? Sometimes I think I must be reincarnated."

SUMMARY OF INTRAPSYCHIC REACTIONS

Tourette's syndrome, then, is more than its behavior manifestation in motor and phonic tics and dystonias. It has profound effect on patients' thoughts, affects, and attitudes, the way they look at life and themselves, their successes and failures. The basic problem with impulse control leads to conscious struggles at control of these impulses, with obsessive conscious, mental images of the emerging vocalizations or motor acts (Cohen, 1980; Cohen, Detlor, Shaywitz and Leckman, 1982). When tension must be released there is a feeling of being overwhelmed. The unacceptable thinking and behavior evoke guilt and there is constant battle between the good and acceptable and the bad and unacceptable. Depression and anxiety may be by-products of these ceaseless conflicts and/or result from the biological substrate, the pathophysiology of Tourette's syndrome, which attenuates the stimulus barrier. Anxiety is seen by day in school refusal, in resistance to change, in extreme rigidity, in infantile demands; by night in sleep disturbance, inability to fall asleep, and when finally sleep occurs the agony of dreams of being attacked and overwhelmed. The stimulus barrier is attenuated, and impulses and drives that normally are more or less mastered erupt in Tourette's syndrome virtually undisguised, adding again to guilt and furthering anxiety. Their self-image is low, and many fear deterioration of their brain. This psychiatric profile may be found, in spite of the heterogeneous nature of the overt clinical manifestations. In addition most suffer from visual–motor problems with consequent difficulty in time-limited written assignments at school. Similar frustrations are also encountered as these children strive to complete assignments at home.

INTERVENTION

The first step in management of children with Tourette's syndrome is understanding them and their world. Detailed comprehensive evaluation is in order. At the least this includes psychiatric, neurological, psychological, neuropsychological, educational, and family study. Routine laboratory work should include an electroencephalogram. What, we must understand, are the content, dynamics, genesis, and structure of these children's thoughts and wishes; the nature of their conflicts, and the way they deal with the anxiety inherent in loss of motor and phonic control and in the attenuation of the stimulus barrier? What about the level of maturation and the integration of the central nervous system function? What about the presence of soft signs, the possibility of subclinical seizures, the nature and extent of perceptual defects, the cognitive abilities and disabilities, the academic successes and failures? How appropriate is school placement? What are the attitudes of teachers and school administrators to these children's problems? Are they receiving appropriate and sufficient remedial education and tolerance for their visual–motor difficulty? Finally, what is the family dynamic? How supportive and understanding are parents and siblings? How are the parents managing their own guilt, frustration, and anger at their problem children? When all these data are obtained, problem areas may be identified and appropriate intervention offered.

Intervention is thus more than the management of tics and vocalizations. Management becomes comprehensive, responding to each problem as uncovered in the evaluation. Teachers, parents, siblings, neurologists, pediatricians, psychologists and psychiatrists—the skills of all may be needed. Unfortunately with so many disciplines involved, management may become fragmented, one professional not appreciating what the other is doing and all, in spite of sincere efforts of each, creating confusion in parents and exacerbating anxiety in the child. What is needed is a central coordinator, an ombudsman, someone to whom the parents and the child may turn as problems arise; someone with knowledge and ability to coordinate the efforts of the various disciplines and agencies as they affect the child. Just what professional or even knowledgeable lay person may serve in this coordinating function is not the issue.

My own preference, however, is to offer my services as coordinator, dealing with medication, psychotherapy, parental guidance; interpreting the problems to the school, heightening its awareness of perceptual defects, interpreting the manifestations of Tourette's syndrome, suggesting how they may relieve anxiety in the child and in themselves, and develop the assets of the particular child. Following comprehensive study, therefore, a meeting with parents helps clarify the issues, identifies their own reactions, outlines the proposed treatment, and supplies them with someone who is available to them throughout the years. A similar meeting is held with the child, another with the teachers and resource people at the child's school.

Other chapters in this volume deal with specific management issues relating to school, family, and social institutions. The task of the physician and psychiatrist, in addition to the coordinating role described, is to aid the patient in control of impulses, decrease anxiety and fears, and promote optimal self-image and development of assets. While a basic aid in impulse control is medication, haloperidol, pimozide, and even clonidine may obtund but do not completely relieve the intrapsychic and reactive conflicts nor strengthen the stimulus barrier induced by Tourette's syndrome. Search for more effective drugs must obviously continue, and the use of families of drugs compatible with the basic ones is suggested. As an example, James who was receiving 4 mg daily of pimozide, with fair control of tics, continued to be hyperactive, unable to sleep at night, had severe fears of burglars coming in and killing him, checked the doors seven times each night, and was beset with nightmares. Alprazolam at bedtime was helpful in cutting through the night phobia so that he could rest well enough to get to school in the morning and permit his mother some rest at night. Similarly the presence of paroxysmal spikes in the electroencephalogram of William suggested the addition of phenytoin to the haloperidol he was receiving.

Equally important, however, is psychotherapy with these children.

Seeing them once each month for medication follow-up is simply not enough. Because Tourette's syndrome appears to be an organic disease in the sense of pathophysiology this does not make these children immune to the psychological problems of growing up. Actually the presence of Tourette's makes the resolution of the stage-specific conflicts incomplete and contributes to the development of psychological defenses such as obsessions and compulsions, which make social adjustment more difficult. A clear explanation of the disease to the child, consistent with his or her own level of comprehension and emotional strength, is the first step in psychotherapy. The level and depth of the therapy, just as with any child, depends upon the child's capacity to deal with his or her emotions and ability to resolve the conflicts as they are uncovered. Therapy may proceed from support in the face of cathartic expression of feelings, through the awareness of insight, to resolution of persistent conflicts. The effectiveness of insight may be seen with Robert, who was able to understand that he identified with the "insane guy." The hard-won realization that it was himself whom he feared did much to quell his night terrors and the frustration of his parents.

The sometimes bizarre, disruptive, and startling behavioral manifestations of Tourette's syndrome and the specific visual–motor problems evoke reactions in the child's environment: bewilderment, guilt, frustration, anger in parents, impatient demands in school, intolerance, sometimes ridicule, in peers. In turn, the reactions of family, teachers, and friends may contribute to the attitudes and behavior of the child. Management is thus a complex and interprofessional task.

REFERENCES

Bliss, J. Sensory experiences of Gilles de la Tourette Syndrome. (1980). *Archives of General Psychiatry. 37,* 1343–1347.

Cohen, D.J. (1980). The pathology of the self in primary childhood autism and Gilles de la Tourette Syndrome. *Psychiatric Clinics of North America. 3,* 383–402.

Cohen, D.J., Detlor, J., Shaywitz, B.A., Leckman, J.F. (1982). Interaction of biological and psychological factors in the natural history of Tourette Syndrome. In A.J. Friedhoff & T.N. Chase (Eds.) *Gilles de la Tourette Syndrome.* New York: Raven Press, 32–40.

Hagin, R.A., Beecher, R., Pagano, J., & Kreeger, H. (1982). Effects of Tourette syndrome in learning. In A. J. Friedhoff & T. N. Chase (Eds.), *Gilles de la Tourette Syndrome.* New York: Raven.

CHAPTER FOURTEEN

Psychotherapeutic Interventions with Tourette's Syndrome

Emanuel C. Wolff

PSYCHODYNAMIC UNDERSTANDING

It is not surprising that historically TS would be treated by that branch of medicine that concerns itself with intra- and interpersonal difficulties. This is an affliction whose major objective symptoms (with only the rare occurrence of physically dangerous tics) are an array of *socially* disturbing tics. Clinicians familiar with TS patients' stories often recount that apart from a hoped-for "cure" or at least a diminution of socially disabling motor and vocal tics to a tolerable level, the greatest global improvement the TS sufferer experiences is psychotherapeutic relief from the burden of unearned guilt, low self-esteem, and, oftentimes, social and familial scorn and condemnation for being bad, weak willed, attention seeking, and so on.

Shamans and physicians over the centuries have contributed to the TS sufferer's burden—from the Dominican friars of Sprenger & Kraemer's (1948) description in the *Malleus Maleficarum* (1489) of a priest exorcised of a demon that manifested his presence with motor and phonic tics to the psychopathological explanation of TS that held sway until the mid-1970s. The adjuration to physicians "above all do no harm" often has been breached by those professionals who have attempted to treat TS sufferers by strictly psychological means. It was implicit in their treatment philosophy that the TS patient was "responsible" for his or her syndrome. Such psychological treatment, conducted in an atmosphere in which the patient's psychopathology was responsible for the manifest disease, has, of late, given psychological and psychotherapeutic interventions a bad name, even among leaders in the rational scientific research on TS. Statements of the sort that "psychotherapy never has been shown to be helpful in TS treatment" are often heard. This appears to be an overkill phenomenon—a backlash against the historical, admittedly erroneous, notion of a strictly psychopathological etiology of TS. However, to dismiss psychological explorations and interventions in the evaluation and treatment of a TS patient and his or her symptoms is throwing the baby out with the bath water, since psychological and psychotherapeutic efforts may be of value in the care of patients with TS.

Mahler's and others' (Ferenczi, 1971; Gerard, 1946; Mahler, 1944; Mahler & Rangell, 1943) extensive early research of psychodynamic evaluation and treatment of children with tics preceded by several decades the discovery of the neuropathological component of TS. Their orientation toward tics clearly was psychopathological and, because of this, might seem at first glance to be of no current value. However, these descriptions of the psychological state of some children with tics and their family systems are still instructive. Furthermore, Mahler proposed in like fashion to Freud (1905) that a complemental series, that is, an interlocking of inheritance and experience, was at work in the TS child. Mahler (1949) stated that "research on the phenomenon of tics revealed that 'motor neurosis' often originates through the interactions of hereditary, or constitutional factors and certain typical environmental attitudes" (p. 279f). Our current understanding of TS represents a quantitative—not a qualitative—shift from this earlier hypothesis. The fact that currently TS tics are considered completely involuntary (when they "break through" conscious suppression) does not mean that the phenomenon of tics never serves a psychopathological function. Mahler's (1949) postulation of a "trigger effect of a sudden threat or trauma, or actual inner conflict in order to produce the crystallization of true tic" (p. 284f) is a notion currently accepted as part of the clinical disease-precipitating mechanism in many TS patients. Early psychoanalytically oriented TS researchers may well have reversed cause and effect—tics and psychodynamics—but these elements of TS remain inextricably linked. It is spurious to believe one can address one of these elements in a person without addressing the other.

Many skilled TS clinicians base their decision whether to medicate a TS patient not on the objective presence or degree of severity of a patient's tics but rather on the social and psychological degree of adaptation to the symptoms by the patient and the patient's systems. With the exception of rare extremes of symptomatology, severity of motor and vocal tics may correlate only loosely with social and personal adjustment. Psychotherapy often is useful in the treatment of the psychological sequelae of any chronic illness, that is, guilt, depression, anxiety, and so on. In the instance of psychotherapy for TS, however, psychotherapy may contribute to some degree to an amelioration of tics themselves— a parallel to the often-made observation that psychological stress may contribute to the exacerbation of or even initially precipitate TS symptoms—the recognition of the natural waxing and waning of symptoms of TS notwithstanding.

Psychological factors have been well studied in relation to the course of other childhood-onset disorders, such as diabetes and end-stage renal disease, and even in relation to cancer. The confluence of findings from such work strongly supports the view that control of anxiety, improved relations with care givers, and other behavioral factors clearly are related to the state of the disorder (e.g., reduced hypoglycemic episodes) and longevity.

Experienced diabetologists often see patients who alter their medication or diet to produce, not always with full consciousness, exacerbations of their disorder to avoid anxiety-filled situations. Parallel to this observation is the way in which Arnold, a young man with moderately severe TS symptoms but fairly well controlled with Haldol, discontinued his medication with resultant return of moderately severe vocal and motor tics. This so put off his fiancee, to whom he shortly was to be married, that the engagement was broken off. He explained his non-compliance with the Haldol regimen to his physician by saying that he "didn't want to take Haldol because [he] was getting married and taking medicine made [him] feel like a patient—ill." He wanted to start marriage with a "clean slate"—as a nonpatient. Arnold's physician accepted the patient's psychodynamic self-formulation without question. It did not occur to either Arnold or his highly skilled (in the pharmacological treatment of TS) physician that the patient could have predicted the consequences of discontinuation of the Haldol and that if the patient insisted on going off medication, a time could have been chosen in which to take a drug holiday without jeopardizing his engagement. It seems much more likely that Arnold, who had been on Haldol for quite some time and knew a great deal about TS, was acting out his ambivalence—not just about identifying himself as "ill" but probably also about his would-be bride and perhaps the idea of marriage itself—a stressful transition for anyone with or without a chronic illness. Perhaps the broken engagement was the intended result of this Haldol misman-agement. Psychodynamic evaluation and ongoing monitoring, perhaps in a course of exploratory psychotherapy, might well have avoided this painful experience—one that further lowered this unfortunate man's self-esteem and added unnecessarily to the large library of interpersonal horror stories that makes the rounds of TS sufferers.

Every TS sufferer and family or support network deserve a very careful and complete psychological evaluation and, where indicated, psychotherapeutic intervention. The evaluation should be as routine a part of the initial workup for TS as a neurological examination. Furthermore, even in those instances where initial psychological evaluation suggests the presence of healthy coping mechanisms and adaptive functioning, the clinician must have the skill to be attuned to shifts in the TS patient—shifts of what Karl A. Menninger (1963) has called "the patient's vital balance" (p. 81). The psychological appraisal of a TS patient ideally is accomplished by someone who is both medically trained, with clinical experience of TS, and psychodynamically sophisticated. The indications for, and conduct of, a psychotherapy are the same for TS as for other disabling medical illnesses, although TS symptoms usually are much more socially disabling that those of many other chronic diseases. The various psychotherapies—analytic, expressive, supportive, family, conjoint, group, or residential placement—any of which may be indicated with one TS patient or another, are skills learned over an extended period of time and then often imperfectly. The following examples may illustrate clinically the point that a psychological understanding of the individual TS sufferer and his symptoms will dictate the need for, type of, and direction of psychotherapeutic intervention.

Psychotherapeutic treatment of TS is not generally the mainstay of treatment, but there are instances in which, despite excellent medical care, the difference between a horrendous clinical course and an acceptable quality of life rests with the successful addressing of psychodynamic issues. The observation that TS waxes and wanes no longer remains a valid criticism of the effectiveness of psychological intervention if certain psychological, and only psychological, variables are changed repeatedly and the patient's response is immediately striking and predictable. The following case illustrates the point that the best medical (psychopharmacological) care of a severe TS patient may be ineffective in the absence of treatment for the patient's psychopathological configurations. The psychodynamics described in this and subsequent cases are not "typical" in that there are no typical psychodynamics for TS any more than there are typical psychodynamics for anyone with a chronic illness. Certain *symptoms* often are present in sufferers from chronic illnesses—symptoms such as depression, anxiety, guilt, and so on that cut across psychodynamic boundaries. The "typical psychodynamics" of TS (e.g., those described by Mahler of an overprotective mother, a withdrawn father, the tic—an autoerotic symptom of inhibited aggression) have not withstood the light of experience. Psychological profiles of TS patients are not different from those of psychiatric outpatients—something that may well be a sequela of being chronically ill.

ABE: TWO DECADES OF TS AND DEVELOPMENTAL DISTURBANCE

Abe, now 28 years old, developed clinically severe signs and symptoms of TS during his school years. Regrettably, as was the case so often two decades ago, his diagnosis of TS was not made until his teens, by which time severe personal, family, and social psychopathological maladjustments had become firmly entrenched. Prior to the correct diagnosis and pharmacologic and psychotherapeutic treatment, Abe and his father had been involved in multiple altercations with one another. Often father's attempts to discipline Abe led to violent verbal and physical confrontations. By the time the correct diagnosis was made and appropriate treatment instituted, both the family and Abe's school–social system had "had it." The modest improvement in Abe's TS symptoms was, in and of itself, insufficient to allow all the participants in this chronic, rancorous struggle to forgive, forget, and move on. Despite the fact that much guilt on all sides had been diminished by the making of the diagnosis of TS and the explanation of the "involuntary" aspect of the simple and complex behavioral symptoms of TS, the pathological defenses that had become part of Abe's character armor remained in place. Abe's defenses consisted primarily of denial, projection, mercurial regression in thinking and behavior, and pathological narcissism manifested by grandiosity with respect to his body image that bordered on the delusional. Even when Abe was not plagued by socially disruptive symptoms, his paranoia was always close to the surface—"What are you looking at?—Yeah, take a good look," and so on. Such comments were offered to complete strangers passing him on the street if they so much as gave Abe a second glance. At this time Abe's tics were actually quite mild, consisting of arching of his back or neck as if stretching. Provocations at home, both real and imagined, and chronic, mutually pathological family interactions were so prevalent and ingrained that massive intervention in the form of residential (boarding school) placement for Abe was necessary in order to avoid, both literally and figuratively, the further spilling of blood.

Abe's placement was in a school for emotionally disturbed boys—a residential treatment setting that provided psychotherapy, milieu therapy, special education, and a psychiatric staff experienced in the psychotherapeutic and pharmacotherapeutic treatment of TS. Abe's neuroleptic regimen was essentially the same as prior to his residential placement and continued under the same team's supervision. After a lengthy period of testing limits at school, Abe began to feel trusting and trusted. The psychiatrist–psychotherapist pointed out to Abe early in his psychotherapy something that initially angered, but secretly pleased, Abe—that Abe could control many aspects of his behavior that were not "involuntary" and were not TS. (It must be noted that making such clinical distinctions in a psychotherapy of a TS patient is hazardous and is best left to clinicians with much experience of TS symptoms and concurrent character pathology.) "Punching so-and-so in the nose is you, Abe, and not uncontrollable Tourette's" was a typical psychotherapy intervention. Abe often responded, "I've never used Tourette's as a crutch—I never have and I never will" (a phrase that Abe might then repeat three or more times). Abe had, of course, been using TS as a crutch in an effort to decrease some of the enormous guilt he felt over his own disinclination to control his angry outbursts at his ambivalently loved family. The enormity of Abe's rage was stated clearly in his oft-repeated remark that he would "kill anyone who said anything against my parents."

Psychotherapeutic interpretation of Abe's disinhibition never could have been made successfully, that is, "heard," by Abe if he had remained at home. It was crucial that Abe be withdrawn from the system that continued to reinforce its own pathological interactions. Psychotherapy had been tried in the past with limited success—psychotherapy in a residential placement was key. When positive transference feelings became established in the psychotherapy, Abe began to reveal the depression, low self-esteem, and anxiety that he had hidden beneath his angry, defensive, paranoid exterior. With no change in Abe's pharmacotherapy, tears now frequently seemed to take the place of temper (and, to some extent, tics). At this point, the psychotherapeutic work began to proceed along more classical lines. The psychoanalytically oriented psychotherapy involved interpretation of transference material contents, occasionally some support, and, most important, working through. Abe felt better now than he had since developing TS. Not only had his objective signs of TS diminished to an all-time low, but, perhaps even more important, Abe had won acceptance from his milieu and felt happy in it. Such a marked change in someone's quality of life goes quite beyond the waxing and waning expected in the course of TS. Striking was the observation that, after Abe had an infrequent weekend at home or even a telephone call from his parents, prompt but temporary regression to his earlier psychopathological behavior and defensive operations appeared. Motor and vocal tics, both simple and complex, reappeared. Pharmacological manipulation at these times appeared to be ineffective. Invariably, however, within a few days after such a family "blowup," Abe would have a cathartic experience in his psychotherapy; he would talk about "a bad weekend at home" and then begin to feel and act better. It did not take long for Abe to gain the painful insight that despite how much he and his family "all loved" one another—"They'd do anything for me and I for them"—that there was another side, as Abe stated, "We [the family] have trouble getting along because so much [negative] stuff has happened in the past."

Abe voluntarily began to decrease his contacts with home, and Abe's clinical course of psychological and somatic functioning remained quite good. Abe, who now was 16 years old, was in better shape continuously than at any time since the onset of his TS a decade earlier. (As an interesting aside, it was a year later that the psychiatrist–psychotherapist treating Abe at the residential center learned that during several months of Abe's period of best health at the school, Abe actually had been on no medication whatsoever. Abe had been part of a double-blind study of which he was unaware.)

When Abe was 18 years old and a senior at the residential school, he realized that he soon would graduate, and anxiety began to reappear, quickly followed by reinstitution of some of the older, more pathological defenses, such as projection, denial, and narcissism. This was accompanied by a resurgence of mild-to-moderate motor and vocal tics. Again, manipulation of medication at this time did not help. The psychotherapy began to focus on Abe's separation anxiety (from the school, from the therapist, etc.), and he began to feel somewhat better, at least psychologically, accompanied by subjectively modest improvement in tic frequency and severity. Abe graduated from the school, moved back to the city, moved in with his parents, and began at a modest, unskilled job. Abe's pharmacological treatment continued in the same hands as over the last 10 years, but a further, rapid decline in Abe's clinical condition occurred, nonetheless. Abe's tics became severe. His behavior became explosive—projection bordering on psychotic paranoia; all of these contributed to Abe losing his job, an event into which, regrettably, he had absolutely no insight. Finally, Abe began to demonstrate simple and complex forms of both psychologically and physically self-destructive behavior. He became very depressed and very angry and began to hit himself, eventually in so severe a fashion that hospitalization and ultimately four-point restraints became necessary.

During this hospitalization, a whole new array of psychoactive drugs was tried (in addition to the usual TS drugs). One of the neuroleptic trials even resulted in Abe's becoming transiently psychotic. The psychotherapist–psychiatrist who had followed Abe's case for years at the residential school believed that Abe's presence in the "city" had stirred up so much in the way of ambivalent feelings in Abe and his family that he simply would not "get well" in the city—regardless of the heroic pharmacological efforts being made in his behalf. Abe was transferred to a hospital out of town, quite near his former residential school, an area of the country with which he had been quite familiar, a place where Abe had felt and been as well as he ever had in his life following the onset of TS. This hospital was of sufficient distance from Abe's home city such that his and his family's need to minimize their contacts with one another (for psychodynamic reasons) could be accomplished without the ensuing guilt—the rationalization being the geographic distance they were from one another.

Despite Abe's protestations of how much he "hated it" in "the sticks," he got well. His medication dosage was reduced. Intensive psychotherapy was reinstituted by Abe's former psychiatrist, along with skilled nursing and physical therapy interventions (a physical therapist found physical exercises that helped "drain" Abe). In the formal psychotherapy, again, the depression and anger that Abe felt about his family resurfaced. Abe barely could speak of his enormous dependency on, and anger at, his parents. Abe became aware of his need to be away from home, away from the city, in order to "get well" and proceed with his life. He couldn't tolerate this insight inasmuch as it cast doubt on his protestations of how much he and his family loved one another. Abe rationalized away this need to be away from his family, to be in "the sticks," by substituting the notion that he needed to be near his treating physicians—a team he felt was much more skilled than any other he had been treated by. Arrangements for Abe's living and working in this "hick" community were worked out. Abe's anger at not being able to go home now was displaced onto his chronic condemnation of the "hick" community that was full of people (employers) who did not appreciate his abilities or girls who were "too stupid" to appreciate his looks and masculinity. Abe's TS continued to improve symptomatically until once again he achieved his best level of postmorbid functioning. Abe again began to accept suggestions from his psychotherapist. Abe felt this was someone he could "check things out with"—a far cry from his earlier "They're all against me—no one understands." Abe was angry at, but accepting of, the therapist's counsel that Abe not return to the city precipitously or leave one job before he had another. Abe had converted physical acting out into verbal activity. Psychotherapy continued, during which Abe briefly tried to deal with the painful, but necessary, acceptance of his own very real intellectual and physical limitations. Abe longed to be a high-level business executive like his father; he barely could complete a high school business math class. Abe longed to be a professional wrestler; he was of average height and weight. Although these narcissistic fantasies remained, Abe did not act on them in any self-defeating ways. They provided (and continue to provide) him with relief from his ever-present preconscious notion of himself as "defective."

The narcissistic defense in Abe manifested itself, in part, by hypochondria. Such "compensatory" eroticization of the body often is seen and first was described in tic syndrome by Ferenczi (1921). (Hypochondria also may be understood, in many instances, as part of the obsessive–compulsive diathesis of TS.) After approximately a year back in "the sticks," Abe felt well again—so well, in fact, that he did what so many patients do whose health is returning: He discontinued the medical regimen that had helped restore healthy functioning. Abe again felt he would try to return to the city with the new proviso that he would not live at home. Regrettably, the entire train of previous disastrous events repeated itself one more time with fairly rapid social, vocational, and TS symptom decompensation. Again, Abe lost his job, his apartment, and his health. Reluctantly, Abe returned to "the sticks" and shortly thereafter again made a clinical recovery to his best postmorbid level of functioning. Unfortunately, the cycle repeated itself again and again.

Abe's case illustrates, among many things, the impact of psychodynamic issues on clinical functioning and Tourette's symptomatology. Those aspects of Abe's behavior that were physically self-destructive determined the highest priority of psychotherapeutic goals. In psychodynamic terms, this translated itself into addressing Abe's anger and guilt at his ambivalently held parents. Underlying psychodynamics that feed into TS symptoms (which we understand to have concurrent psycho- and physiopathological etiology) dictate the nature of the psychotherapeutic interventions, that is, expressive or supportive, individual and/or family therapy, and so on. Abe's level of ego strength varied continually, as did the severity of his pathological defensive structures. Abe's hitting himself clearly was TS, but its precipitance and persistence and perhaps its degree of severity seemed to be modifiable through the addressing of psychodynamic issues. Clearly, Abe had not been dealing very well over the years with his hostility toward family members. In contrast to Abe's preconscious anger at his family, he had the conscious need to perpetuate the myth that he was one member of a happy, intact family. Despite long-term psychotherapeutic efforts, Abe could never allow himself to admit to any but the most sterilized comments about the negative side of his feelings toward his parents and siblings. Wild, pseudoanalytic interpretations that Abe really wanted to hit his father could precipitate an attack of Abe pummeling himself until he was bloody. On the other hand, when the psychotherapist acknowledged in the psychotherapy the severity of the beating Abe already had given himself and how much he (Abe) must be suffering, Abe stopped hitting himself. Abe was "beating up" introjects. When he was "told"—staying strictly within the metaphor—that these introjects had been beaten enough, Abe was able to stop. On another level, when Abe—again in the metaphor—was informed that his passive–aggressive behavior had had the desired effect, that is, that all the witnesses to his beating himself also were feeling beaten up by their inability to help him, Abe stopped.

To be sure, generalizing from this type of clinical material concerning a disorder with an unpredictable clinical course must be with caution. Yet in this instance, the therapist could consistently predict the effect that a psychotherapeutic intervention or tack would have on Abe's clinical course—helping it or worsening it—and not just with respect to Abe's psychological state, but also with respect to objective signs of TS. Among other things, the psychotherapy allowed for a catharsis of some of Abe's anger. It also allowed for the development of a primitive ambivalent transference neurosis, particularly with respect to the negative side of the transference that manifested itself in Abe's seeing the therapist, another Godlike figure, who, like father, was imperfect—"he also had feet of clay." The negative things about father that Abe never could bring himself to say he displaced onto the therapist. The therapist was "fat, stupid, didn't dress well, had no talent, was clumsy, never played sports," and so on. (One also hears, of course, a reflection of Abe's self-image in this projection.) Abe could "act in" in the therapy—berating and ridiculing the therapist–father one moment and expressing undying friendship and affection the next.

The next case illustrates the usefulness of psychotherapy at the opposite end of the spectrum of severity of TS. This case illustrates the finding that psychotherapy may be the only treatment a patient with TS needs, since fairly troubling psychological disability as a consequence of objectively mild TS is not an unusual finding.

This is the case of a young adolescent. The advent of adolescence is a troubled time in and of itself for many youngsters. It is especially so for the TS child, given the ubiquitous adolescent concerns about body image, sexual matters, peer acceptance, and so on. These hurdles of passage, coupled with the oft-seen exacerbation of TS during puberty, make this a period of time fraught with pitfalls of psychological malad-aptations, which, if not recognized and treated early, often lead to personality malformations. This is an especially tragic development in that it is preventable. Personality malformations may be out of proportion to degree of TS severity.

ROD: AN ADOLESCENT WITH TS

Rod was a very intelligent, handsome 16-year-old high school student of whom one would have thought: "He has everything going for him." Everyone who met Rod felt that he was a terrific kid with a bright future—good looking, intelligent, engaging personality, loving, support-ive parents, socioeconomically advantaged—everything. The fly in the ointment was TS. Perhaps "fly" is an appropriate metaphor in that the objective severity of Rod's TS symptoms was minuscule—almost subvo-cal grunts that were concealed well and occasional motor tics consisting of head jerking—again, not particularly noticeable to anyone but skilled observers. Rod, however, was very distressed by his symptoms and felt his tics were quite noticeable. Rod was, in fact, somewhat obses-sional about his concerns. (The obsessionality may, of course, have been a part of his TS diathesis.) Perhaps Rod would have been as worried and upset over acne, but he worried about his tics. He believed, "Kids won't like me—I can never tell anyone—how can I ever get a girl-friend—what if we get close and I wanted to kiss her and I ticced," and so on. Those readers with experience in treating (or raising) adolescents hear echoes of ubiquitous adolescent concerns in Rod's worries—con-cerns that, however, have focused in this instance on TS. Psychodynami-cally, Rod's TS can be looked upon most usefully as a psychologically overdetermined perception of himself as having a "defect."

Rod's perception of himself as unattractive (but focused on Tou-rette's) should be seen in the same light as such oft-voiced adolescent concerns as "The boys won't like me because my neck is too long—the girls won't like me because my hair sticks up—I'm too tall—I'm too short, too fat, too thin—I should have been a blonde," and so on. Rod, like all other teenagers, felt his imagined defect (in its degree of sever-ity) very deeply, and no amount of reasoning or reassurance on the part of friends (those who knew of his TS), parents, or doctors could relieve his anxiety, obsessional worries, and depression. Analytically oriented, expressive psychotherapy was instituted with the goal of exploring the underlying conflicts that were camouflaged by the TS. Rod certainly

had TS, and its "real" presence in his life lent itself all too easily to
hiding considerable, but typical, age-appropriate concerns about other
conflicts. A minimally directive approach was used in the psychotherapy, and the content of Rod's sessions began to move away from his
bemoaning his Tourette's and toward his worries about sexual issues,
the search for identity, dependency conflicts, and so on—in short, "normal," adolescent, preconscious concerns.

Under other circumstances (i.e., a child without TS), such "normal"
adolescent findings would not prompt psychotherapeutic intervention.
For a patient with chronic disease, however, psychotherapeutic intervention to help resolve even "normal" conflicts allows that amount of
energy involved in dealing with these struggles to be available to promote higher-level adaptation to the presence of the illness. Classical
analytic psychotherapy addressed Rod's predominantly aggressive and
rivalrous conflicts (oedipal derivatives) and some of his dependency
concerns. It looked under the surface of his anxieties about some issues
of adolescent development. The issues that now dominated therapy sessions were related to Rod's concerns about going out on a single—
rather than a double—date, going steady, and striking a reasonable balance between homework and play (as opposed to his earlier total
"grind" status). Not surprisingly, as Rod felt some easing of anxiety
about his adolescent passage, and these milestones had been negotiated
successfully, he felt that his TS was, in fact, much better—that he "hardly
noticed it any more." Rod was reassured tremendously when, upon
vouch-safing with considerable trepidation his "shameful secret" of TS
to a few close friends and a newly acquired girlfriend, he learned that
they had been minimally, if at all, aware of it. His tics long ago had
blended into the overall perception people had of him—namely, that
of a "nice guy." It was a confirmation of something clinicians have often
seen—that a healthy personality makes the individual's physical defect
"disappear," interpersonally speaking. Rod's defect had achieved that
kind of invisibility as far as the outside world was concerned. It remained for Rod to discover that he was not viewed as defective by anyone other than himself. It is important to add that, thoughout Rod's
psychotherapy, objective signs of TS remained generally at their minimal-to-mild level. At the end of his psychotherapy, however, Rod perceived himself to be improved with respect to his tics and changed his
own subjective classification from mildly or moderately impaired by tics
to minimally impaired. Rod's self-perception finally was in accord with
long-term objective observation.

Psychotherapy for TS sufferers who have objectively minimal-to-mild
tics, but who present with a maladaptive psychological response, often
helps such individuals with their emotional and/or personality difficulties. Such patients after a course of psychotherapy often perceive the

tics to be much improved and therefore are happier and more successful, better adjusted, less depressed. Objectively speaking, there actually
may be little, if any, variation in the tics. Many TS patients, like Rod,
fall into this trap of unnecessary suffering because of neurotic misperceptions of their disease or body image. Psychotherapy may effect a
subjective improvement or even "social cure" that exceeds tic improvement with pharmacological regimen. (Perhaps it was for this reason that
reports appeared in the scientific literature until the mid–1970s of the
treatment of TS by exclusively psychological means.) Psychopathological parallels appear in other organic disabilities, for instance, the so-
called cardiac cripple, who may, indeed, have cardiovascular disease,
perhaps even be post–myocardial infarction but, for neurotic reasons,
suffers the belief that his life is hanging by a thread and so consequently
constricts his activities and enjoyment of life as if he were bedridden in
imminent danger of cardiac arrest. With the very rare exception of severe motor and vocal tics, being "crippled" by TS is a psychological,
rather than a physical, sequela.

BEN: MIDDLE-AGED DEPRESSION AND ANGER, A "TS CRIPPLE"

Ben was a 45-year-old man with moderately severe TS since schoolage.
When he was in high school, he was very shy and kept to himself because
of his numerous motor and vocal tics. There was another student in
Ben's high school class whom he regarded as having motor and vocal
tics much more severe than his own. Ben was amazed that this other
boy was the star pitcher of the high school baseball team. "When you're
the pitcher, everyone is looking at you." Ben's diagnosis of TS was not
made until his late thirties. Ben's conclusion as an adolescent about this
other student with severe tics was that he had "nervous habits." Ben
recalls that, as an adolescent, he felt that this pitcher "must have had
terrific parents to give him so much self-confidence" despite his "very
noticeable" affliction. Ben, by contrast, a still unhappy, still seclusive,
angry, depressed 45-year-old TS sufferer, continues to struggle with the
severe neurotic residue of childhood pathological family dynamics. Ben
has been treated for several years pharmacologically with very gratifying results, if measured on the scale of frequency and disruptiveness of
motor and vocal tics. His social and vocational life remains, however, a
tragic disaster. Unresolved wishes to avenge himself violently against his
father unconsciously contaminate most of his relationships with men, in
general, and with his job supervisor, in particular. Ben stated that, in
terms of quality of life, he would have been happier with the even more
severe tics of his childhood peer, the baseball pitcher, if the trade-off
could have included the pitcher's apparently successful psychological
adaptation. Despite Ben's seemingly insightful observation of his need

for healthier psychological adaptation, he remained, psychologically speaking, a TS cripple enmeshed in ancient battles. Years earlier, Haldol "cured" Ben's tics but not the person. Regrettably, Ben had had a falling out with his psychotherapist of many years when the therapist, upon being informed by Ben that a diagnosis of TS (finally) had been made, looked up TS in an out-of-date textbook and pronounced TS as strictly psychological in origin—thus (according to Ben) "blaming" Ben for his disruptive behavior. Ben then saw the therapist as he had similarly seen his father many years earlier—someone who blamed him for something he could not help. Ben had believed for many years that psychotherapy meant looking for the unconscious complex that, when found, would "cure" him. Ben was now justifiably dubious of this psychotherapeutic goal (and psychotherapist).

By contrast, a successful adaptation to TS symptoms as severe as Ben's was demonstrated by a 12-year-old boy, who stated that his tics were part of "what makes me me." In his psychotherapy he came up with the idea that adapting to his tics makes him stronger—it shows he has more "character." He even developed a healthy play fantasy of a character he calls Tourette's Man—an obvious analogy to, of course, Superman. (It will be recalled that Superman also has idiosyncracies—he is faster than a speeding bullet, can leap tall buildings at a single bound, etc.)

CONCLUSIONS: TS AND THE WHOLE PERSON

To summarize: (1) The TS patient's suffering, with the exception of rare instances of physically hurtful tics, is experienced in an interpersonal field. (2) The degree of suffering is not at all necessarily proportional to an objective measurement of tics. (3) The psychological damage that may have occurred in the developing personality because of TS symptoms usually is not undone by relief from symptoms through pharmacological means. (4) A careful, skilled, psychodynamic evaluation of someone with TS or TS diathesis always is indicated in any workup for these conditions. (5) The need for psychotherapeutic treatment is indicated by the presence of maladaptive psychological defense mechanisms or the development of personality distortions. In psychologically troubled TS patients, anger, depression, distorted body image, and schizoid and/or paranoid personality behavior disorders (over and above TS complexes) are typical findings. (6) Psychotherapeutic intervention must be flexible and geared to the psychodynamic findings. This may encompass treatment modalities ranging from individual to family therapy, from psychoanalysis to supportive therapy. The psychotherapy is offered not as a treatment for TS symptoms, per se, but for the consequences of the intra-and interpersonally disruptive aspect of the disease. (7) The TS patient may suffer from any or all of the usual neurotic complaints of life. The TS patient, because he or she has a chronic disease, may have less ego strength to deal with the neuroses of everyday life. Treatment of these ordinary, perhaps even subclinical (under other circumstances) neuroses may result in the TS patient's feeling better, may improve his or her sense of the positive quality of life, and even decrease the disruptive index of symptoms. Treatment may also decrease that portion of TS symptoms that are triggered psychologically. (The psyche well may affect the soma.) (8) Psychotherapy of the TS patient is best left in the hands of practitioners skilled in both psycho- and physiopathology of TS. This is particularly important for the psychotherapeutic task of helping the TS patient distinguish between TS symptoms and behavioral phenomena of other than TS origin. Like any other chronic illness or congenital or acquired "defect," TS can be incorporated into an individual's character armor. The very real presence of TS symptoms can be used by the person in the service of pathological character structures. (This is what Freud referred to in his paper "The Exceptions [1916] and Eric Berne [1962] described in his book *Games People Play* as the "wooden leg syndrome.") (9) A psychotherapeutic approach may be a necessary, but not sufficient, condition for a subjective "cure" of a TS patient. Psychotherapy, in skilled hands, is, at best, potentially very helpful and, at worst, if not misrepresented, harmless. At the least, psychotherapy may bring the patient into an ongoing relationship with a therapist who will see him or her as a full person and not just a "case" with symptoms. From this, the patient may improve or regain his or her sense of himself or herself as a person. After years of overconcern about tics, medications to manage the tics, medication to "control" medication side effects, and physical examinations and treatments of other types, psychotherapy may help the individual with TS refocus on living his or her own life.

REFERENCES

Berne, E. (1962). *Games People Play.* New York: Grove.

Ferenczi, S. (1952). Psychoanalytic observations on tics. In : Selected Papers, Vol. 2: E. Jones (ed.). *Further Contributions to the Theory and Technique of Psychoanalysis.* New York: Basic Books.

Freud, S. (1957). Three essays on the theory of sexuality. In J. Strachey (Ed. and Trans.), *The Standard Edition of the Complete Psychological Works of Sigmund Freud.* (Vol. 7, pp. 239–240). London: Hogarth Press. (Original work published 1905)

Freud, S. (1957). Some character types met in psychological work. In J. Strachey (Ed. and Trans.), *The Standard Edition of the Complete Psychological Works of Sig-*

mund Freud (Vol. 14, pp. 311–315). London: Hogarth Press. (Original work published 1916)

Gerard, M.W. (1946). The psychogenic tic in ego development. *Psychoanalytic Study of the Child, 2,* 133–162.

Mahler, M. (1944). Tics and impulsions in children: A study of motility. *Psychoanalytic Quarterly, 13*(4), 430–444.

Mahler, M. (1949). A psychoanalytic evaluation of tics in psychopathology of children: Symptomatic tic and tic syndrome. *Psychoanalytic Study of the Child, 3/4,* 279–310.

Mahler, M., & Rangell, L. (1943). A psychosomatic study of maladie des tics (Gilles de la Tourette's disease). *Psychiatric Quarterly, 17,* 579–603.

Menninger, K. (1963). *The vital balance.* New York: Viking.

Sprenger, J., & Kraemer, H. (1948). *Malleus Maleficarum* (Montague Summers, Trans.) London: Pushkin. (Original work published 1489).

CHAPTER FIFTEEN

School Problems Associated with Tourette's Syndrome

Rosa A. Hagin
John Kugler

It is a child's business to learn. So deeply is this capacity ingrained in human beings that some students of human behavior have speculated that our specialization as a species is a specialization for learning (Bruner, 1966). While other species begin their learning anew with each generation, humankind has devised the educational process in order to conserve and transmit past learning to each succeeding generation. Schools have been given major responsibility for the formal process of education. Thus the opportunity to attend school and to learn has come to be regarded as a fundamental human right.

For children and youth with Tourette's syndrome, education has a special importance. Not only is schooling a significant aspect of their clinical management, but it may also be a major rehabilitative strategy in planning for their adjustment in adult life. Unfortunately, Tourette's syndrome presents many barriers to these youngsters as they attempt to secure the benefits of an appropriate education.

BARRIERS TO LEARNING

Children and youth with Tourette's syndrome may experience educational problems at a number of different levels. There are primary problems implicit in the disorder itself. The underlying pathology responsible for Tourette's syndrome may impair learning at biochemical and physiological levels. Indirect effects of the disorder can result in impaired attention, behavioral difficulties, and problems in social adjustment when other people fail to understand the nature of the symptoms.

However, not all youngsters experience the effects of these barriers to learning to the same degree. In fact, with many youngsters it is surprising that they have learned as well as they have, considering the interferences they must deal with.

The purpose of this chapter is to describe the learning strengths and deficits of youngsters with Tourette's syndrome, to delineate the effects on schooling, and to suggest some positive approaches to their education.

SOURCES OF DATA

The data base for this chapter consists of three samples: (1) a sample of 10 youngsters with Tourette's syndrome who represent positive adjustment in terms of school achievement and resolution of the family crises regarding diagnosis (referred to hereafter as the *recruited sample*); (2) a sample of 16 youngsters and young adults who sought the services of the School Consultation Center at Fordham University-Lincoln Center (referred to hereafter as the *referred sample*); and (3) a sample of 72 families who responded to a questionnaire about school practices (referred to hereafter as the *questionnaire sample*).

The recruited sample was drawn in order to identify positive educational practices for the schooling of children with Tourette's syndrome. Ages ranged from 7 to 13 years with a median age of 10 years. All children were attending school, 8 in regular classes, 1 in a special class for neurologically impaired children, and 1 in a residential school. IQs earned on the Wechsler Intelligence Scale for Children—Revised were above average with a mean Full Scale IQ of 111 ± 19, a mean Verbal IQ of 114 ± 22, and a mean Performance IQ of 106 ± 17. Diagnostically, the group was found to consist of 10 children with Tourette's syndrome and 1 with an additional diagnosis of learning disability.

Each of the youngsters of the referred group came to the Center with specific questions to be answered. The original referral problems involved school placement issues (5 referrals), underachievement at school (3 referrals), problem behavior at home and/or at school (4 referrals), and impaired life adjustment (4 referrals). Age range was wider, spreading from 11 years to young adulthood (median age 15 years), and intellectual functioning was closer to the average range and more widely dispersed than that of the recruited sample, with a mean Full Scale IQ of 100 ± 12, a mean Verbal IQ of 102 ± 13, and a mean Performance IQ of 99 ± 13 found on the Wechsler scales. In addition to the original diagnosis of Tourette's syndrome, some individuals in the referred sample presented developmental and emotional problems. These included learning disability (6 youngsters), conduct disorder (3 youngsters), severe stuttering (1 youngster), depression (3 youngsters), and overanxious disorder (2 youngsters).

The combination of the two samples presents a wider range of functioning than either sample taken separately. Thus the combined clinical samples permit consideration of a broad spectrum of school problems encountered by individuals with Tourette's syndrome.

The questionnaire sample consisted of 72 respondents who replied to our request for information about positive school practices. The questionnaire had been enclosed in a regular issue of the *Tourette Syndrome Association Newsletter*. Responses came from 19 states, Canada, Australia, and Korea. Individual responses were read as they were received, then reread as a group to highlight recurrent issues. They were then coded in terms of general categories: (1) educational settings; (2) educational practices; and (3) sources of support.

These three samples provided information about the cognitive functioning, academic and neuropsychological skills, and social adjustment of children and adolescents with Tourette's syndrome.

COGNITIVE FUNCTIONING

Data from the combined clinical groups indicate that all of the young-sters in the samples possessed intellectual strengths. Means on the ap-propriate levels of the Wechsler scales placed at 104 ± 16, 106 ± 18, and 102 ± 15 for Full Scale, Verbal, and Performance IQs respectively. These measures of central tendency obscure a trend toward greater than ex-pected interscale variability in the clinical groups.

Verbal–Performance IQ differences of 15 points or more are consid-ered "important" (Wechsler, 1974, p. 34). By this standard 35 percent of the group had significantly higher Verbal IQ scores and 12 percent had significantly higher Performance IQ scores. Although this trend is significant only at a 5 percent level ($\chi^2 = 7.38$), it suggests greater var-iability than might be expected. However, it should be noted that the variation appears in both directions.

Variability was also assessed in terms of abnormal scatter among the Wechsler subtest scores using the rules of Seltz and Reitan (1979). Based on relationships between ranges and means of subtest scores, 36 per-cent of the combined sampled demonstrated an increased degree of scatter. This proportion differs significantly from what might be ex-pected ($\chi^2 = 18.75$; $p < .001$). The fact that the incidence of abnormal scatter did not differ between the referred and the recruited groups suggests that increased variability may be a general characteristic of Tourette's syndrome, rather than being related to unsuccessful school achievement.

Further analysis located the source of the increased scatter seen among the Wechsler subtests for the combined samples. Based on the standard errors of measurement of the subtests, Wechsler (1974, p. 34) has offered a rule of thumb that values of more than 3 scaled score points may be considered in analyses of subtest differences. Differences of this magnitude were calculated in terms of mean scaled scores for each of the youngsters. The results of this analysis appear in Table 15.1. As can be seen from the table, although there is considerable variation among subtest scores, for most subtests no consistent pattern emerges; some youngsters earn scores above and others earn scores below the mean of their scaled scores. These scores suggest that there is no "typi-cal" test pattern for children with Tourette's syndrome, but rather that youngsters must be considered in terms of their own patterns of strengths and needs in the interpretation of individual tests of intelli-gence.

Only the Coding subtest presents a contrasting picture with 40 per-cent of the scores falling significantly below the individual's mean scaled scores. This is understandable when one considers the task re-quirements of Coding. The test taps speed and accuracy in associating

Table 15.1. Significant Deviations of Wechsler Subtests

Subtest	Percentage High[a]	Percentage Low[b]	χ^2	p value
Information	8	8	2.94	NS
Similarities	12	12	.75	NS
Arithmetic	4	4	6.62	<.05
Vocabulary	8	12	1.78	NS
Digit Span	20	8	1.31	NS
Picture Completion	24	8	2.00	NS
Picture Arrangement	8	8	2.94	NS
Block Design	12	4	3.44	NS
Object Assembly	8	12	1.78	NS
Coding	0	40	16.78	<.001

[a]Percentage of subjects earning scores more than 3 scaled score points above their mean scaled scores.
[b]Percentage of subjects earning scores more than 3 scaled score points below their mean scaled scores.

symbols. These associations are completely arbitrary, with no logical relationships among them. The possibility of reversal errors is present in several of the symbol pairs. The pressure of time adds stress. Finally, because the test requires written responses, it has a strong motor component. While every member of the group did not have serious trouble with this subtest, a substantial proportion found it difficult. These findings are in keeping with results of some previous studies. For example, Golden's (1984) review of higher cerebral functions in Tourette's syndrome cited eight studies in which motor control was found to be impaired, in contrast to four studies in which it was found to be normal.

SCHOOL ACHIEVEMENT

In order to relate levels of cognitive functioning to schooling, individual educational expectancies based on chronological age and levels of functioning on the Wechsler scales were computed for each member of the combined samples according to the Harris formula (Harris, 1970). These expectancy estimates permitted comparisons with actual grade placements and with educational achievement.

All youngsters placed in graded classrooms demonstrated educational expectancies appropriate to the grade level represented. Two youngsters in the samples were enrolled in ungraded classrooms in order to receive special education services for their learning disabilities. A visit to one of the classrooms indicated a fine working atmosphere and appropriate challenge and assistance in the classroom. This was not the case with the second ungraded class placement, where the setting in a class of children with severe conduct disorders prevented effective remediation of the boy's specific learning disability. Although the usual special education designation is "other health related conditions," youngsters with Tourette's syndrome may require a range of classroom settings in order to meet their varied educational needs.

Individual educational expectancies for each youngster in the sample were used as a standard against which to compare scores earned on tests of educational skills. Educational skills were assessed in the following areas: oral reading and spelling (Wide Range Achievement Test); reading comprehension (Reading Cluster of the Woodcock-Johnson Psychoeducational Battery); mathematics (Mathematics Cluster of the Woodcock-Johnson Psychoeducational Battery). In addition, some members of the sample received a group test of reading (Metropolitan Reading Achievement Test for elementary grade children, Diagnostic Reading Tests for high school students). Scores for these tests were compared with individual expectancy estimates to determine whether each youngster's scores placed at, above, or below expectancy. These results appear in Table 15.2. In each case the proportion of scores in each of the three categories, (above, at, or below expectancy) was compared with the proportion expected in these categories in a normal distribution of scores. When evaluated by the chi-square statistic, the proportions observed in the combined sample were significantly different from expected proportions in all academic areas.

Strengths were seen in word attack skills as judged from tests of oral reading on which 84 percent of the sample scored at or above expectancy. These youngsters have learned a variety of decoding skills and use them successfully in reading aloud. Reading comprehension as assessed on an individual reading test was also handled effectively by a proportion greater than that expected in a normal distribution. However, the proportion of youngsters earning comprehension scores at or above expectancy was somewhat smaller than the successful proportion on the oral reading test.

The sample's response to group tests of reading shows a decidedly different picture from that seen when reading was tested individually. The group reading tests are representative of the standardized achievement tests typically given in group testing programs in schools. A high proportion (68 percent) of the combined sample earned scores below expectancy on this measure, despite the fact that many of them showed adequate reading skills on the individual comprehension and oral reading tests.

Because of this striking difference occurring in the assessment of the

Table 15.2. Comparison of Educational Expectancy and Achievement

Test	Expectancy[a]			χ^2	p value
	Above	At	Below		
Oral reading	68%	16%	16%	52.19	<.001
Individual reading comprehension	50%	10%	40%	23.51	<.001
Group reading comprehension	18%	14%	68%	38.89	<.001
Spelling	28%	20%	52%	30.97	<.001
Mathematics	32%	12%	56%	40.53	<.001

[a]Percentage of combined sample earning scores above, at, or below expectancy on each of the educational skills as compared with a normal distribution of scores for these skills.

same skill, some consideration of test requirements is in order. The group tests require sustained work over an extended period of time. The youngster must work independently, sustaining focus on the task on his or her own. In contrast, the individual tests like the Woodcock-Johnson Psychoeducational Battery use an easel format to present a few items at a time. The youngster does not have to sustain attention to a single test booklet and an answer sheet, because the examiner records responses with individual tests. Finally, the examiner sets the tempo for presentation of test items in terms of the previous responses. These differences suggest that it may be difficult for youngsters with Tourette's syndrome to demonstrate their reading skills on group tests because of problems with the test format, rather than solely because of skill deficiencies.

Scores for the spelling test show that less than half (48 percent) of the combined sample achieve at or above expectancy in this area. This discrepancy in encoding skills is unexpected in view of the strong decoding skills the group showed in the oral reading test. This may be another example of the difficulties youngsters with Tourette's syndrome experience when they attempt to demonstrate what they have learned. It may be, for example, that with some youngsters basic motor problems result in slow, inconvenient, and illegible handwriting. Because these children write as infrequently as possible, they do not receive enough practice with written work to make spelling skills automatic. Mathematics represents another area of need for the sample as a whole, with 56 percent of the group earning scores below expectancy in this area, a proportion significantly different from that of the expected distribution.

POSITIVE APPROACHES TO EDUCATION

The questionnaire sample provided considerable information about the day-to-day school experiences of youngsters with Tourette's syndrome. Coding of the 72 responses resulted in three broad content areas.

Educational Settings

Questionnaire responses emphasized the importance of a moderate degree of structure in classrooms for these children. Items concerning classroom structure, however, elicited a variety of responses. Thirteen replies mentioned specifically a *less* structured setting as being more beneficial than more traditional settings. The ideal setting is one in which children are permitted the freedom of physical movement when their symptoms require it, but one that also offers appropriate environmental cues to guide learning.

In contrast to the moderate structure that was mentioned frequently, 2 responses favored highly structured boarding schools in which "every hour of the day is programmed." These parents mentioned such programming as crucial to their children's learning. An additional 7 parents mentioned small independent schools with "therapeutically oriented" and "humanitarian" approaches to pupils.

While some parents advocated special class placements, a number of families firmly supported the mainstream class in which children have opportunities for special provisions in resource rooms, but also work for the major part of the school day with other children of ages similar to their own.

An especially important provision was some kind of refuge that the youngster might go to when the symptoms become severe. The opportunity to leave the classroom at any time without seeking special permission is a helpful arrangement between the youngster and the teacher. Refuges such as resource rooms, school clinics, and nurses' offices are the kinds of provisions mentioned. One young adult said he did his best work near a noisy heater in the back of the school library. One family described an inventive teacher who suggested "errands that give the child the opportunity to leave the classroom in a purposeful fashion." A physician who had to deal with a very rigid school placement for his patient finally resorted to a prescription that read: "This child must go to the bathroom every hour," thus assuring the child of the possibility of refuge, despite the school's rules and regulations.

While the physical and organizational climate of the school is important, the psychological climate is equally important. Questionnaire responses mentioned over and over again the need for concerned and active efforts to assist the child to develop his or her full potential. One parent mentioned "a teacher who never gave up on my son." Another parent mentioned the need for the kind of teacher who emphasizes the number of correct answers, rather than the number of errors. Teachers need to learn to ignore the tics and focus on the child.

Specific Instructional Suggestions

Some specific ideas were directed toward improving instruction.

One-to-One Help. Individual tutoring with reading and mathematics is frequently essential. This help may be received in a program for children with learning disabilities or in some remedial programs. Whatever the source of the instruction, it should emphasize perceptual cues, sound–symbol associations for word attack, and a decoding approach to reading.

Reasonable Goals. Small segments of work are preferable because they present reasonable goals. Strong efforts should be made for mastery of these small segments before the youngster goes on to more complex work. When goals are met, praise is an essential part of the learning process. This praise should be specific to the task. Praise is a strong motivator, and all youngsters like to have good work recognized.

Timing. The timing of schoolwork is a critical matter. Like most of us, youngsters with Tourette's syndrome need to work at their own speed. Rigid emphasis on timing increases stress.

Help with Directions. Most youngsters need some help in following directions. Parents and teachers can help by underlining significant words in written directions to draw attention to a sequence of steps. Verbal rehearsal can help youngsters deal effectively with oral directions.

Help with Handwriting. Some families have solved this problem by requesting that the child be allowed to print. A limit on the requirements for written work also helps. Typing may be a solution for some youngsters, although it has been found to be a source of stress for others. It would depend upon the nature and intensity of tics and whether control would be possible as the youngster learns the typewriter or word processor keyboards. The use of a buddy system to cut down on the amount of writing by asking classmates to write the list of homework assignments with a sheet of carbon paper in the notebook was also suggested. The use of guidelines, color cues, and plastic pencil wedges all appear to be reasonable suggestions that may be helpful for some youngsters.

Examinations.   Tests and examinations represent a critical issue for most older youngsters with Tourette's syndrome. Taking important examinations like the Scholastic Aptitude Test in private, untimed administration is one possibility worth consideration. Another solution with in-school tests is to allow the youngster to take a rest break between parts of the examination.

Sources of Support

A number of parents described ways of informing school staff members about Tourette's syndrome. Fifteen respondents mentioned school staff meetings as a method for such work. Films like *The Sudden Intruder* and *Stop It—I Can't* were used as the focus of discussions, and publications of the Tourette Syndrome Association were distributed. The importance of an appropriate explanation to the peer group is not to be underestimated.

Negative points appeared in the discussion of school adjustment. These points are helpful instruction in avoiding the pitfalls they imply. Mentioned most frequently was the isolation many children with Tourette's syndrome experience in the classroom. Occasionally, outright rejection occurs in the form of verbal abuse. A more subtle kind of rejection can be seen in the gratuitous advice from school personnel who attribute the symptoms to the parents' high expectations.

Teacher support for the youngster with Tourette's syndrome was mentioned repeatedly. One wise parent wrote: "Good teachers don't pity, pamper, or patronize." A young adult warned: "Don't let a kid cop out in school; I should have been in college prep." The responses showed general acceptance of the idea that school is a most important element in planning for the future of a youngster with Tourette's syndrome. In many reports of good school adjustment, there was evidence of mature, supportive parents in the background. These parents encouraged peer acceptance, but also made sure that there was adult supervision as needed during unstructured times at school.

A variety of school personnel were mentioned as having contributed to good school adjustment. The teacher is a key person in this respect, but a number of respondents mentioned school nurses, guidance counselors, school psychologists, resource room teachers, vice principals, and school secretaries.

Several respondents mentioned the need for careful interpretation of medication effects to school personnel, as well as the need for adjusting homework assignments for children who may be relatively symptom free during the school day.

Ultimately, the parent has the basic role in the support system. All parents should be well informed about the provisions of Public Law 94–142, the Education for All Handicapped Children Act. Knowledge of these provisions is a useful tool in securing the best education possible for the children.

IMPLICATIONS OF TOURETTE'S SYNDROME FOR EDUCATION

Children and youth with Tourette's syndrome may experience educational problems at a number of different levels. There are primary problems implicit in the disorder itself. The underlying pathology responsible for Tourette's syndrome may impair learning at biochemical and physiological levels.

Direct Effects of the Tics

Direct effects of the tics upon the performance of specific learning tasks are apparent with such school activities as handwriting or public speaking. Fine motor tasks may be difficult to perform when a tic can cause the pencil to fly out of the writer's grasp. Writing rapidly enough to keep up with the instructor's lecture or directions may also present problems to the student with Tourette's syndrome. Slow writing can result in gaps in note taking, missed details in homework assignments, or failure to finish tests with time limits. The stress of speaking to an audience may exacerbate tics, so that these youngsters may avoid active participation in class discussions. These direct effects of the symptoms on written and oral expression are particularly frustrating in that they keep the learner from demonstrating what he or she has learned.

Indirect Effects of the Disorder

Attempts to inhibit the symptoms in the classroom present another barrier to learning. Informal reports of these symptoms were confirmed in a study that contrasted the number of tics manifested during clinical interview with the number manifested during a similar period of observation by an anonymous observer in the child's own school room (Hagin, Beecher, Pagano, & Kreeger, 1980). In the group studied the mean number of tics observed during psychiatric interview was 9, in contrast to the mean of 2.5 tics observed in the classrooms. The physical and psychological effects on children's inhibiting tics are not well understood. Bruun (1984) reported two contrasting opinions expressed by adults: Some feel that such inhibition of symptoms in public indicates that they are coping well, while others feel that the resulting inner tension takes a heavy toll. In the classroom one cannot assess the gaps in information processing and interferences in attention that occur at the cost of the temporary suppression of symptoms, even though the families report all too vividly the children's release of symptoms within the privacy of their homes.

The fact that symptoms can be inhibited for short periods of time adds to confusion about the nature of the disorder. This cannot continue indefinitely, for eventually the tension mounts and finds motor or vocal expression. Such suppression of symptoms can be confusing to diagnosticians who base their assessments of the learning problems on a time-limited sample of behavior. This confusion could result in the conclusion that the child is malingering and the symptoms are a figment of the parents' imagination. Such a diagnostic conclusion could result in a decision to withhold special educational provisions that are in actuality badly needed by the child.

Generalized Learning Difficulties

More generalized learning difficulties resulting from individual behavioral symptoms associated with the puzzling and unpredictable disorder, such as attention deficits, hyperactivity, compulsions, obsessional thinking, irritability, low thresholds for frustration, and impulsive behavior, can also constitute barriers to school learning. While the motor and vocal tics are the most obvious manifestations, some investigators regard them as often the least disabling aspects of the disorder. Cohen, Detlor, Shaywitz, and Leckman (1982) suggest that it is more useful to view Tourette's syndrome as a disorder of psychomotor inhibition with pervasive effects upon all aspects of the personality. Whether these behaviors are regarded as primary manifestations of Tourette's syndrome or as attempts of the organism to reestablish equilibrium in response to a neurological disorder, they must be dealt with if the child is to benefit from schooling. Whatever their origin, the implication of these behaviors for appropriate classroom participation and the effective completion of learning tasks is obvious.

Side Effects of Medication

While the only proven effective treatment for Tourette's syndrome is pharmacologic, side effects of the medication used to control the symptoms may affect school learning. For some children such side effects as lethargy, cognitive blunting, anxiety, school-phobic reactions, and depression may interfere with educational productivity and even with regular school attendance.

Social Isolation

Education is more than an isolated teaching–learning process. Occurring as it does within the social system of the school, it involves a complex of motivational, interpersonal, administrative, economic, and legal forces that influence learning outcomes to a significant extent. The social isolation that may result from the bizarre symptoms of the disorder can decrease the youngsters' involvement in school activities and their motivation with schoolwork. Vocal tics may be perceived as disturbances to the concentration of classmates; coprolalia may be regarded as a violation of behavior standards of the school. The social isolation resulting from nonacceptance, rejection, and ridicule by classmates represents a serious barrier to school achievement, particularly for the adolescent with Tourette's syndrome.

Not all youngsters experience the effects of these barriers to learning. In fact, with many youngsters it is surprising that they have learned as well as they have, considering the learning interferences they must deal with. Effects on individuals depend upon the youngsters themselves and their families' resources for coping with the disorder. The extent to which school staff members are informed about Tourette's syndrome also may be a crucial factor in school adjustment.

REFERENCES

Bruner, J.S. (1966). *Toward a Theory of Instruction.* Cambridge, MA: Belknap Press of Harvard University Press.

Bruun, R.D. (1984). Gilles de la Tourette's syndrome: An overview of clinical experience. *Journal of the American Academy of Child Psychiatry,* 2, 126–133.

Cohen, D.J., Detlor, J., Shaywitz, B.A., & Leckman, J.F. (1982). Interaction of biological and psychological factors in the natural history of Tourette syndrome: A paradigm of childhood neuropsychiatric disorders. In A.J. Friedhoff & T.N. Chase (Eds.), *Gilles de la Tourette Syndrome.* New York: Raven Press.

Durost, W.N., Bixler, H.H., Hildreth, G.H., Lund, K.W. & Wrightstone, J.W. (1959). *Metropolitan Achievement Tests: Reading Tests.* New York: Harcourt, Brace & World.

Golden, G.S. (1984). Psychologic and neuropsychologic aspects of Tourette's syndrome. *Psychological and Neurologic Clinics,* 2, 91–102.

Hagin, R.A., Beecher, R., Pagano, G., & Kreeger, H. (1980). *Final Report to the Gatepost Foundation.* Mimeo.

Harris, A.J. (1970). *How to Increase your Reading Ability.* New York: McKay.

Jastak, J.F., & Jastak, S. (1978). *Wide Range Achievement Test.* Wilmington, DE: Jastak Associates.

Selz, M., & Reitan, R.M. (1979). Rules for neuropsychological diagnosis: Classification of brain function in older children. *Journal of Consulting and Clinical Psychology, 47,* 258–264.

Triggs, F.O., Bear, R.M., Spache, G.D., Townsend, A., Traxler, A.E., & Westover, F.L. (1976). *Diagnostic Reading Tests, Survey Section Form A.* Mountain Home, NC:

Wechsler, D. (1974). *Manual for the Wechsler Intelligence Scale for Children -Revised.* New York: Psychological Corporation.

Woodcock, R.W. & Johnson, M.B. (1977). *Woodcock-Johnson Psychoeducational Battery.* Boston: Teaching Resources Corporation.

CHAPTER SIXTEEN

Behavior Therapy for Tourette's Syndrome and Tic Disorders

Nathan H. Azrin
Alan L. Peterson

Tourette's syndrome (TS) and related tic disorders are influenced greatly by psychological factors, as evidenced by the very definition of TS patients as individuals who have the "ability to suppress movements voluntarily for minutes to hours" (APA, 1980). Behavior therapy has been employed in numerous studies of TS and tic disorders. This chapter reviews the research literature on behavioral treatment approaches to these disorders. It is unclear whether the various tic disorders—transient tics of childhood, chronic motor tic disorders, and TS—exist in a continuum or are distinct nosological entities. Some of the leading TS researchers (e.g., Shapiro & Shapiro, 1982) believe that the disorders exist in a continuum, with the mild transient tics of childhood on one end and the severe tics of TS on the other. Although the primary focus of this chapter is on TS, the treatment of other tic disorders (i.e., transient tic disorders, chronic motor tic disorders) is also reviewed. This chapter also provides fairly specific details on one of the recommended behavior therapy procedures for the treatment of TS and tic disorders.

METHODOLOGICAL CONSIDERATIONS

In reviewing the treatment outcome literature on behavioral approaches to TS and tic disorders, certain methodological criteria have been emphasized. Perhaps the most important methodological criterion is the method of measurement of the symptoms. Ideally, the measurement should be as objective as possible and involve direct frequency counts of the tics from either videotapes, direct observation, or self-recordings. The research studies should adequately describe the measurement modalities employed, provide the summary data on changes in tic frequency, and describe the changes in tic frequency. In addition to frequency, the tics may change in severity, intensity, or disruptiveness as a result of treatment. The major problem in attempting to delineate such changes in symptoms is that subjective ratings are required that are difficult to interpret. Several rating scales have been developed to characterize the severity, intensity, or disruptiveness of tics, including the TS Symptom Checklist (Cohen, Detlor, Young, & Shaywitz, 1980) and the TS Global Scale (Harcherik, Leckman, Detlor, & Cohen, 1984). (See Chapter Four, this volume.)

Another important factor is to ensure measures are taken both in the clinical experimental setting and in the patient's natural environment. Changes observed in the clinical setting are frequently different than those found in outside settings. Additionally, the studies should have an experimental design that controls for individual differences, the passage of time, and other possible extraneous factors.

BEHAVIORAL TREATMENTS OF TOURETTE'S SYNDROME

Numerous behavioral approaches have been used in treatment out-come studies of TS, including massed negative practice, contingency management, relaxation training, self-monitoring, and habit reversal. Thirty-one studies have been identified that have employed behavioral therapy as the primary treatment for TS, many of which have found behavioral treatment to be effective. Several methodological strengths exist in the studies that have been conducted. Virtually all behavioral studies of TS have used objective measures of tic frequency from video-tapes or direct observation. A second noteworthy feature is that several studies have taken measures in both the experimental and the natural setting (Azrin & Peterson, 1987; Billings, 1978; Doleys & Kurtz, 1974; Varni, Boyd, & Cataldo, 1978), a practice rarely used in pharmacological studies. Another positive characteristic of behavioral studies is the em-phasis on within-subject design. All of the behavioral studies of TS con-ducted to date have employed within-subject designs that allow compar-isons without the confounds that exist in between-subject comparisons. Several studies used multiple-baseline (Feldman & Werry, 1966; Hutzell, Platzek, & Logue, 1974; Thomas, Abrams, & Johnson, 1971) or reversal (Franco, 1981) designs. As is also the case in most pharmacological stud-ies of TS, long-term follow-up in behavioral studies has not been the norm, and only three studies reviewed conducted follow-ups for longer than 6 months after treatment (Azrin & Peterson, 1987; Hutzell et al., 1974; Varni et al., 1978). No group study evaluating between-subject dif-ferences has been conducted using behavioral treatment approaches to TS. Therefore, a systematic review of the case studies is warranted to attempt to determine the general efficacy of behavioral treatments for TS.

Massed Negative Practice

The most frequently employed behavioral treatment approach for TS has been massed negative practice. In massed negative practice, the pa-tient deliberately performs the tic movement as quickly and effortfully as possible. The patient performs the movement for a specified period of time (e.g., 30 minutes) interspersed with brief periods of rest (e.g., 4 minutes of exercise, 1 minute of rest). Theoretically, the patient be-comes "tired" of performing the movement and develops reactive inhi-bition, leading to a decrease in tic frequency. Eighteen case studies have been conducted (including a total of 24 subjects), using massed negative practice as the sole or a major component procedure. Ten of the studies (12 subjects) found that the frequency of tics decreased at the end of treatment (Browning & Stover, 1971; Clark, 1966; Miller, 1970; Nicassio, Liberman, Patterson, Raminez, & Saunder, 1972; Savicki & Carlin, 1972; Storms, 1985; Tophoff, 1973; Walton, 1961, 1964; Yates, 1958), whereas the remaining eight studies did not obtain a decrease in symptoms (Barr, Lovibond, & Kasaros, 1972; Canavan & Powell, 1981; Feldman & Werry, 1966; Hollandsworth & Bausinger, 1978; Lahey, McNees, & Mc-Nees, 1973; Sand, 1973; Teoh, 1974; Turpin & Powell, 1984). Several of these studies indicated a negative therapeutic effect, the frequency of tics actually increasing (Feldman & Werry, 1966; Hollandsworth & Bausinger, 1978; Teoh, 1974; Turpin & Powell, 1984), a former tic reappearing in one case (Feldman & Werry, 1966), and the clarity of coprolalia increasing in another case (Hollandsworth & Bausinger, 1978). Of the seven studies that found reductions in tics using massed negative practice and conducted systematic follow-ups (Miller, 1970; Nicassio et al., 1972; Savicki & Carlin, 1972; Storms, 1985; Tophoff, 1973; Walton, 1961, 1964), five studies showed maintained improvement (Miller, 1970; Storms, 1985; Tophoff, 1973; Walton, 1961, 1964), and two showed a return to the baseline frequency levels (Nicassio et al., 1972; Savicki & Carlin, 1972). Two studies conducted a follow-up for longer than 6 months (Miller, 1970; Walton, 1961). The results of the first study (Miller, 1970) are clouded, however, in that in addition to massed negative practice other procedures were used such as reinforcement for tic-free periods, contingency contracting, and relaxation training, and no direct measures of the reduction in tic frequency were reported. The findings from the second study (Walton, 1961) are also difficult to evaluate because of lack of objective measures of treatment outcome and the concurrent use of psychotropic medication. Long-term maintenance of the benefits is therefore uncertain.

Five of the studies that resulted in reductions in tic frequency from massed negative practice provided sufficient quantitative data to determine the precise degrees of effectiveness (Browning & Stover, 1971; Clark, 1966; Nicassio et al., 1972; Savicki & Carlin, 1972; Storms, 1985). These studies either used massed negative practice as the sole procedure or employed a design that allowed for the independent evaluation of the effectiveness of the procedure. The studies reported reductions in tic frequency of 55, 68, 38, 44, and 86 percent, respectively, for an overall average of 58 percent reduction in tic frequency. Similar conclusions were arrived at in a literature review (Turpin, 1983) regarding the use of massed negative practice in the treatment of tic disorders in general, not specifically TS. In this review it was found that, out of 22 studies employing massed negative practice, 3 indicated successful outcomes as assessed at long-term follow-up (> 6 months).

In summary, massed negative practice for the reduction of TS tics has been demonstrated to be a somewhat effective treatment modality for many subjects. About half of the studies conducted have reported decreases in tic frequency. At the current state of knowledge, massed negative practice in the treatment of TS shows definite therapeutic benefit, but that benefit is limited to some persons and averages about 58 percent reduction in tics for those persons.

Contingency Management

Contingency management has been the second most frequently employed behavioral treatment approach for TS. This approach is based on operant learning theory and posits that behaviors are maintained by the consequences that follow them. Individuals have been positively reinforced using praise, monetary reward, preferred activities, and so on for not performing tics or for performing alternative behaviors.

The use of positive reinforcement has been limited to studies of children with TS. Nine case studies have been conducted employing positive reinforcement (Barr et al., 1972; Browning & Stover, 1971; Doleys & Kurtz, 1974; Hollandsworth & Bausinger, 1978; Miller, 1970; Rosen & Wesner, 1973; Shulman, 1974; Tophoff, 1972; Varni et al., 1978). One study included two subjects (Browning & Stover, 1971); all others included a single subject. None of the studies used positive reinforcement as the sole behavioral intervention. Nevertheless, all of the studies except one (Hollandsworth & Bausinger, 1978) reported decreases in tic frequency at the end of treatment. At follow-up, six out of the seven studies maintained their improvement (Browning & Stover, 1971; Doleys & Kurtz, 1974; Miller, 1970; Tophoff, 1972; Varni et al., 1978; Wesner, 1973). Because none of the studies evaluated the independent effectiveness of positive reinforcement, the actual percentage of reduction in symptoms specifically attributable to contingency management cannot be determined. For children, at least, positive reinforcement for the absence of tics seems effective for almost all subjects when used in combination with other procedures.

Punishment has been employed as a behavioral treatment component in seven studies in the form of electric shock (Barr et al., 1972; Clark, 1966), white noise (Doleys & Kurtz, 1974), or time-out (Browning & Stover, 1971; Canavan & Powell, 1981; Lahey et al., 1973; Varni et al., 1978). Six out of the seven studies showed decreases in tic frequency at the end of treatment. Two out of the four studies that conducted follow-ups indicated that the improvement was maintained (Doleys & Kurtz, 1974; Varni et al., 1978).

In three of the studies using punishment (Barr et al., 1972; Canavan & Powell, 1981; Lahey et al., 1973), the authors noted that the decreases in tics were temporary and that there was difficulty in generalization. For example, one study (Barr et al., 1972) indicated that tics were only reduced when a shock electrode was connected to the subject's finger. When the electrode was removed, tics returned to baseline frequencies. Similarly, another study (Lahey et al., 1973) found that coprolalia was reduced in a school setting when time-out was implemented. In this study the child was immediately placed in a time-out room for a minimum of 5 minutes and until he was quiet for at least 1 minute. However, the coprolalia quickly returned to baseline levels when the contingencies were removed.

In summary, positive reinforcement and punishment have both been demonstrated to be somewhat effective in reducing the frequency of tics of TS. The results are somewhat clouded in that these procedures have been used as part of multicomponent treatment programs and have not been evaluated as individual treatment components. This is somewhat understandable in that virtually all behavioral treatment approaches to TS employ forms of praise from the experimenters or family members, whether explicitly stated or not. Positive reinforcement such as praise and encouragement is highly recommended for use in the treatment of any patient with TS, especially children. It may be that positive reinforcement in and of itself does not lead to reductions in frequency of tics, but increases the patient's motivation to use self-control or to employ some specifically prescribed treatment procedure. The use of aversive punishment such as electric shock has been demonstrated to reduce TS tics; however, these procedures raise ethical questions and cannot be highly recommended as a treatment prescription based on the available data.

Relaxation Training

Relaxation training has also been frequently used as a component in multimodal behavioral treatment approaches to TS. *Relaxation training* is a generic term that may involve many procedures, such as muscular tensing and relaxing (Jacobson, 1938), deep breathing (Cappo & Holmes, 1984), visual imagery (Suinn, 1975), and verbalizations or self-statements of relaxation (Schultz & Luthe, 1959). Different types of relaxation procedures may lead to different kinds of relaxed states.

Relaxation training has been used as a behavioral intervention component in eight case studies of TS (Azrin & Peterson, 1987; Canavan & Powell, 1981; Franco, 1981; Friedman, 1980; Rosen & Wesner, 1973; Savicki & Carlin, 1972; Tophoff, 1972; Turpin & Powell, 1984). Jacobsonian progressive muscular relaxation (Jacobson, 1938), which is achieved by the systematic tensing and relaxing of specific muscle groups, has been the most frequently used relaxation technique in studies of TS (Azrin & Peterson, 1987; Franco, 1981; Friedman, 1980; Rosen & Wesner, 1973; Tophoff, 1972). The other studies have not specified the relaxation procedures employed (Canavan & Powell, 1981; Savicki & Carlin, 1972; Turpin & Powell, 1984). In each of the eight studies conducted using relaxation training, tic frequencies were significantly reduced and were frequently nonexistent during the relaxed state. However, the reductions were usually rather temporary, with tics returning to baseline levels after a few minutes or hours.

In summary, relaxation training appears to be an effective method of reducing the tics of TS for short periods. Because no studies have been conducted using relaxation training as the sole intervention strategy, the specific efficacy of the procedure cannot be determined.

Self-Monitoring

Self-monitoring is frequently used in TS studies as a method of obtaining data on tic frequencies outside the experimental setting. Subjects are instructed to use a wrist counter, small notebook, or other device to record the frequency of their tics for a specified period of time. Some evidence exists that this procedure alone can lead to reductions in the frequency of tics. Three case studies have been conducted in which self-monitoring has been used as either the primary treatment procedure (Billings, 1978; Hutzell et al., 1974) or a major treatment component (Thomas et al., 1971). All three of these studies resulted in significant reductions in tic frequency. In the first study (Billings, 1978), the patient used a wrist counter; the self-monitoring led to a 75 percent reduction in tics outside the clinic setting. Direct observation and frequency counts in the clinic showed the tics to be reduced 100 percent. At a 6-month follow-up, tics were found to be further reduced outside the clinic setting. Researchers in the second study (Hutzell et al., 1974) also used direct observation and frequency counts in a clinic setting and found self-monitoring to lead to a 69 percent reduction in tics in the clinic. Self-report data indicated the tics were also reduced in the home setting. The improvements were maintained at a 1-year follow-up. The third study (Thomas et al., 1971) was conducted in an inpatient hospital setting and found that self-monitoring led to a 90 percent reduction in tics based on direct observation data and frequency count. However, the interpretation of these effects is complicated by the concurrent use of positive reinforcement and relaxation training.

In summary, self-monitoring has been demonstrated in three case studies to be effective in reducing the tics of TS. Exactly why this simple procedure works is unclear. Self-monitoring may result in the patient becoming keenly aware of the high frequency of tics, thereby leading to some unknown type of self-control procedure by the patient to control the tics.

Habit Reversal

The use of habit reversal (Azrin & Nunn, 1977; Azrin, Nunn, & Frantz, 1980) has been shown to be very effective in treating tic disorders, and some support is available that this procedure is also effective in treating individuals with TS (Azrin & Peterson, 1987; Finney, Rapoff, Hall & Christopherson, 1983; Franco, 1981; Zikis, 1983). Habit reversal is a composite procedure that is distinctive in its use of competing responses to prevent the occurrence of tics. In addition, it includes awareness training, self-monitoring, contingency management, and relaxation training. The competing response for many tics is the isometric tensing of muscles opposite to the tic movements. The opposing muscles are contracted for approximately 2 minutes contingent on the emission of, or urge to have, a tic. Habit reversal is somewhat similar to massed negative practice in that both require the practice of specific responses; however, while massed negative practice requires the practice of the actual tic, habit reversal requires the practice of incompatible movements that will not allow tics to occur. Habit reversal is also somewhat related to punishment in that performing the competing reaction can be aversive in that it requires a concerted effort by the subject.

Two individuals with TS were treated in one study (Franco, 1981) using habit reversal in which 10-minute videotapes were taken to record tic frequency. A component analysis of several of the habit reversal procedures was conducted using a reversal design. Results indicated the greatest reduction in tics occurred when the entire habit reversal procedure was implemented (awareness training, relaxation, isometric tensing). Only a partial reduction was found with relaxation training and awareness training. Tics were reduced by 99 percent in both subjects at the end of treatment. This study is limited, however, because: (1) only the major tic was treated in each subject and secondary tics were not recorded; (2) the measures were limited to the experimental laboratory setting; and (3) no systematic follow-up was conducted.

In another study (Finney et al., 1983), habit reversal was employed to treat an 11-year-old boy with multiple tics similar to those found in TS. The researchers used a multiple-baseline across-behaviors design and took 10-minute videotapes of the child in his natural home setting to measure changes in tic frequency. Habit reversal reduced the tics by an average of 85 percent at the end of 18 weeks of treatment. At 1-year follow-up, all tics were absent.

Habit reversal was also used in a case study (Zikis, 1983) to treat a 10-year-old boy with TS who exhibited a total of 19 different tics. Habit reversal treatment began after 1 year of unsuccessful treatment with drugs and brief insight psychotherapy. Eight weekly sessions of 2 hours' duration were conducted in a hospital outpatient department as well as

1-hour sessions daily for 10 weeks at home. Tics began to decrease during the third session and continued to decrease for the duration of the treatment. A major limitation of this case study is that, although frequency counts of tics were apparently taken, no data on percentage of reduction of tic frequency were reported and the subject was simply described as "much improved."

A study was recently completed by the authors (Azrin & Peterson, 1987) in which habit reversal was used to treat three adult males with TS. Frequency counts and severity measures were obtained in the clinic setting using videotapes and at home using unobtrusive direct observations by the subjects' spouses. Tic frequency was reduced for all three subjects over a 6- to 8-month period by 90 to 97 percent in the clinic setting and by 64 to 99 percent in the home setting, with a concurrent decrease in severity.

In summary, habit reversal also appears to be a very effective method for treating TS. However, the empirical evidence for this is based on a small number of case studies of individuals with TS. Although some extrapolation is required, the group study conducted by Azrin and co-workers (Azrin et al., 1980) may also lend support to the effectiveness of habit reversal in the treatment of TS. This is especially true if stereotypic movement disorders do indeed exist in a continuum from the mild transient tics of childhood to the severe tics of TS.

BEHAVIORAL TREATMENTS ON NON-TOURETTE'S TIC DISORDERS

Numerous behavioral approaches have been employed to treat transient and chronic motor tic disorders, including massed negative practice, contingency management, relaxation training, self-monitoring, and habit reversal. These are the same procedures reviewed earlier for TS. All but a single study (Azrin et al., 1980) have been case studies. These behavioral procedures have all been shown to reduce somewhat the frequency of tics. Turpin (1983) conducted an excellent review of the behavioral management of tic disorders and arrived at the same conclusions.

One group study has been conducted (Azrin et al., 1980) that resulted in a dramatic reduction of tics and provides strong research support for the use of a specific behavioral approach for the treatment of tic disorders. In this study 22 subjects were included who exhibited a wide range of simple and complex motor and vocal tics. Habit reversal was used to treat each subject's major or most disruptive tic. A between-groups design was employed in this study and subjects were randomly assigned to either a habit reversal or a massed practice group. In this study, habit reversal resulted in an 84 percent reduction in tics on the first day as reported from patients' direct frequency count outside the office setting. At an 18-month follow-up, there was a 97 percent reduction in tics and 80 percent of the patients were tic free. Massed practice led to a 33 percent reduction in tics, and at a 4-week follow-up, only 2/ 12 patients were tic free. Habit reversal has been employed in several other case studies and has obtained similar results (Azrin & Nunn, 1973; Finney et al., 1983; Franco, 1981; Ollendick, 1981; Zikis, 1983).

In summary, habit reversal has been demonstrated to be very effective in the treatment of tic disorders and is considered by many to be the treatment of choice (Adams & Sutker, 1984).

RECOMMENDED BEHAVIOR THERAPY PROCEDURES FOR TOURETTE'S SYNDROME AND TIC DISORDERS

The following sections of this chapter include the recommended behavior therapy procedures for treating individuals with TS and tic disorders. The foundation for the recommended procedures is the treatment outcome studies that have been conducted on these disorders. The sections are written to provide fairly detailed descriptions of the basic procedures required to employ the recommended behavior therapy procedures.

As noted above, the habit reversal method is a multicomponent treatment program that incorporates several of the procedures that have been demonstrated to be effective: self-monitoring, relaxation training, contingency management, and competing response training. These procedures are currently being used to treat tics and TS by the present authors in a research program at Nova University in Fort Lauderdale.

Self-Monitoring and Awareness Training

The initial procedure used when employing habit reversal is *awareness training,* which focuses on increasing the patient's awareness of: (1) frequency and severity of the tics; (2) environmental variables influencing symptoms; and (3) the specific movements involved in the tics. *Self-monitoring,* or the recording of tic frequency, is the initial assignment conducted by the patient. In addition to providing initial baseline data, self-monitoring has been demonstrated to reduce somewhat the frequency of tics. The patient is instructed to record the incidence of each tic for a specified duration each day. Each tic is recorded separately because it helps to identify which tics are most frequent and because different habit reversal procedures may be used for each tic. The duration of the recording period must be adjusted depending on the frequency of tics. For high-frequency tics, a 10-minute period each day will usually suffice. For low-frequency tics, patients can keep records for the entire day. Tics may be recorded in several ways. One of the simplest methods is the use of a wrist counter; however, only one total can be aggregated at a time, which limits the recording to either the total of all tics or the total of an individual tic. Another method is to record tics in a notebook or on a recording sheet. To simplify the recording process, a code can be developed for each patient, such as "H" for head shake, "S" for eye squint, "A" for arm jerk, and so on. The patient then records the code for each tic as it occurs (e.g., HHSAHH). After the recording period, the patient counts the total of each individual tic and records it on the record sheet. Recordings are also taken by an additional individual such as a parent or spouse, to provide supplementary data.

The second part of awareness training is the *response description procedure*. The patient describes the details of each tic to the therapist, using a mirror or videotape if necessary. This procedure helps ensure that the patient is aware of all of the tics currently being exhibited and the specific movement involved in each. Sometimes patients are reluctant to view themselves on a videotape or in a mirror; however, being able to control tic symptoms effectively requires the patient to be keenly aware of all tic movements. Having to observe oneself on videotape or mirror can also help increase the patient's motivation to perform the required treatment procedures. In the third part, the *response detection procedure,* the therapist teaches the patient to detect the occurrence of each tic by alerting the patient when an instance of the tic occurs. The fourth part is the *early warning procedure,* wherein the patient is given practice in detecting the earliest sign or sensory precondition (Bliss, 1980; Bullen & Hemsley, 1983) of a tic. The fifth procedure is *situation awareness training,* which focuses on helping the patient become more aware of the situations in which tics are most frequent or severe. Information gathered during self-monitorings is helpful in implementing this procedure. The patient identifies the situations, persons, and places in association with which symptoms are better or worse. By being aware of the situations in which tics are more severe, patients can be prepared to implement the appropriate procedures immediately upon entering them or even shortly prior to doing so.

Relaxation Training

Patients with TS and tic disorders should be taught relaxation training as a general procedure to help reduce tension and decrease the frequency and severity of tics. Several procedures have been demonstrated to be effective in producing relaxation or eliminating anxiety, including progressive muscular relaxation (Jacobson, 1938), deep breathing (Cappo & Holmes, 1984), visual imagery (Suinn, 1975), and self-statements of relaxation (Schultz & Luthe, 1959). It is recommended that all of these procedures be introduced and taught to the patient. Brown (1978, pp. 257–264) and Padus (1986, pp. 249–267) provide excellent reviews of the procedures used for several different types of relaxation exercises. Jacobsonian progressive muscular relaxation involves systematically tensing and relaxing specific muscles for approximately 10 to 15 seconds each and focusing on the differences in sensations perceived when the muscles are tense versus relaxed.

Using imagery (Suinn, 1975), the patient imagines he or she is in the ideal location for relaxation. The patient is directed by the therapist to try to imagine seeing all the colors, hearing the sounds, and smelling the aromas. If the patient has difficulty imagining this type of scene or has difficulty concentrating on relaxing, he or she should be directed to try to imagine and focus on some inanimate object that does not have any special meaning to the patient (e.g., candle, red ball, etc.). By focusing on this object, the patient may avoid anxiety-producing intrusive thoughts.

Deep breathing is another relaxation technique that has been demonstrated to be effective in reducing anxiety (Cappo & Holmes, 1984). The patient is taught to breathe very deeply, inhaling and exhaling slowly without pausing. The best effects have been found when the exhalation is slightly longer than the inhalation.

One final method of relaxation that has been shown to be effective is self-statements of relaxation (Schultz & Luthe, 1959). During the relaxation exercises, the patient is directed to repeat subvocally words or phrases relating to the achievement of the relaxed state. *Relax* or *calm* are some of the most effective words that can be used.

These procedures can and should be used in conjunction with each other. The patient is taught the relaxation procedures during the first treatment session. For the initial home assignment, the patient sits in a comfortable chair, preferably with a headrest, in a quiet room and practices the procedures at least once per day for a period of 10 to 15 minutes. The patient is also instructed to employ the relaxation procedures, or as many procedures as possible, on a cue-controlled basis. The effects of relaxation training have been shown to be enhanced when the procedures are employed on a cue-controlled basis (Goldfried, 1973). Any time the patient begins to feel anxious or emits a tic, the procedures should be implemented for a period of 1 to 2 minutes. The extent to which all of the procedures may be employed will depend on the environmental conditions; however, some of the procedures, such as deep breathing and self-statements, can be employed in virtually any setting.

The patient is instructed that the full effects of the relaxation procedures will not be noticed for approximately 2 weeks. It takes this long for the patient to become proficient at implementing the cue-controlled relaxation. Once he or she is proficient, the cue-controlled relaxation provides the patient with the opportunity to achieve a relaxed, tic-free state at times other than during scheduled practice sessions.

Competing Response Training

The primary habit reversal component is the *competing response procedure.* The goal is to identify some competing response that is antithetical to a tic, or will not allow the tic to occur. The competing response is designed to have the characteristics of (1) being opposite to the tic movement, (2) being capable of being maintained for several minutes, and (3) being socially inconspicuous and easily compatible with normal ongoing activities but incompatible with the tic.

The competing response that can be used for many motor tics is the isometric tensing of the muscles that are opposite to the tic movement. The patient tenses the muscles just tight enough so that the tic movement cannot occur, even when he or she is instructed to attempt to perform the tic movement intentionally. Some tics require competing responses other than isometric tensing of muscles, such as the use of a specific breathing pattern for vocal tics or an eye-blinking technique for eye tics. For peculiar tics the therapist must sometimes "brainstorm" with the patient, trying several procedures until the competing reaction that will stop the tic can be identified. To employ the competing response procedure, the patient implements the specific incompatible procedure for about 2 minutes whenever there is an urge to have a tic or immediately after the actual occurrence of a tic.

Brief descriptions of some of the competing responses that have been found to be effective with tics are as follows:

Backward head jerking

The isometric contraction of the neck flexors (sternocleidomastoid group), while pulling the chin slightly down and in, and maintaining the head in an eyes-forward position.

Shoulder jerking

Isometric contraction of the shoulder depressors to strengthen the muscles that work in opposition to the upward jerking movement.

Head shaking

Slow isometric contraction of the neck muscles with the eyes forward until the head can be maintained perfectly still.

Forward shoulder jerking

Pushing hands down and backward against some object, such as the chair arms while sitting, or against the thigh if standing.

Eye squint

Systematic voluntary, soft blinking consciously maintained at a rate of one blink per 3 to 5 seconds. Frequent downward shifting of gaze about every 5 to 10 seconds.

Barking

Slow rhythmic deep breathing through the nose while keeping the mouth closed. Exhalation should be slightly longer than inhalation (e.g., 5 seconds of inhalation, 7 seconds of exhalation). The flow of air should not stop at any point other than when shifting from inhalation to exhalation and vice versa.

The tic that is the most frequent or most disruptive is treated first. At least one treatment session is devoted to training the individual to employ the competing response procedure both during the session and during the following week in the patient's natural home setting. In subsequent sessions, each different type of tic is treated one at a time until a specific competing response has been established for every one. By treating the major tics first, it is frequently found that the effects generalize and other tics are reduced as well.

The patient is actively involved in trying to determine the specific competing response that will work for each tic. The patient is also instructed on how to generalize the competing response procedure to new tics should they arise. This is an important feature considering that waxing, waning, and changing of symptoms are common in TS.

Contingency Management

Little success will result from the behavior therapy procedures if the patient is only casually interested in eliminating the tics. Contingency management helps ensure that the patient is as motivated as possible to perform all of the procedures. The patient should be reinforced by family and close friends who comment favorably on the improved appearance of the patient when they notice tic-free periods or significant reductions. The patient's motivation can be further increased by using the *habit inconvenience review*, in which the therapist and patient review in detail the inconveniences, embarrassment, and suffering that resulted from emitting the tics. The therapist and patient then review the positive aspects and advantages of reducing or eliminating tics. The information on inconveniences of emitting tics and positive aspects of controlling tics is then written on an index card for the patient. This card is carried by the patient and reviewed frequently as a cognitive strategy to increase the patient's motivation to perform the exercises. It is also a means of increasing self-reinforcement and positive self-statements.

Contingency management is especially important with children, who may not be as motivated to rid themselves of tics. The child's family members and teachers are instructed to praise the child for performing the exercises and for improved appearance. For unmotivated, uncooperative children, a token economy (Ayllon & Azrin, 1968) is developed to provide a complete contingency management program. Parents and teachers can also prompt the child by manually guiding the child through the required exercises whenever the child fails to initiate the exercises himself or herself.

As patients improve, they are encouraged to participate in enjoyable social activities that were previously avoided because of the social disruptiveness of their tics. For many individuals, this is the strongest natural reinforcer available for reducing or eliminating tics.

Generalization Training

During each treatment session, the patient is given practice and instruction on how to control the tics in everyday situations. First the patient practices the specific procedure in the session until it can be correctly executed. To teach the patient to be aware of tics in situations outside the office setting, the *symbolic rehearsal procedure* is used in which the client imagines being in common and tic-eliciting situations and detecting the urge to emit a tic, and then performs the required exercise. This rehearsal utilizes the list of situations obtained previously from the patient in the situation awareness procedure. Additionally, after the cue-controlled relaxation or competing response procedure has been taught to the patient, the procedures are employed by the client for the duration of each treatment session. If the patient fails to detect a tic or self-initiate a procedure, the therapist prompts the patient to implement the appropriate procedure.

CONCLUSION

Behavior therapy plays an important role in the effective treatment of TS and tic disorders. Chronic motor tics have been demonstrated to be very effectively treated using behavioral interventions. Habit reversal has been demonstrated to produce a greater than 90 percent reduction in tic frequency and is recommended as the treatment of choice for chronic motor tics. Behavior therapy is also highly recommended for the treatment of TS. All of the behavior therapy procedures reviewed in this chapter—massed negative practice, contingency management, relaxation training, self-monitoring, habit reversal—have been found to reduce the frequency of TS tics. Behavior therapy is recommended as the treatment of choice for TS patients who are nonresponders to drug treatment or who experience unwanted side effects. Concurrent pharmacotherapy and behavior therapy are also recommended. Many individuals taking TS medication still have symptoms or would like to decrease dosage levels; behavior therapy can help these individuals. In a brief review of the advances in treatment and research of TS, Cohen and Leckman (1984) stated: "Today, TS stands as a good example of the way in which multidisciplinary research can illuminate a clinical syndrome" (p. 124). Similarly, the most efficacious treatment of TS and tic disorders can be achieved through an interdisciplinary approach involving medical and behavioral procedures. Behavior therapy has much to offer in the effective treatment of TS and tic disorders.

REFERENCES

Adams, H.E., & Stuker, P.B. (Eds.). (1984). *Comprehensive Handbook of Psychopathology*. New York: Plenum.

Ayllon, T., & Azrin, N.H. (1968). *The Token Economy: A Motivational System for Therapy and Rehabilitation*. New York: Appleton-Century-Crofts.

American Psychiatric Association. (1980). *Diagnostic and Statistical Manual of Mental Disorders* (3rd ed.). Washington, DC: Author.

Azrin, N.H., & Nunn, R.G. (1973). Habit-reversal: A method of eliminating nervous habits and tics. *Behavior Research & Therapy, 11*, 619–628.

Azrin, N.H., & Nunn, R.G. (1977). *Habit Control in a Day*. New York: Simon & Schuster.

Azrin, N.H., Nunn, R.G., & Frantz, S.E. (1980). Habit-reversal vs negative practice treatment of nervous tics. *Behavior Therapy, 11*, 169–178.

Azrin, N.H., & Peterson, A.L. (1987). *Habit Reversal for the Treatment of Tourette Syndrome*. Manuscript submitted for publication.

Barr, R.F., Lovibond, S.H., & Katsaros, E. (1972). Gilles de la Tourette's syndrome in a brain-damaged child. *Medical Journal of Australia, 2*, 372–374.

Billings, A. (1978). Self-monitoring in the treatment of tics: A single-subject analysis. *Journal of Behavior Therapy & Experimental Psychiatry, 9*, 339–342.

Bliss, J. (1980). Sensory experiences of Gilles de la Tourette syndrome. *Archives of General Psychiatry, 37*, 1343–1347.

Brown, B.B. (1978). *Stress and the Art of Biofeedback.* New York: Bantam.

Browning, R.M., & Stover, D.O. (1971). *Behavior modification in child treatment: An experimental and clinical approach.* Chicago: Aldine-Atherton.

Bullen, J.G., & Hemsley, D.R. (1983). Sensory experience as a trigger in Gilles de la Tourette's syndrome. *Journal of Behavior Therapy & Experimental Psychiatry, 14,* 197–201.

Canavan, A.G.M., & Powell, G.E. (1981). The efficacy of several treatments of Gilles de la Tourette's syndrome as assessed in a single case. *Behaviour Research & Therapy, 19,* 549–556.

Cappo, B.M., & Holmes, D.S. (1984). The utility of prolonged respiratory exhalation for reducing physiological and psychological arousal in non-threatening and threatening situations. *Journal of Psychosomatic Research, 28,* 265–273.

Clark, D.F. (1966). Behaviour therapy of Gilles de la Tourette's syndrome. *British Journal of Psychiatry, 112,* 771–778.

Cohen, D.J., Detlor, J., Young, J.G., & Shaywitz, B.A. (1980). Clonidine ameliorates Gilles de la Tourette syndrome. *Archives of General Psychiatry, 37,* 1350–1357.

Cohen, D.J., & Leckman, J.F. (1984). Tourette's syndrome: Advances in treatment and research. *Journal of the American Academy of Child Psychiatry, 23,* 123–125.

Doleys, D.M., & Kurtz, P.S. (1974). A behavioral treatment program for the Gilles de la Tourette syndrome. *Psychological Reports, 35,* 43–48.

Feldman, R.B., & Werry, J.S. (1966). An unsuccessful attempt to treat a ticquer by massed practice. *Behavior Research & Therapy, 4,* 111–117.

Finney, J.W., Rapoff, M.A., Hall, C.L., & Christopherson, E. R. (1983). Replication and social validation of habit reversal treatment for tics. *Behavior Therapy, 14,* 116–126.

Franco, D.D. (1981). Habit reversal and isometric tensing with motor tics. *Dissertation Abstracts International, 42,* 3418B.

Friedman, S. (1980). Self-control in the treatment of Gilles de la Tourette's syndrome: Case study with 18-month follow-up. *Journal of Conferences in Clinical Psychology, 48,* 400–402.

Goldfried, M.R. (1971). Systematic desensitization as training in self-control. *Journal of Consulting & Clinical Psychology, 37,* 228–234.

Harcherik, D.F., Leckman, J.F., Detlor, J., & Cohen, D.J. (1984). A new instrument for clinical studies of Tourette's syndrome. *Journal of the American Academy of Child Psychiatry, 23,* 153–160.

Hollandsworth, J.G., & Bausinger, L. (1978). Unsuccessful use of massed practice in the treatment of Gilles de la Tourette syndrome. *Psychological Report, 43,* 671–677.

Hutzell, R.R., Platzek, D., & Logue, P.E. (1974). Control of symptoms of Gilles de la Tourette's syndrome by self-monitoring. *Journal of Behavior Therapy & Experimental Psychiatry, 5,* 71–76.

Jacobson, E. (1938). *Progressive relaxation.* Chicago: University of Chicago Press.

Lahey, B.B., McNees, M.P., & McNees, M.C. (1973). Control of an obscene "verbal tic" through time out in an elementary classroom. *Journal of Applied Behavioral Analysis, 6,* 101–104.

Miller, A.L. (1970). Treatment of a child with Gilles de la Tourette's syndrome using behavior modification techniques. *Journal of Behavior Therapy & Experimental Psychiatry, 1,* 319–321.

Nicassio, F.J., Liberman, R.P., Patterson, R.L., Raminez, E., & Saunder, N. (1972). The treatment of tics by negative practice. *Journal of Behavior Therapy & Experimental Psychiatry, 3,* 281–287.

Ollendick, T.H. (1981). Self-monitoring and self-administered overcorrection: The modification of nervous tics in children. *Behavior Modification, 5,* 75–84.

Padus, E. (1986). *The Complete Guide to Your Emotions and Your Health: New Dimensions in Mind/body Healing.* Emmaus, PA: Rodale Press.

Rosen, M., & Wesner, C. (1979). A behavioral approach to Tourette's syndrome. *Journal of Canadian Clinical Psychology, 41,* 303–312.

Sand, P.L., & Carlson, C. (1973). Failure to establish control over tics in the Gilles de la Tourette syndrome with behavior therapy techniques. *British Journal of Psychiatry, 122,* 665–670.

Savicki, V., & Carlin, A.S. (1972). Behavioral treatment of Gilles de la Tourette syndrome. *International Journal of Child Psychotherapy, 1,* 97–109.

Schulman, M. (1974). Control of tics by maternal reinforcement. *Journal of Behavior Therapy & Experimental Psychiatry, 5,* 95–96.

Schultz, J., & Luthe, W. (1959). *Autogenic Training: A Psychophysiologic Approach in Psychotherapy.* New York: Grune & Stratton.

Shapiro, A.K., & Shapiro, E. (1982). Tourette syndrome: History and present status. In A.J. Friedhoff & T.N. Chase (Eds.), *Gilles de la Tourette Syndrome.* New York: Raven.

Storms, L. (1985). Massed negative practice as a behavioral treatment for Gilles de la Tourette's syndrome. *American Journal of Psychotherapy, 39,* 277–281.

Suinn, R.M. (1975). Anxiety management training for general anxiety. In R.M. Suinn & R.G. Weigel (Eds.), *The Innovative Psychological Therapies: Critical and Creative Contributions.* New York: Harper & Row.

Teoh, J.L. (1974). Gilles de la Tourette's syndrome: A study of the treatment of six cases by mass negative practice and with haloperidol. *Singapore Medical Journal, 15,* 139–146.

Thomas, E.J., Abrams, K.S., & Johnson, J.B. (1971). Self-monitoring and reciprocal inhibition in the modification of multiple tics of Gilles de la Tourette's syndrome. *Journal of Behavior Therapy & Experimental Psychiatry, 2,* 159–171.

Tophoff, M. (1973). Massed practice, relaxation and assertion training in the treatment of Gilles de la Tourette's syndrome. *Journal of Behavior Therapy & Experimental Psychiatry, 4,* 71–73.

Turpin, G. (1983). The behavioral management of tic disorders: A critical review. *Advances in Behavior Research & Therapy, 5,* 203–245.

Turpin, G., & Powell, G.E. (1984). Effects of massed practice and cue controlled relaxation on tic frequency in Gilles de la Tourette's syndrome. *Behaviour Research & Therapy, 22,* 165–178.

Varni, J.W., Boyd, E.F., & Cataldo, M.F. (1978). Self-monitoring, external reinforcement, and time-out procedures in the control of high rate tic behaviors in a hyperactive child. *Journal of Behavior Therapy & Experimental Psychiatry, 9,* 353–358.

Walton, D. (1961). Experimental psychology and the treatment of a ticquer. *Journal of Child Psychology & Psychiatry, 2,* 148–155.

Walton, D. (1964). Massed practice and simultaneous reduction in drive level: Further evidence on the efficacy of this approach to the treatment of tics. In H.J. Eysenck (Ed.), *Experiments in behaviour therapy.* London: Pergamon.

Yates, A.J. (1958). The application of learning theory to the treatment of tics. *Journal of Abnormal Social Psychology, 56,* 175–182.

Zikis, P. (1983). Habit reversal treatment of a 10-year-old school boy with severe tics. *The Behavior Therapist, 6,* 50–51.

CHAPTER SEVENTEEN

Social Issues
of Tourette's Syndrome

Abbey S. Meyers

Social issues that can have a major impact upon persons with Tourette's syndrome (TS) are numerous. They can be placed into two major categories: (1) attitudinal and behavioral barriers, and (2) services.

ATTITUDINAL AND BEHAVIORAL BARRIERS

The scientific argument as to which common behavioral patterns are an integral part or a symptom of TS and which occur as a consequence of having TS will probably continue for decades to come. There is no question, however, that TS is a socially stigmatizing disorder, and that a physician's authoritarian role can do much to alleviate negative social impact.

If behaviors such as impulsivity, hyperactivity, and obsessive-compulsive personality traits that are often cited in the literature are components of TS, this would imply that people with TS are probably extensively handicapped by their inability to cope with environmental stresses. On the other hand, the unfamiliar and sometimes bizarre symptoms of TS often create attitudinal barriers in strangers, peers, employers, teachers, and others central to the patient's development. Therefore, people with TS, no matter how healthy their emotional status is, are often not afforded a chance to be independent and productive.

The physician can help to minimize these attitudinal barriers by clearly defining the disorder and explaining symptoms that affect the patient *at the present time.* Letters to insurers, employers, teachers, and so on should avoid detailed descriptions of the broad array of symptoms the patient may never get. Most important, explanations about the involuntary nature of TS to people in the patient's environment will allow the patient to be understood and accepted rather than feared or ridiculed.

Some patients and families may try to hide the existence of TS. It is not uncommon for a TS student to be denied special education services (and consequently to be treated as a behavior problem in the classroom) simply because the parents will not tell school administrators of the child's diagnosis. Nor is is uncommon for an adult to be fired from a job as a result of TS symptoms, and then admit that he or she never told the employer about TS. Some physicians reinforce this concept of secrecy. However, Tourette's syndrome cannot be hidden like controlled epilepsy. Symptoms are often visible or audible, and in the absence of an explanation they are commonly misperceived as unnatural or bizarre.

While a complete understanding of TS is often essential in school, the workplace, and especially at home, there are some behaviors associated with TS symptomatology that can be very crippling. In youngsters, hyperactivity and learning disabilities may indicate placement out of the mainstream. Adults with TS who suffer from obsessive–compulsive or ritualistic behaviors can sometimes take hours to complete a task. These problems appear to be intrinsic to the disorder. Thus the attitudes of onlookers, employers, or teachers may not be the primary barrier to normal functioning, but rather, the disorder itself can render a patient disabled.

SERVICES

The physician would do well to familiarize himself or herself with available services in the community that can be used as a referral source for TS patients and families. These services can be found within the scope of any program available to handicapped or disabled people.

Special Education and Related Services

The TS student having difficulties in school can be referred by a parent, teacher, or physician for psychoeducational evaluation. The physician can have input into subsequent placement of the student in an appropriate learning environment. A letter to the school principal, teacher, or guidance counselor may initiate this process. *In the absence of a physician's written diagnosis, it is extremely difficult to obtain special education for a child.*

Special education can be provided in a mainstream classroom (i.e., allow a child to use a calculator for math or to dictate written work), a resource room (one or two class periods in a separate room with a tutor and only two or three other students), a self-contained classroom (in a public or private school), or residential school. In all cases, there should be no cost to the parents as long as the school and family agree on the appropriate placement. Physicians can advise parents to request the Tourette Syndrome Association's (TSA) booklet, *Know Your Rights: Facts You Should Know About Your Rights to Free Appropriate Education.* Additionally, many local TSA chapters will provide advocates to accompany parents to school meetings.

The input and suggestions of a physician to the school team are essential to the design of an appropriate educational program. For example, the cognitive effects of medication must be considered during the program's implementation.

Once a child is identified as "handicapped" by the school team, he or she will be eligible for additional related services. These may include psychological counseling, family counseling, year-round programming, and so on. In essence, many of the services needed by a TS child (except medical services) can be provided at no cost to parents if the school agrees that the child needs them.

Employment and Vocational Issues

Vocational choices for people with TS may be limited as a result of: (1) the socially unacceptable nature of TS symptoms (particularly vocalizations); (2) learning disabilities, perceptual problems, and/or poor motor coordination; (3) level of education and intelligence; and (4) emotional complications. In general, anecdotal reports indicate that many people with TS have difficulty getting jobs, remaining employed, or receiving promotions and raises at the same rate as their peers. Until recently, the only documentation of these problems was a study by Jagger (1982) in which adult respondents to the Yale questionnaire indicated that they had difficulty getting a job (25 percent) or reported problems holding a job (34 percent).

During the spring of 1982 a well-designed questionnaire was disseminated by the University of Cincinnati to all diagnosed TS patients known to the Tourette Syndrome Association (TSA) in Ohio. The response rate was more than 80 percent, and of those, 114 were adults over 19 years of age who were not in school. Of these, 36 percent were employed full-time, 14 percent part-time, and 48 percent were unemployed. At the time of the survey Ohio's official unemployment rate was 12.8 percent for the general population.

Interestingly, the severity of TS symptoms had little relation to a TS patient's employability. That is, a high percentage of patients who described their symptoms as mild or moderate were unemployed, although a higher percentage of those with severe symptoms were unemployed. Only 4 of the respondents were receiving social security benefits, although 9 of them had never worked at all.

Only 12 percent of Ohio adult responders indicated that they had received vocational rehabilitation (VR) services, and only one-half of those felt that that VR services were effective. Since VR counselors are commonly unfamiliar with TS and remedial techniques, this finding is not surprising.

Comparing the educational levels of these TS adults to their employment picture was somewhat revealing. Some college work, graduation from college, or graduate study had been attained by 46.5 percent, and an additional 31.6 percent had graduated from high school. This high rate of educational accomplishment in the TS population would indicate that there is a problem of *under*employment of people with TS. A total of 40 percent of adults reported job discrimination, and only 8.9 percent indicated that their employer had made special accommodations for them on the job.

TSA receives substantial requests for information and/or assistance related to vocational issues for the TS population. Although the results of the Ohio questionnaire may not be completely accurate for the entire nation, we sense that supports are available to offer TS children a free appropriate education, and accommodations can be made in colleges and technical schools that may allow people with TS to benefit from vocational training, but the end result of these supports and services must be *employment*. This is not being accomplished. Even among those who reported full-time employment, many with college degrees are employed as laborers and blue-collar workers. Therefore, the physician must determine whether the patient cannot work because the symptoms of TS interfere with task performance or whether he or she is being prevented from working because of attitudinal barriers created by employers or coworkers.

Social Security

The question of when a person with TS can be defined as disabled and thus become eligible for Social Security Disability (SSD) or Supplementary Security Income (SSI) is best answered by a patient's physician. The Social Security Administration does not include Tourette's in its *Medical Criteria Listing*. Therefore, the Social Security Administration relies heavily upon the physician's written testimony about the patient's condition.

It is insufficient to state in a letter that "the patient has Tourette's syndrome and is disabled." The physician must explain TS, the symptoms the patient has, and how those symptoms interfere with the patient's daily functioning. Prognosis is also important; if one explains that the patient has just begun a trial of medication and is expected to improve, social security benefits may be denied. It is more helpful to explain that medication is being tried, and you are hopeful that symptoms may improve by a percentage (e.g., 50 percent). The physician should state whether a 50 percent improvement is expected to make the patient employable, or whether he or she will still be disabled after this improvement. Patients are eligible for social security only if their disability is expected to last more than one year.

It is common for people with TS to be initially denied SSD or SSI. Many patients have to appeal, and cases are commonly won on appeal if the physician's written testimony is precise and accurate.

Insurance

Life Insurance. Many life insurance companies will deny policies to people with any chronic condition. The physician can be helpful by informing insurance companies about TS, that it is not fatal or degenerative, and explaining the manner in which TS affects the particular patient. Sometimes a good explanation of the disorder results in the awarding of a life insurance policy, and sometimes it does not. Patients should be referred to the Tourette Syndrome Association for names of insurance companies that offer life insurance policies at noninflated rates to people with TS.

Health Insurance.   Many health insurance companies deny coverage to people with any preexisting condition. More commonly, health insurers tend to categorize TS as a mental rather than a neurological illness. The majority of health insurance policies contain language that makes "nervous and mental disorders" ineligible for reimbursement (or reimbursable at reduced rates). This has caused severe hardships for many TS families, and can be a major obstacle to proper medical care.

If coverage is denied by a health insurer, the physician can be helpful by writing a letter to the insurance company explaining that TS is a neurological disorder, not a mental illness. It is wise to explain the type of service you provide to the patient. For example, if you titrate medication the treatment provided would be chemotherapy. Insurers are more likely to reimburse for medication titration than for psychotherapy. Psychotherapy is not an accepted treatment for TS. It is viewed as adjunctive for coping or adjustment problems.

Many times coverage for treatment of TS will be provided by health insurers after a physician has written a clear explanatory letter on behalf of the patient. However, some companies will not reverse their decision despite Herculean efforts by the physician. To counter this, some states have created high-risk health insurance pools. People with preexisting conditions can purchase health insurance (although at inflated rates) through these pools. Patients should contact their state insurance department to determine whether a high-risk health insurance policy is available in their state. If it is not, it would be incumbent upon the physician to reinforce the fact that TS is a nondegenerative neurological disorder that does not affect a patient's general health, and at the very least a health insurer should provide medical coverage for health conditions not related to TS.

Driver's License

There are no state laws that prohibit people with TS from obtaining a driver's license. Laws that govern licensing usually cover disorders in which a loss of consciousness is symptomatic of the illness. People with TS can postpone symptoms for a variable period of time. Therefore a tic can usually be inhibited during those driving instances when it may present a danger.

Military

The Department of Defense has a strict policy against allowing people with TS into the military. Sometimes youngsters with TS who want to enter the military will not tell recruiters about their diagnosis.

Periodically, the military screens soldiers for drug and alcohol abuse. If traces of drugs are found in the blood or urine, this is grounds for instant dismissal. Soldiers who are not taking drugs for control of TS can also be discovered through routine physicals, or by the appearance of symptoms during particularly stressful periods.

Other patients may have entered the military before they were diagnosed. Very often, appearance of symptoms while under stress may lead to a psychiatric misdiagnosis with discharge. A number of these patients may be eligible for veterans' disability benefits if they can show that military service exacerbated their condition.

Housing

Housing for people with loud vocalizations can be a seemingly insurmountable problem. However, there are certain programs for which patients may be eligible based upon their handicapping condition, Tourette's syndrome:

1. Community residences or intermediate care facilities are housing programs funded by states under their developmental disabilities programs. These programs can provide highly structured supervised living environments for severely afflicted patients. The major problems with these programs are that they are usually reserved for mentally retarded people and that there are commonly long waiting lists for admission.
2. The Section 8 program offered by the Department of Housing and Urban Development (HUD) provides rent subsidies for disabled people who meet financial criteria. Other HUD programs provide funds to landlords who make their apartments accessible to the handicapped. If a person is mobility impaired, these funds can be used to construct a ramp into the building. If a person has TS, the funds may be used to install sound-absorbing materials. These may include a thick rug, acoustic tiles on walls and ceilings, a soundproof door, and so on. With these accommodations, people with loud vocalizations can live comfortably without disturbing their neighbors.

Miscellaneous

In general, the problems people with TS face daily should be approached with commonsense solutions. The problems—like the symptoms of TS—will wax and wane, changing over time. If loud vocaliz-ations are the problem today, sound-absorbing materials at home, or sound-absorbing office partitions in the workplace, may alleviate the problem. In a few months, the vocalizations may improve, but the pa-tient may find himself or herself stamping loudly on the floor. Placing a piece of rug beneath the chair or desk may similarly reduce the dis-turbing impact of this tic.

During times of severe tic exacerbation, the patient may have great difficulty performing tasks. Reading may be problematical as a result of eye tics. For a time, recorded books supplied by the Library for the Blind may circumvent this problem. Tape recorders may minimize the impact of not being able to write, or a patient may find that he or she can concentrate better when screening out all visible stimuli by closing the eyes during lectures.

However, many of these adaptive techniques may require physician intervention. For example, the student who closes his or her eyes during lectures may be reprimanded for sleeping in class, or a landlord may try to evict a tenant whom he considers to be disruptive. Often the phy-sician tends to address these problems as medical issues, and decides that a medication adjustment is the only course of action. To the con-trary, there are many interventions available to physicians that may en-able the patient to cope better, or at the very least, to tolerate an exacer-bation until the next waning period offers relief.

REFERENCES

Cohen, D.J., Leckman, J.F., & Shaywitz, B.A. (1984). The Tourette syndrome and other tics. In D. Shaffer, A.A. Ehrhandt, & L. Greenhill (Eds.), *A clinical guide to child psychiatry*. New York: Free Press.

Hagin, R.A. (1984). *Tourette syndrome and the school psychologist*. New York: Tourette Syndrome Association.

Jagger, J., Prusoff, B., Cohen, D.J., Kidd, K.K., Carbonari, C., & John, K. (1982). The epidemiology of Tourette's Syndrome. *Schizophrenia Bulletin, 8,* 267–278.

Meyers, A.S. (1984). *Serving clients with Tourette syndrome: A manual for service provid-ers*. New York: Tourette Syndrome Association.

Ort, S. (1984) *Tourette syndrome and the school nurse*. New York: Tourette Syndrome Association.

Stefl, M.E. (1974). Mental health needs associated with Tourette syndrome. *Amer-ican Journal of Public Health, 74,* 1310–1313.

Stefl, M.E., & Rubin, M. (1985). Tourette syndrome in the classroom: Special problems, special needs. *Journal of School Health, 5,* 72–75.

Part IV

Pharmacotherapy

CHAPTER EIGHTEEN

Treatment of Tic Disorders with Haloperidol

Arthur K. Shapiro
Elaine Shapiro

This chapter provides a clinical guide for the management and treatment of tics and Tourette's disorder (TS) with haloperidol. Conclusions about its use are based on clinical reports and controlled studies in the literature, 22 years of experience in the evaluation, observation, or treatment of over 1600 patients with tic disorders, and a recently completed comprehensive and detailed study of our large sample of TS patients (A. Shapiro, E. Shapiro, Young, & Feinberg, 1987).

HISTORY OF TREATMENT

Most medicinal, surgical, psychological, and other therapeutic modalities have been used unsuccessfully at one time or another to treat TS (A. Shapiro, E. Shapiro, Bruun, & Sweet, 1978; A. Shapiro et al., 1987). Neurologists began to attribute disorders of unknown origin to psychological conflicts at the end of the nineteenth century. This trend culminated in a massive overpsychologizing in medicine and the use of psychotherapeutic treatment for TS, which varied from psychoanalysis to est (A. Shapiro et al., 1978; A. Shapiro et al., 1987).

It was inevitable that neuroleptics would be used after their introduction in the early 1950s. Haloperidol was first reported as effective in single patients with TS by Seignot (1961) and Caprini and Melotti (1961), in 2 patients by Challas and Brauer (1963), in 3 patients by A. Shapiro and E. Shapiro (1968), and subsequently 34 patients (A. Shapiro, E. Shapiro, & Wayne, 1973) and 80 patients (A. Shapiro et al., 1978).

SPONTANEOUS, NONSPECIFIC, AND PLACEBO EFFECTS

Placebo, spontaneous changes, and other nonspecific effects are frequently associated with the use of new drugs (A. Shapiro, 1978; A. Shapiro & E. Shapiro, 1985; A. Shapiro et al., 1987) and have characterized the treatment of TS (A. Shapiro, 1976; A. Shapiro et al., 1978; A. Shapiro et al., 1987). For example, in a double-blind, crossover study of 20 TS patients treated for 6 weeks with pimozide or placebo, 30 percent of patients on placebo were rated as improved at end point on various measures of improvement (A. Shapiro & E. Shapiro, 1984). In addition, patients change to a new drug usually at a time when symptoms are maximum and subsequent improvement may be due to spontaneous waning of symptoms. Moreover, 97 percent of patients report spontaneous changes in the severity of their symptoms, 96 percent report spontaneous changes in the type or location of their symptoms, and 27 percent report spontaneous remission of their symptoms lasting from a month to more than 7 years (A. Shapiro & E. Shapiro, 1982; A. Shapiro et al., 1987). Additionally patients may feel better after discontinuing neuroleptics that induce adverse effects and misinterpret the absence of adverse effects as improvement. Patients treated with high dosages of haloperidol for a prolonged period of time may fear exacerbation of their symptoms if they reduce the dosage or discontinue treatment, thus making it difficult to evaluate whether the sustained improvement is caused by medication or spontaneous waning of symptoms. After treatment with a new medication, symptom reduction may be erroneously interpreted as improvement, but again may reflect spontaneous change. To address these methodological problems, large-scale, well-controlled, double-blind studies are required to determine which drugs are effective for the treatment of tic disorders. Early studies of treatment were limited to open studies because of the small number of identified TS patients.

GENERAL CONSIDERATIONS ABOUT TREATMENT OF TIC DISORDERS

Our clinical impression and provisional hypothesis is that all of the tic disorders (transient tic disorder, chronic motor or vocal tic disorder, and Tourette's syndrome) have an undetermined organic central nervous system etiology (A. Shapiro, E. Shapiro, Wayne and Clarkin, 1973; A. Shapiro et al., 1978; A. Shapiro et al., 1987; E. Shapiro & A. Shapiro 1986), and that treatment should be directed primarily at reducing the motor and vocal tics of TS.

The controversy about whether behavioral problems and psychopathology are etiologically related to the onset of TS has been evaluated elsewhere (A. Shapiro et al., 1987) and is discussed in other chapters of this volume. Papers in the literature proposing a relationship between psychopathology and TS are largely uncontrolled clinic reports or opinions with few poorly controlled retrospective studies.

Our predictive studies indicate that TS patients without attention deficit disorder (ADD) do not differ significantly from a carefully matched normal control group on measures of psychopathology, whereas TS patients with ADD have significantly more psychopathology than TS patients without ADD and a normal control group and are similar to a sample of patients referred to mental health facilities.

Our conclusion is that the frequency of behavior problems, psychopathology, and ADD, including obsessive-compulsive disorder and symptoms, in TS patients is no greater than that in the general population.

We have, therefore, concluded that the treatment of TS should be directed primarily at reducing tic symptoms with medication. Other as-

sociated problems, psychopathology, and learning or attentional problems may require other types of remediation.

INDICATIONS FOR TREATMENT

The indications for treatment of tics are more obvious at the extremes.
Pharmacological treatment is recommended if the symptoms impair
psychosocial, educational, and occupational functioning. Since treatment is palliative, however, it is usually unnecessary if the symptoms
are mild, do not elicit comments and curiosity by outside observers, and
do not interfere with psychosocial functioning. Treatment of patients
with mild to moderate symptoms is elective and should be determined
by the patient based on the degree of distress caused by the tics.

GENERAL PRINCIPLES OF TREATMENT
WITH NEUROLEPTICS

An important principle of treatment with neuroleptics is that the dosage has to be individually titrated to achieve maximum effectiveness
with minimal adverse effects. Dosage is determined by pragmatic clinical trial and error. The clinically effective dosage of neuroleptics used
to treat TS patients is much lower than that for patients with psychoses.
Functioning TS patients report more bothersome and impairing adverse effects with lower dosages than is commonly reported by psychotic patients treated with higher dosages. Unfortunately, blood levels
of medication are largely unassociated with age, weight, sex, severity,
clinical response, or adverse effects (A. Shapiro, E. Shapiro, & Sweet,
1981; A. Shapiro et al., 1987). Neuroleptics generally have a long half-
life and tend to accumulate in the body so that the same dosage over
time results in higher cumulative blood levels. A steady state blood level
is reached in about 4 days. Thus the clinical effect should be evaluated
on the fourth day during initial titration, and the dosage should be
changed appropriately on the fifth day. The elimination of the drug
takes about 4 days during initial acute treatment, and ranges from 4 to
30 days, usually averaging 2 weeks, with chronic treatment. With acute
withdrawal, adverse effects tend to decrease and disappear before the
tics reappear at their preexisting level. Because neuroleptics have a long
half-life, the total dosage can be administered at bedtime for most patients. Akinesic or sedative effects may increase after intake and are
often better tolerated by patients during sleep. Once-a-day, nighttime
administration contributes to ease of administration and improves com-

pliance. Occasional patients have a better response and fewer adverse effects if medication is administered at intervals throughout the day.

EFFECTIVENESS OF HALOPERIDOL

Haloperidol is the only butyrophenone used for the treatment of tic disorders. Abuzzahab and Anderson (1973) conducted an exhaustive search of the world's literature and described the results for approximately 600 treatments of various types received by 430 patients. The percentage of improvement, without regard to length of treatment, was 89 percent for haloperidol, 48 percent for other neuroleptics, 20 percent for other chemotherapy, 22 percent for various somatotherapies, and 35 percent for assorted psychological treatment. A. Shapiro and colleagues (1978) reviewed the results of treatment with haloperidol for 144 patients reported in 41 publications between 1961 and 1975. The results suggested that treatment with haloperidol improved 78 to 91 percent of patients; only 8 to 22 percent failed to improve. A retrospective study of the treatment of 34 consecutive patients was described by A. Shapiro (1973), and extended to the first 80 consecutive patients treated for 7 months to 8.5 years from 1965 to 1974 (A. Shapiro et al., 1978). Patients treated with an average dosage of 5.0 mg/per day of haloperidol had an average of 80 percent (median 90 percent) decrease of symptoms compared with 24 percent (median 0 percent) in the non–haloperidol-treated group (p <.001). Improvement of at least 50 percent was reported in 97 percent of patients treated with haloperidol and in 40 percent by the non–haloperidol-treated group (p<.005). The amount of improvement variance accounted for by haloperidol was 44 percent. Other uncontrolled studies report improvement in 62 to 84 percent (Nee, Caine, Polinsky, Eldridge & Ebert, 1980), 73 percent (Wassman, Eldridge, Abuzzahab & Nee, 1978), 70 percent (Nomura & Segawa, 1982), and 90 percent (Golden 1978). However, some clinicians report less favorable results (Cohen, Detlor, Young, & Shaywitz, 1980; Ford & Gottlieb, 1969; Leckman, Cohen, Detlor, Young, Harcherik, & Shaywitz, 1982; Tibbetts, 1981; van Woert, Rosenbaum, & Enna, 1982). Nevertheless, because of the largely favorable clinical reports, haloperidol has become the drug of choice for the treatment of TS.

Our conclusion, based on a review of the literature and clinical experience, is that haloperidol is an effective treatment for the symptoms of TS. Our results indicate that 25 percent of patients have at least 70 percent reduction of symptoms at a low dosage without significant adverse effects. Another 50 percent of patients develop adverse effects when treated with therapeutic dosages of haloperidol, but these can be successfully managed over time. The remaining 25 percent are treatment failures because adverse effects nullify therapeutic benefits.

However, there are no carefully controlled, randomized double-blind studies supporting the effectiveness or superiority of haloperidol over placebo or other medications. Moreover, not all patients respond adequately, and adverse effects limit its usefulness. Therefore, controlled studies are necessary to develop more effective drugs with less adverse effects (A. Shapiro et al., 1987).

TREATMENT REGIMEN

We have recommended for many years that for most functioning patients the starting dosage should be low such as 0.25 mg of haloperidol at bedtime. To prevent acute dystonia, which occurs in 5 to 9 percent of patients within 72 hours, and akinesia, which occurs in 25 percent of patients usually within the first 2 weeks of treatment, the anticholinergic drug benztropine mesylate, at a dosage of 0.5 mg at bedtime, is used by us routinely at the beginning of treatment. Dosage of haloperidol is increased 0.25 mg every 5 days until either symptoms decrease 50 to 70 percent without adverse effects, adverse effects occur without symptomatic benefit, or symptoms decrease and adverse effects occur at the same time. The last possibility is the usual response. If adverse effects are minimal and do not interfere with functioning, such as dry mouth and slightly increased sedation at bedtime and on awakening, dosage should not be increased until adverse effects disappear. If adverse effects interfere slightly with functioning, dosage should be decreased 0.25 mg/per day per week. If adverse effects are severe, dosage should be reduced 50 percent immediately. Titration should be reinstituted more slowly at intervals varying from 7 to 30 days after disappearance of severe adverse effects. Although the dosage ranges from 2 to 10 mg/per day and ultimately averages 5 mg/per day, higher doses are required by some patients. More rapid titration, 0.25 to 1 mg every day or even every hour, is feasible in patients with very severe TS.

The goal of treatment is to reduce tics at least 70 percent in school, at work, with strangers, and in social situations. Symptoms are usually more severe at home, especially in the evening, and while it is possible to control symptoms at home, by increasing the dosage, to do so usually results in increased adverse effects.

Some patients achieve only 50 to 60 percent reduction of tics, while others have 90 to 99 percent reduction of symptoms without adverse effects. The dosage is constantly titrated over time as the symptoms spontaneously vary. Constant and flexible titration results in lower dosages and minimal adverse effects and enhances the physician's ability to detect spontaneous decreases or remission of symptoms. Our general impression is that for most patients symptom severity is the same before and during adolescence in 65 percent of patients and is reduced in adolescence in 35 percent of patients. Most patients have a reduction of symptoms and less waxing, waning, or fluctuation of symptoms in adulthood. Occasional patients experience periods of severe, brief, or prolonged exacerbation, sometimes in adulthood.

RECOGNITION AND MANAGEMENT OF FREQUENTLY ENCOUNTERED ADVERSE EFFECTS

Although the discussion of adverse effects focuses on the treatment of tic disorders with haloperidol, these adverse effects occur with all neuroleptics.

Acute Dystonia

Acute dystonia involves sustained, occasionally intermittent contraction of unilateral or bilateral muscles usually of the upper body, particularly the head, neck, shoulders, and back, resulting in mandibular and oculogyric spasms, speech and swallowing difficulties, torticollis, hyperextension of the neck and truck, and torsion spasm. It occurs in 5 to 9 percent of TS patients treated with haloperidol, usually within 48 to 72 hours after initial treatment, and is unrelated to dosage. Fatal acute dystonia has been reported in patients with laryngeal spasm. Administration of benztropine mesylate, 0.5 mg/per day concomitant with haloperidol, will prevent its occurrence in most patients. Acute dystonia can be immediately and completely controlled by intravenous antiparkinson drugs, such as benztropine mesylate, followed by oral administration of the antiparkinson agent, without discontinuing treatment with haloperidol. Acute dystonia almost never occurs subsequently even after discontinuing anticholinergic medication.

Akinesia

Akinesia is characterized by muscular weakness and aches and pains in muscles or joints and can result in apathy, depression, regression, dependence, and motivational and cognitive dulling. Children become irritable, fearful, and cling to their mother, may develop school phobias, and often seem uninterested in their work. These symptoms can occur acutely during the first 2 weeks of treatment and are unrelated to dosage. Subsequently, akinesic effects are associated with dosage and are usually readily controlled with the use of anticholinergic drugs or dosage reduction. Anticholinergic medication can usually be discontinued after 3 to 8 months of treatment. Persistent akinesic effects may require the use of stimulants.

Akathisia

Akathisia is characterized by motor restlessness, which can range from a mild jitteriness to severe pacing, as well as an inability to concentrate for longer than moments and insomnia, and is often experienced as anxiety. It usually, but not always, disappears within 3 months. If severe, the dosage of benztropine mesylate is increased or small doses of benzodiazepines may be used temporarily.

Extrapyramidal Parkinson-like Adverse Effects

These adverse effects are frequent, temporary, reversible, and related to dosage. In addition to acute akinesia, which develops within 2 weeks of initial treatment, a subtle adverse effect is slight evening akinesia, which may cause patients to retire somewhat earlier than usual or have difficulty with morning awakening. As dosage is increased other symptoms may appear: tremors, rigidity, depressed-looking expression, drooling, flattened facial folds, shuffling gait, loss of associated movements, cogwheeling, and akinesia experienced as daytime sedation. Patients may nap during the day and experience interference with academic and occupational functioning. These adverse effects can occasionally be detected early in treatment by observing the patient's handwriting, which becomes constricted and jerky. Reduction of dosage and the use of antiparkinson agents are effective in reducing these adverse effects, which usually decrease or disappear after 3 to 4 months of treatment.

Cognitive Impairment

Cognitive impairment, which may involve impaired attention, motivation, memory, or response time, is a subtle and major limitation of the use of haloperidol, especially in children. It occurs at dosages that vary from 2 to 10 mg/per day. School grades begin to fall and motivation in children and adults is impaired. Management requires constant titration to the minimal dosage required for maximum improvement outside the home and possibly the prudent use of anticholinergic and stimulant drugs (A. Shapiro et al., 1978; A. Shapiro et al., 1987; A. Shapiro & E. Shapiro, 1981; E. Shapiro, A. Shapiro, & Levine, 1984).

Tardive Dyskinesia

Patients and physicians are justifiably concerned about long-term effects such as tardive dyskinesia (TD) and covert dyskinesia (CD). These movements may be difficult to differentiate from tics except by physicians experienced with both movement disorders. TD appears or breaks through while the patient is on various medications, such as haloperidol, lasts longer than 3 months, may slowly disappear over years or be permanent. CD appears only after reduction of dosage, and the clinical course is similar to that of TD. Withdrawal dyskinesia (WD) appears only after rapid dosage reduction or sudden discontinuation of medication, and the symptoms disappear within 3 months.

None of the patients with tic disorders treated by us with haloperidol has developed TD, probably because of the use of low dosages of haloperidol. Although nine cases of haloperidol-induced TD in Tourette's patients have been reported (Caine, Margolin, Brown, & Ebert, 1978; Caine & Polinsky, 1981; Golden, 1985; Mizrahi, Holtzman, & Tharp, 1980; Riddle, Hardin, Towbin, Leckman, & Cohen, 1987), our review of these cases suggests that only one of them had TD (E. Shapiro & A. Shapiro 1982), the more recent reports notwithstanding. The difficulties of differential diagnosis are comprehensively discussed elsewhere (A. Shapiro et al., 1978; A. Shapiro et al., 1987; E. Shapiro & A. Shapiro, 1982). Nevertheless, patients should be monitored carefully because of the possible development of TD.

Anticholinergic Adverse Effects

Anticholinergic adverse effects, such as xerostomia, mydriasis, impaired accommodation for near objects, and constipation, are related to dosage, associated with both haloperidol and most anticholinergic or antiparkinson drugs, and their effects are additive. They are usually not troublesome and can be managed by reduction of dosage, change to another drug, or the use of various corrective measures.

Endocrinological Adverse Effects

These adverse effects tend to be related to dosage and are usually associated with elevated prolactin levels. They include galactorrhea, breast engorgement, menstrual irregularities, gynecomastia, decreased libido, and hyperglycemia.

Depressive, Dysphoric, and Phobic Adverse Effect

These effects are related to dosage but may occur at very low dosages in susceptible individuals. Patients frequently complain of nonspecific dysphoric effects or become aware of them after discontinuing the neuroleptic. We have been unable to identify premorbid characteristics that predispose patients to the development of depression. Phobias and separation anxiety, including school phobias in children, are somewhat related to dosage, but they may occur on low dosage in susceptible individuals (Linet, 1985; Mikkelson, Detlor, & Cohen, 1981; A. Shapiro & E. Shapiro 1980). Management may require dosage reduction or the use of stimulants or tricyclic antidepressants such as desipramine.

Use of Anticholinergic Medication

Anticholinergics, such as benztropine mesylate, are frequently effective in controlling or minimizing extrapyramidal symptoms (EPS). Anticholinergics generally have a long half-life, are usually excreted after 24 hours, and can be administered once a day at bedtime. The effective dosage for mild EPS ranges from 1 to 3 mg/per day, occasionally 6 mg/per day. Dosage should be titrated 0.5 mg/per day until the EPS are controlled, or anticholinergic adverse effects appear without benefit on EPS. Dosage should be reduced 0.5 to 1 mg/per day to the minimal effective dosage without adverse effects, or discontinued entirely if there is no beneficial effect. Anticholinergics are usually more effective early in treatment and usually can be discontinued after 6 to 8 months of chronic treatment.

Decreasing Dosage

If the patient experiences mild interference with academic, occupational, and psychosocial functioning, dosage of haloperidol should be reduced by 0.25 mg every 5 to 7 days until adverse effects decrease or disappear. If adverse effects become severe, the dosage is halved immediately; that is, a dosage of 4 mg/per day is lowered to 2 mg/per day or even less. After adverse effects disappear, dosage can be increased very slowly, 0.25 mg/per day every 1 to 4 weeks, until adequate symptomatic control is achieved.

Use of Stimulants to Treat Adverse Effects

The use of stimulants to treat patients with tic disorders is controversial (see discussion by Comings & Comings in Chapter 8, and an alternative view by Golden in Chapter 22). A thorough examination of the evidence about this controversy is made elsewhere (A. Shapiro et al., 1987). Some authors, based on retrospective reports, have concluded that stimulants can cause tics, worsen or permanently exacerbate tics, or precipitate TS (Golden, 1974, 1977; Lowe, Cohen, Detlor, Kremenitzer, & Shaywitz, 1982). Others have concluded that high dosages of stimulants may cause a temporary increase in tics, but that stimulants do not precipitate TS (Comings & Comings, 1984; Erenberg, 1982; A. Shapiro & E. Shapiro, 1981b). Some physicians recognize that patients with TS-ADDH may in fact require a trial on stimulants if the ADDH is severe (Erenberg, 1982; Golden, 1984; A. Shapiro & E. Shapiro, 1981a). In our opinion, there is inadequate evidence that stimulants precipitate or permanently exacerbate TS. This conclusion is supported by a study by Comings and Comings (1984) of patients with ADD who later developed TS. They reasoned that, if stimulants were associated with the development of TS, ADD patients treated with stimulants would develop TS earlier than patients who were not treated with stimulants. They found, however, that ADD patients treated with stimulants developed TS at a significantly later age than patients not treated with stimulants. Further support for the hypothesis is provided in a study of six identical twins with TS and ADD (Price, Leckman, Pauls, Cohen and Kidd, 1986) in which one twin, but not the other, was treated with stimulants. Both twins developed TS whether they were pretreated with stimulants or not.

We have had experience with more than 100 TS patients who have used stimulants. Some were treated with stimulants prior to the onset of TS or treatment with haloperidol. Others with TS and hyperactivity were treated successfully with neuroleptics and stimulants concomitantly. Stimulants have been used successfully in many patients to manage akinesic adverse effects of neuroleptics such as lethargy, dysphoria, depression, and impaired cognition and motivation. Tics may increase in susceptible patients, especially at higher dosages. However, the increase in tics is short-lived and the potential benefits of stimulants often outweigh their disadvantages.

We consider stimulants to be necessary agents in the treatment and management of children with TS and clinically significant hyperactivity. The pattern of effective therapeutic and adverse effects suggests that stimulants and butyrophenones are not simply antagonistic but have overlapping and different effects on tics and on the adverse effects of haloperidol.

Methylphenidate is given at an initial dosage of 2.5 mg and subsequently titrated in daily increments of 2.5 mg/per day, to a dosage that varies from 5 to 40 mg/per day. The results are often dramatic. If tics increase, they readily subside within 8 hours after reduction of dosage. An added benefit is decreased appetite and loss of weight. Other stimulants, such as pemoline, a long-lasting stimulant, can be administered once daily, titrated up or down at weekly intervals, the dosage varying at 18.75 to 150 mg/per day.

CONCLUSION

Clinical studies and experience indicate that neuroleptics such as haloperidol, pimozide, penfluridol, and fluphenazine are the most effective drugs for the treatment of tics and Tourette's Syndrome. Each of these drugs has helped some patients who fail on other drugs. The effectiveness, indications, adverse effects, treatment, and management of adverse effects are essentially similar for all neuroleptics, although the dosages are different. Although we now have several drugs, in contrast to the past, that can help patients with tic disorders, more effective medications with fewer adverse effects and greater ease of use by nonspecialists are necessary.

In evaluating drugs for tic disorders, however, it is important to remember that about 30 percent of patients improve, 30 percent remain unchanged, and 30 percent are worse when treated with placebos, that severity of symptoms spontaneously varies in 97 percent, type and location of symptoms change in 96 percent and 27 percent report spontaneous remissions lasting 1 month to more than 7 years. These problems indicate that open or poorly controlled studies require confirmation with carefully controlled, double-blind studies, adequate samples, and other methodological safeguards.

REFERENCES

Abuzzahab, F.S., & Anderson, F.O. (1973). Gilles de la Tourette's syndrome. *International Registry, 56,* 492–496.

Caine, E.D., Margolin, D.I., Brown, G.L., & Ebert, M.H. (1978). Gilles de la Tourette's syndrome, tardive dyskinesia, and psychosis in an adolescent. *American Journal of Psychiatry, 135,* 241–242.

Caine, E.D., & Polinsky, R.J. (1981). Tardive dyskinesia in persons with Gilles de la Tourette's disease, *Archives of Neurology, 38,* 471–472.

Caprini, G., & Melotti, V. (1961). Un grave sindrome ticcosa guarity con haloperidol. *Riv. Sper. Freniat, 85,* 191–197.

Challas, G., & Brauer, T. (1963) Tourette's disease: Relief of symptoms with R–1625. *American Journal of Psychiatry, 120,* 283–284.

Cohen, D.J., Detlor J., Young J.G., & Shaywitz, B.A. (1980). Clonidine ameliorates Gilles de la Tourette syndrome. *Archives of General Psychiatry, 37,* 1350–1357.

Comings, D.E., & Comings, B.G. (1984). Tourette syndrome and attention deficit disorder with hyperactivity—Are they due to the same gene? *Journal of American Academy of Child Psychiatry 23,* 138–146.

Erenberg, G. (1982) [Letter to the editor.] *Journal of the American Medical Association, 248,* 1062.

Ford, C.V., & Gottlieb, F. (1969). An objective evaluation of haloperidol in Gilles de la Tourette's syndrome. *Diseases of the Nervous System, 30,* 328–332.

Golden, G.S. (1974). Gilles de la Tourette's syndrome following methylphenidate action. *Developmental Medicine and Child Neurology, 16,* 76–78.

Golden G.S. (1978). Tics, twitches and habit spasms. *Current Problems in Pediatrics, 8,* 29–41.

Golden, G.S. (1977). The effect of central nervous system stimulants on Tourette syndrome. *Annals of Neurology, 2,* 69–70.

Golden, G.S. (1984). Comments in abstracts. J.D.B.P., *5,* 226–227.

Leckman, J.F., Cohen, D.J., Detlor, J., Young, J.G., Harcherik, D., & Shaywitz, B.A. (1982). Clonidine in the treatment of Tourette syndrome: A review of data. In A.J. Friedhoff & T.N. Chase (Eds.), *Gilles de la Tourette's syndrome.* New York: Raven.

Linet, L. (1985). Tourette syndrome, pimozide and school phobia: The neuroleptic separation anxiety syndrome. *American Journal of Psychiatry, 142,* 613–615.

Lowe, T.L., Cohen, D.J., Detlor, J., Kremenitzer, M.W., & Shaywitz, B.A. (1982). Stimulant medications precipitate Tourette's syndrome. *Journal of the American Medical Association, 247,* 1168–1169.

Mikkelsen, E.J., Detlor, J., & Cohen, D.J. (1981). School avoidance and social phobia triggered by haloperidol in patients with Tourette's disorder. *American Journal of Psychiatry, 138,* 1572–1575.

Mizrahi, E.M., Holtzman, D., & Tharp, B. (1980). Haloperidol-induced tardive dyskinesia in a child with Gilles de la Tourette's disease. *Archives of Neurology, 37*(12), 780.

Nee, L.E., Caine, E.D., Polinsky, R.J., Eldridge, R. and Ebert, M.H., (1980). Gilles de la Tourette's syndrome: Clinical and family study in 50 cases. *Annals of Neurology 7,* 41–49.

Nomura, Y., & Segawa, M. (1979). Gilles de la Tourette's syndrome in Oriental children. *Brain Development, 1,* 103–111.

Price, A.R., Leckman, J.F., Pauls, D.L., Cohen, D.J. and Kidd, K.K. (1986). Tics and central nervous system stimulants in twins and non-twins with Tourette syndrome. *Neurology, 36,* 232–237.

Riddle, M.A., Hardin, M.T., Towbin, K.E, Leckman, J.F., & Cohen, D.J. (1987). Tardive dyskinesia following haloperidol treatment in Tourette's syndrome [Letter to the editor]. *Archives of General Psychiatry, 44,* 98–99.

Seignot, M.J.N. (1961). Un cas de maladie des tics de Gilles de la Tourette gueri par de R–1625. *Annales Médico-Psychogiques (Paris), 119,* 578–579.

Shapiro, A.K. (1976). Psychopharmacology. In R.G. Grenell & S. Gabay (Eds.), *Biological Foundations of Psychiatry.* New York: Raven.

Shapiro, A.K. (1978). The placebo effect. In W.G. Clark & J. Del Guidice (Eds.), *Principles of Psychopharmocology.* New York: Academic.

Shapiro, A.K., & Shapiro, E. (1968). Treatment of Gilles de la Tourette's syndrome with haloperidol. *British Journal of Psychiatry, 114,* 345–350.

Shapiro, A.K., & Shapiro, E. (1980). *Tics, Tourette syndrome and other movement disorders: A pediatrician's guide.* New York: Tourette Syndrome Association.

Shapiro, A.K., & Shapiro, E. (1981a). The treatment and etiology of Tourette syndrome. *Comprehensive Psychiatry, 22,* 193–205.

Shapiro, A.K., & Shapiro, E. (1981b). Do stimulants provoke, cause or exacerbate tics and Tourette syndrome? *Comprehensive Psychiatry, 22,* 265–273.

Shapiro, A.K., & Shapiro, E. (1982). Tourette syndrome: Clinical aspects, treatment and etiology. *Seminars in Neurology, Movement Disorders, 2,* 373–385.

Shapiro, A.K., & Shapiro, E. (1984). Controlled study of pimozide vs. placebo in Tourette's syndrome. *Journal of the American Academy of Child Psychiatry, 23,* 161–173.

Shapiro, A.K., & Shapiro, E. (1985). Patient-provider relationships and the placebo effect. In J.D. Matarazzo, N.E. Miller, S.M. Weiss, & J.A. Herd (Eds.), *Behavioral Health: Handbook of Health Enhancement and Disease Prevention.* New York: Wiley.

Shapiro, A.K., Shapiro, E., Brunn, R.D., & Sweet, R.D. (1978). *Gilles de la Tourette Syndrome.* New York: Raven.

Shapiro, A.K., Shapiro, E., & Sweet, R.D. (1981). Treatment of tics and Tourette syndrome. In A. Barbeau (Ed.), *Disorders of Movement.* Lancaster, England: MTP Press.

Shapiro, A.K., Shapiro, E., & Wayne, H.L. (1973). Treatment of Gilles de la Tourette syndrome with haloperidol: Review of 34 cases. *Archives of General Psychiatry, 28,* 92–96.

Shapiro, A.K., Shapiro, E., Wayne, H., & Clarkin, J. (1973). Organic factors in Gilles de la Tourette syndrome. *British Journal of Psychiatry, 122,* 659–664.

Shapiro, A.K., Shapiro, E., Young, J.G., & Feinberg, T.E. (1987). Gilles de la Tourette syndrome. Second edition. New York: Raven.

Shapiro, E. & Shapiro, A.K. (1982). Tardive dyskinesia and chronic neuroleptic treatment of Tourette patients. In A.J. Friedhoff & T.N. Chase (Eds.), *Gilles de la Tourette Syndrome.* New York: Raven.

Shapiro, E., & Shapiro, A.K. (1986). Semiology, nosology and criteria for tic disorders. *Revue Neurologique, 142,* 824–832.

Shapiro, E., Shapiro, A.K., & Levine, R. (1984). The effect of pimozide on cognition. Presented to the American Academy of Child Psychiatry, Toronto, Canada.

Tibbits, R.W. (1981). Neuropsychiatric aspects of tics and spasms. *British Journal of Hospital Medicine, 25,* 454, 456–457.

van Woert, M.H., Rosenbaum, D., & Enna, S.J. (1982). Overview of pharmocological approaches to therapy for Tourette syndrome. In A.J. Friedhoff & T.N. Chase (Eds.), *Gilles de la Tourette syndrome.* New York: Raven.

Wassman, E.R., Eldridge, R., Abuzzahab, F.S. and Nee, L.E., (1975). Gilles de la Tourette syndrome: Clinical and genetic studies in a midwestern city. *Neurology, 28,* 304–307.

CHAPTER NINETEEN

Pimozide in the Treatment of Tourette's Syndrome

Harvey Moldofsky
Paul Sandor

The etiology of Tourette's syndrome is unknown at this time (Shapiro & Shapiro, 1982). We know, however, that 80 to 90 percent of patients respond favorably to treatment with dopamine receptor antagonists such as haloperidol (Shapiro, Shapiro, & Bruun, 1978) and pimozide (Ross & Moldofsky, 1978).

Pimozide, a diphenylbutylpiperidine, has more specific dopamine receptor blocking activity than haloperidol (Seeman & Lee, 1975). Pimozide is also known to have calcium channel blocking properties (Gould, Murphy, Reynolds, & Snyder, 1983). Furthermore, pimozide has a low potential for inducing adverse effects (Ayd, 1971; Chouinard & Steinberg, 1982; Morris, MacKenzie, & Masheter, 1970). While pimozide was initially recommended for the management of chronic schizophrenic patients, recent evidence suggests that it is also effective in controlling the symptoms of Gilles de la Tourette's syndrome (Ross & Moldofsky, 1978).

PHARMACOKINETICS

Studies in schizophrenic patients suggest that pimozide has a slow absorption time (4 to 12 hours) and a rather long plasma-elimination half-life (50 to 60 hours) (McCreadie, et al., 1979). Sallee and colleagues (1986) found much longer elimination half-life after a single dose of pimozide in three adults (103 ± 15 hours) than in four children ages 8.5 ± 3 years (25.5 ± 10.5 hours). We determined pimozide pharmacokinetics in five adult patients with Tourette's syndrome. Absorption was slow with peak plasma levels observed 4 to 14 hours following the administration of 1 mg of pimozide orally. The elimination half-life ranged from 15.5 hours to 52 hours (Sandor & Moldofsky, 1985). Because of the long half-life, it is recommended that after an initial oral dose of 1 mg (children) or 2 mg (adults) the drug should be gradually increased by 1 or 2 mg every 10 days. The average dose reported is variable (from 7 to 16 mg daily). Complete elimination of all tics should not be the prime objective. Rather, the least amount of medication should be given that will provide acceptable tic control with minimal untoward drug effects.

Extrapyramidal symptoms may be controlled with the usual drugs (benztropine mesylate, trihexyphenidyl hydrochloride, procyclidine, biperiden hydrochloride, or diphenhydramine).

NEUROENDOCRINE EFFECTS

Dopamine plays an important role in regulation of hypothalamopituitary functions. It has been reported that dopamine stimulates growth hormone release (Pecile & Olgiati, 1978) and reduces prolactin secretion (Gudelsky, 1981). It can be expected that dopamine receptor block-ade by pimozide will produce observable changes in growth hormone and prolactin. In fact, the postulated drop in growth hormone secretion was a cause for avoiding the use of neuroleptics in children for fear that their growth might be impaired. There is now evidence that the growth hormone levels are not affected by pimozide treatment in manic patients (Cookson, Silverstone, & Rees, 1982) or in children with behav-ioral disorders (Suwa, 1984). This is in keeping with our clinical experi-ence that children with Tourette's syndrome, whom we have followed for many years, were not inhibited in their growth despite chronic treat-ment with pimozide (Moldofsky, Musisi, Dorian, & Sandor, 1985).

Elevation of the plasma prolactin during neuroleptic treatment has been well documented (Gruen, 1978). The first author of this chapter suggested that the optimal clinical response to pimozide treatment of Tourette's syndrome occurs when plasma prolactin reaches maximum or plateau response to dopamine receptor blockade (Moldofsky & Brown, 1982). All 10 patients in the study displayed similar patterns. We have studied 5 more male Tourette's syndrome patients in greater detail in hospital and confirmed the results of the previous study. We measured plasma prolactin and pimozide concentration and the fre-quency of motor and phonic tics first after a single 1-mg dose of pimo-zide and 3 days later, on a fixed dosage schedule starting with 1 mg at night and increasing by 1 mg each 10 days to allow steady state to de-velop. Tic frequency was observed by trained observers who counted the number of motor and phonic tics during a specified 5-minute interval unknown to the patient (Sandor & Moldofsky, 1985).

All patients showed a moderate decrease in tic count and elevation of plasma prolactin concentration above the normal range (Table 19.1). In all 5 patients the maximal response as measured by tic count oc-curred at the time when they began to show maximal prolactin eleva-tion. The representative pattern of response is illustrated in Figure 19.1.

These observations lead us to speculate that the dopamine receptors

Table 19.1. Pimozide and Prolactin Concentration in Tourette's Syndrome Patients at Optimal Response

Patient Number	Pimozide Optimal Dose (mg)	Pimozide Concentration (nm/l)	Prolactin Concentration (μg/l)	Tic Count Decrease Relative to Baseline (percentage)
1	3	6.5	32	75
2	2	9.0	50	64
3	2	11.0	42	61
4	2	9.4	43	90
5	2	3.2	34	87

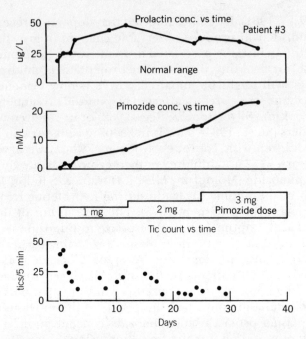

Figure 19.1. Representative pattern of plasma prolactin concentration and tic fre-quency in response to pimozide dosage.

in the hypothalamus involved with the prolactin release regulation and those in the nigrostriatal pathway or in basal ganglia become saturated at the same pimozide concentration. Hence the plasma level of prolactin may become the clinically relevant measure linking the dopaminergic transmission activity on the neuronal level with the pimozide effects on the tic behavior. It seems that increasing the dose of pimozide once maximal prolactin release has been produced is unlikely to produce further symptomatic improvement while increasing the probability of adverse effects.

Clinical Effectiveness

In a double-blind, placebo-controlled, 33-day crossover study, both pimozide and haloperidol significantly and equally decreased tic frequency in nine hospitalized patients, ranging in age from 8 to 28 years (mean = 18.7 years). The initial dose was 2 mg orally and was increased 2 mg every other day to a maximum of 10 to 12 mg over 12 days. Pimozide proved less sedative. Follow-up from 4 to 20 months showed that six of the seven patients who continued with pimozide experienced greater than 75 percent improvement in symptoms. Eight to 30 mg per day with a mean dose of 16 mg was required. Two patients needed benz-tropine mesylate to combat occasional dyskinetic symptoms (Ross & Moldofsky, 1978).

In open, uncontrolled drug trials, one study of pimozide therapy claimed that seven of eight oriental children with Tourette's syndrome showed 87.5 percent improvement. None had any adverse effect, but no drug dosage is mentioned (Nomura and Segawa, 1979). Another study of 31 outpatients who had not favorably responded to haloperidol claimed that 90.3 percent were improved, 3.2 percent were unchanged, and 6.5 percent were worse, compared to no treatment. After abut 12 months (range 3 to 48 months), the patients reported that pimozide was more effective and induced fewer akinesic and phobic side effects than haloperidol. An average of 13 mg (range 1 to 64 mg orally) per day was used (Shapiro, Shapiro, & Eisenkraft, 1983).

We reviewed 33 patients with Tourette's syndrome who were followed for 1 to 15 years. Nine patients received haloperidol, 12 pimozide, and 12 no specific medication. Seventy percent of patients treated with pimozide and 78 percent of those treated with haloperidol reported moderate to marked improvement. Neuroleptic treatment was not beneficial in controlling associated symptoms such as obsessive–compulsive symptoms, attention deficit disorder, and paraphilias (Musisi, Moldofsky, Sandor and Lang, 1987).

A report from Denmark found that 81 percent of 65 patients with Tourette's syndrome experienced good clinical response without side effects. Pimozide dose ranged from 0.5 mg to 9 mg daily (Regeur, Pak-kenberg, Fog, Pakkenberg, 1986). Another early clinical trial also reported beneficial effects of pimozide on 33 children with various types of tics (Debray, Messerchmitt, Lomchamp, 1972). While these open-trial clinical reports appear to confirm the beneficial effects of the drug, the studies are not conclusive because of the variable and unpredictable clinical course of the disorder and the absence of double-blind procedure, random allocation of drugs, crossover design, and the use of reliable and valid measures for assessing the disorder. However, a second double-blind crossover prospective 14-week study comparing pimozide with placebo in 20 outpatients does confirm that this drug is effective in providing improvement (80 percent compared with 10 percent receiving placebo). An average of approximately 7 mg per day was given. Benztropine mesylate was often used prophylactically for the first few weeks to prevent acute dystonic reactions. Ten months later, 11 patients (55 percent) continued treatment. The others stopped the drug because adverse effects offset improvement in 4 patients, 2 had adverse effects without improvement, and 3 had no improvement or adverse effects (Shapiro & Shapiro, 1984).

Altered drug dynamics and/or the heterogeneity of the disorder in its response to dopamine receptor blocking agents might account for the failure in response in some patients (Moldofsky & Brown, 1982).

ADVERSE EFFECTS

Pimozide may induce occasional and unpredictable extrapyramidal symptoms that can be controlled with the usual medications employed with other neuroleptics, such as anticholinergics. The major advantage of pimozide over haloperidol is that it produces less sedation or akinesia. In comparison with placebo, there were single reports of intolerable adverse reactions in the study of 20 patients receiving pimozide. These included extrapyramidal symptoms, impotence, and headaches. In this study, one 12-year-old boy showed ECG changes characterized by U waves and inverted T waves when a dose of 8 mg of pimozide was given. The ECG returned to normal after the drug was stopped (Shapiro & Shapiro, 1984). Our long-term follow-up study showed that pimozide was less likely to induce acute dystonic effects in comparison to haloperidol. Both drugs had similar effects in controlling motor tics and phonic utterances, but pimozide was better in controlling ocular tics (Moldofsky, Musisi, Moldofsky, Sandor, Lang, 1987). In a follow-up study, we compared electrocardiograms of 10 patients treated with pimozide for an average of 3.8 years (range 1 to 7 years), at a mean dose of 9 mg (range 2 to 18 mg per day) to 10 patients treated with haloperidol for an average of 5.3 years (range 2 to 15 years), at a mean dose of 5.5 mg (range 2 to 15 mg per day) (Moldofsky, Musisi, Dorian, & Sandor, 1985). One 53-year-old woman with rheumatoid arthritis who had received 12 mg per day of pimozide for 4 years but was also receiving 75 mg per day of amitriptyline for 2 months showed a left bundle branch block and slightly prolonged QT interval. Another 17-year-old girl with methylmalonic aciduria who had received 16 mg per day of pimozide for 7 years showed nonspecific T-wave abnormalities. Overall there was no evidence of any specific adverse drug effect on EKG in any patient on pimozide at dosages below 20 mg per day.

Other coincidental symptoms reported in some patients include transient depressive disorder (Ross & Moldofsky, 1978). There is a single case report of school phobia in an 11-year-old that appeared after treatment with haloperidol and each of three attempts at treatment with pimozide. The symptoms resolved 3 weeks after discontinuation of pimozide (Linet, 1985). This is similar to the report of emergence of school avoidance and social phobias in 15 patients during treatment with low-dose haloperidol. The phobias were observed in most cases within the first months of starting the treatment (Mikkelsen, Detlor, & Cohen, 1981).

The potential for the development of tardive dyskinesia is a concern in light of recent reports in the literature. However, there is the suggestion of a reduced risk of this disorder with pimozide (Chouinard & Steinberg, 1982; Regeur et al., 1986). Women on high doses of pimozide may develop galactorrhea. Similar caution should be used as with other neuroleptic medications.

DRUG INTERACTIONS

Alcohol, hypnotics, sedatives, and other neuroleptics potentiate CNS depressant effects. Stimulants have been reported to provoke tics in some patients. Anticholinergic drugs will potentiate anticholinergic effects. The response of anticonvulsants may be reduced. Epinephrine should not be used because of the danger of severe hypotension.

SUMMARY

Pimozide is an effective drug for the control of symptoms of Gilles de la Tourette's syndrome. Because it is equally effective but less sedative than the hitherto employed standard drug, haloperidol, pimozide may be preferable. However, caution should be employed pending the outcome of long-term studies.

REFERENCES

Ayd, F.J. (1971). A promising new neuroleptic. *International Drug Therapy Newsletter, 6,* 17–20.

Chouinard, G., & Steinberg, S. (1982). Type I tardive dyskinesia induced by anticholinergic drugs, dopamine agonists and neuroleptics. *Progress in Neuropsychopharmacology and Biological Psychiatry, 6,* 571–578.

Cookson, J.C., Silverstone, T., & Rees, L. (1982). Plasma prolactin and growth hormone levels in manic patients treated with pimozide. *British Journal of Psychiatry, 140,* 274–279.

Debray, P., Messerchmitt, P., Lomchamp, D., (1972). L'utilization du pimozide en pedopsychiatrie. *Nouv Presse Med 1,* 2917–2918.

Gould, R.J., Murphy, K.M.M., Reynolds, I.B., & Snyder, S.H. (1983). *Proceedings of the National Academy of Science. USA, 80,* 5122–5128.

Gruen, P.H., Sachar, E.J., Langer, G., Altman, N., Leifer, M., Frantz, A., & Halpern, F.S. (1978). Prolactin responses to neuroleptics in normal and schizophrenic subjects. *Archives of General Psychiatry, 35,* 108–116.

Gudelsky, G.A. (1981). Tubero-infandibular dopamine neurons and the regulation of prolactin secretion. *Psychoneuroendrocrinology, 6,* 3–16.

Linet, L.S. (1985). Tourette syndrome, pimozide and school phobia: The neuroleptic separation anxiety syndrome. *American Journal of Psychiatry, 142,*(5), 613–615.

McCreadie, R.G., Heykants, J.J.P., Chalmers, A., & Anderson, A.M. (1979). Plasma pimozide profiles in chronic schizophrenics. *Brit J Clin Pharmacol, 7,* 533–534.

Mikkelsen, E.J., Detlor, J., & Cohen, D.J. (1981). School avoidance and social phobia triggered by haloperidol in patients with Tourette's disorder. *American Journal of Psychiatry, 138*(12), 1572–1575.

Moldofsky, H., & Brown, G.M. (1982). Tics and serum prolactin response to pimozide in Tourette syndrome. In T.N. Chase & A.J. Friedhoff (Eds.). *Gilles de la Tourette's syndrome.* New York: Raven.

Moldofsky, H., Musisi, S., Dorian, P. & Sandor, P. (1985), unpublished data.

Morris, P.A., MacKenzie, D.H., & Masheter, H. (1970). A comparative double blind trial of pimozide and fluphenazine in chronic schizophrenia. *British Journal of Psychiatry, 117,* 583–584.

Musisi, S.N., Moldofsky, H., Sandor P. and Lang A. (1987). Gilles de la Tourette's syndrome: A follow-up study (abstract) *Proceedings of American Psychiatric Association 140th Annual Meeting,* p. 233.

Nomura, Y., & Segawa, M. (1979). Gilles de la Tourette's syndrome in oriental children. *Brain Dev, 1,* 103–111.

Pecile, A., & Olgiati, V.R. (1978). Control growth hormone secretion. In S.L. Jeffcoat & J.S.M. Hutchinson (Eds.), *The endocrine hypothalamus.* London: Academic.

Pinder, R.M., Brogden, R.N. Sawyer, P.R., Speight, T.M., Spencer, R., & Avery, G.S., (1976). Pimozide: A review of its pharmacological properties and therapeutic uses in psychiatry. *Drugs, 12,* 1–40.

Regeur, L., Pakkenberg, B., Fog, R. & Pakkenberg, H., (1986). Clinical features and long-term treatment with pimozide in 65 patients with Gilles de la Tourette's syndrome. *Journal of Neurology, Neurosurgery, & Psychiatry, 49,* 791–795.

Ross, M.S., & Moldofsky, H. (1978). A comparison of pimozide and haloperidol in the treatment of Gilles de la Tourette's syndrome. *American Journal of Psychiatry, 135*(5), 585–587.

Sallee, F.R., Pollock, B.G., Stiller, R.L., Stull, S., & Perel, J.M., (1986). Pharmacokinetics of pimozide in patients with Tourette's syndrome. *Clinical Research, 34*(3), 867A.

Sandor, P. & Moldofsky, H. (1985). Unpublished data.

Seeman, P., & Lee, T. (1975). Antipsychotic drugs: Direct correlation between clinical potency and presynaptic action on dopamine neurons. *Science, 188,* 1217–1219.

Shapiro, A.K., Shapiro, E., Bruun, R.D., & Sweet, R.D., (1978). Gilles de la Tourette's Syndrome. New York: Raven.

Shapiro, A.K., Shapiro, E. (1982). An update on Tourette syndrome. *American Journal of Psychotherapy, 36*(3), 379–390.

Shapiro, A.K., Shapiro, E., & Eisenkraft, G.J. (1983). Treatment of Gilles de la Tourette's syndrome with pimozide. *American Journal of Psychiatry, 140,* 1183–1186.

Shapiro, A.K., & Shapiro, E. (1984). Controlled study of pimozide vs. placebo in Tourette's syndrome. *Journal of American Academy of Child Psychiatry, 23,* 161–173.

Suwa, S., Naruse, H., Ohura, T., Tsuruhara, T., Takesada, M., Yamazaki, K., & Miklini, M., (1984). Influence of pimozide on hypothalomo-pituitary function in children with behavioural disorders. *Psychoneuroendocrinology, 9*(1), 37–44.

CHAPTER TWENTY

Clonidine Treatment of Tourette's Syndrome

James F. Leckman
John T. Walkup
Donald J. Cohen

Clonidine was serendipitously discovered to have hypotensive effects in 1962. Since that time, its site and mechanisms of action have been intensively studied. The knowledge of the specific central nervous system effects of clonidine has led to the expanded use of clonidine as a therapeutic agent in other medical and psychiatric disorders.

Clonidine's beneficial effects in Tourette's syndrome (TS) were first reported in 1979. That report has led to widespread use of clonidine in the treatment of TS and has stimulated research into the role of the noradrenergic system in the pathophysiology of TS. Most clinical trials support clonidine's efficacy in TS, yet controversy remains. This controversy has recently been heightened by the failure of a large double-blind trial to demonstrate significant clinical improvement. If clonidine is proven effective, a more complete understanding of central noradrenergic–dopaminergic interactions may lead to improved treatment in TS.

NEUROCHEMICAL STUDIES IN TOURETTE'S SYNDROME

A variety of neurochemical systems have been implicated in the pathogenesis and pathophysiology of TS. Central dopaminergic systems localized in the midbrain are a major focus of research interest. Other neurochemical systems implicated in the pathogenesis of TS include: cholinergic, GABAergic, endogenous opiate, and noradrenergic systems (Leckman, Riddle, Cohen, Chapter 7, this volume).

Theories of altered central noradrenergic function have been advanced to account for the beneficial effects of clonidine in some TS patients. Other evidence of noradrenergic involvement includes reduced levels of urinary 3-methoxy-4-hydroxy-phenylethylene glycol (MHPG) excretion in TS patients (Ang, Borison, Dysken, & Davis, 1982) and reduced clonidine-stimulated growth hormone release (Leckman, Cohen, Gertner, Ort, & Harcherik, 1984). Current hypotheses to explain clonidine's efficacy focus on central noradrenergic–dopaminergic and noradrenergic–serotoninergic–dopaminergic interactions. Evidence supporting these hypotheses includes the concordance of clonidine and haloperidol in a double crossover study of these agents (Borison, Ang, Hamilton, Diamond, & David, 1983) and altered plasma HVA levels after chronic clonidine treatment and withdrawal (Leckman et al., 1986). Studies of the site of this interaction are focusing on the connections between the DA cell groups in the central mesencephalic tegmentum and the noradrenergic neurons in the locus coeruleus (Deutch, Goldstein, & Roth, 1986). Serotonin neurons in the raphe may also be important intermediaries of noradrenergic–dopaminergic interactions (Bunney & DeRiemer, 1982).

CLONIDINE

Clonidine HCL is an imidazoline derivative widely used as a centrally acting antihypertensive agent. It is an alpha-adrenergic agonist that preferentially stimulates alpha$_2$-adrenergic receptors. Stimulation of presynaptic alpha$_2$ receptors in the brain decreases the amount of norepinephrine released into the synapse per nerve impulse, thereby decreasing centrally mediated vasoconstriction of the peripheral circulation, which leads to a reduction in blood pressure. In addition to this effect on blood pressure, clonidine inhibits spontaneous firing in the locus coeruleus, reduces brain norepinephrine turnover, inhibits ACTH and renin secretion, increases growth hormone secretion, and stimulates central histamine H$_2$-receptors. Indirect effects on other neurotransmitter systems have been noted, specifically serotonin (Antelman & Caggiula, 1977) and dopamine (Bunney & DeRiemer, 1982). Long-term treatments with clonidine indicates continued inhibitory effects on norepinephrine release and augmenting effects on dopamine turnover (Martin, Ebert, Gordon, Linnoila, & Kopin, 1984).

These studies of clonidine's multiple effects in the CNS are paralleled by studies that used clonidine as an "adrenergic probe," exploiting its specific alpha$_2$-agonist activity. The adrenergic system has been implicated in a variety of neurological and psychiatric disorders, including schizophrenia, depression, bipolar disorder, anxiety disorders, tardive dyskinesias, withdrawal syndromes, and Tourette's syndrome. These disorders have been treated with clonidine in an attempt to offer symptomatic relief but also to understand the role of the noradrenergic system in these disturbances. This work has resulted in the accepted use of clonidine in the treatment of opiate withdrawal syndromes (Gold, Redmond, & Kleber, 1978).

CLONIDINE IN TOURETTE'S SYNDROME

The beneficial effects of clonidine in the treatment of TS first were reported by Cohen, Young, Nathanson, and Shaywitz (1979). Since that time, there has been widespread use of clonidine in TS. Presently, nearly a third of clinically treated TS patients in the United States have likely received clonidine (Stefl, 1983). The majority of clinical trials completed to date support the efficacy of clonidine in TS, but active controversy remains, as some studies have reported that clonidine is of marginal or no significant benefit to TS patients.

Critical evaluation of the various clinical trials reveals significant problems that limit the inferences that can be drawn from the studies. The lack of well-designed, double-blind, placebo-controlled trials is most evident. Other problems include unaccounted-for differences in: age (adult vs. child), severity of symptoms, the presence or absence of comorbid conditions, variable treatment parameters (low vs. high dose, rapid increases vs. slow increases in dose, short [<6 weeks] vs. long [>12 weeks] treatment trials), and variations in assessment procedures used to describe TS symptom severity, comorbid behavioral patterns, and the outcome of treatments.

Open and Single-Blind Trials

In the past 6 years, more than 15 open or single-blind trials of clonidine in more than 200 TS patients have been reported (Table 20.1). Most studies suggest that clonidine is an effective treatment. Bruun (1984) reported on 72 patients she treated with clonidine. Thirty-four (42 percent) patients experienced at least a 50 percent reduction in symptoms. Eleven patients (15 percent) improved on combined therapy of clonidine and haloperidol. More recently, Singer, Gammon, and Quaskey (1986) treated 30 TS patients and reported that 47 percent achieved a good to fair result. In contrast to these reports, Shapiro, Shapiro, and Eisenkraft in 1983 reported on 68 patients treated with clonidine. They found only 18 (26 percent) patients to have a greater than 50 percent decrease in symptoms.

Double-Blind Trials

Four double-blind trials have been reported. Two of these studies are single-case reports describing one positive response (McKeith, Williams, & Nicol, 1981) and one non-response to clonidine (Dysken et al., 1980). The third study, by Borison and coworkers (1983), involved 22 TS patients in a double-blind crossover trial comparing clonidine, haloperidol, and placebo. Patients received 0.25 to 0.9 mg per day of clonidine and were treated for a minimum of 9 weeks. Assessments were performed rating the frequency and intensity of tics. No information was provided concerning the reliability of these assessments. Fifteen of the 22 (68 percent) patients responded positively to clonidine, and there was a concordance of the response to haloperidol and clonidine in 18 patients (12 positive and 6 negative). The authors concluded that clonidine was as effective as haloperidol and that both agents were superior to placebo ($p < .005$).

A fourth study, by Goetz and colleagues (1987), involved 30 TS patients 8 to 62 years old who were treated with 0.0075 or 0.015 mg/kg per day of clonidine for 12 weeks. "Objective" videotape ratings of anatomical distribution, number, and severity of tics were performed at 3-week intervals. Interrater reliabilities were assessed, ranging between .60 for

Table 20.1. Effects of Clonidine in Tourette's Syndrome

Investigator	Number	Dose (mg per day)	Duration	Efficacy[a] ≥50% (good)	≥25% (fair)	≤25% (poor)
Open and Single-Blind Studies						
Cohen et al. (1979, 1980)	25	0.05–0.4	open	[---	70% ---]	30%
Dorsey (1981)	12[b]	0.3–0.6	2–24 months	[---	75% ---]	25%
Abuzzahab (1981)	10	0.1–0.6	4–52 weeks	[---	20% ---]	80%
Shapiro et al. (1983)	68	0.20–2.0	2–3 months	10%	14%	76%
Bruun (1984)	72	0.1–0.8	5 weeks 9 months	[---	47% ---]	38%
Leckman et al. (1983, 1984, 1986) (short term)	26	0.1–0.35	8–12 weeks	15%	46%	38%
Leckman et al. (1983, 1984, 1986) (long term)	25	0.1–0.3	10–12 months	64%	32%	4%
Singer et al. (1986)	30	0.1–0.8	1–44 months	17%	30%	53%
Double-Blind Studies						
Dysken et al. (1980)	1	0.05–0.6	2–5 week trials	"not improved"		
McKeith et al. (1981)	1	0.2	2 weeks	"improved"		
Borison et al. (1983)	22	0.25–0.9	9 weeks min	[--- 68% ---]		32%
Goetz et al. (1987)	30	0.3–0.6	12 weeks	"no objective improvement"		

[a]Efficacy is measured in percentage of reduction in tic symptoms.
[b]One patient in this group is also in Cohen et al. (1980).

295

anatomic distribution of motor tics and .97 for the number of vocal tics. According to the authors, there was no "objective" evidence for improvement during clonidine treatment. However, 13 patients reported "subjective" improvement while on clonidine, and 16 patients elected to continue treatment with clonidine at the end of the study. Importantly, a substantial "subjective" response to placebo was also reported in 9 subjects. These data seriously challenge the role of clonidine in the treatment of TS.

Currently, a second large double-blind clinical trial (Leckman, unpublished data) is underway comparing clonidine and placebo, which should help resolve the question of clonidine's efficacy in TS.

Indications for Treatment and Patient Selection

The decision to treat the symptoms of TS is related to the level of functional impairment and the subjective distress experienced by the patient. Obviously, the more severe the dysfunction and the distress, the clearer the need for medication. However, the clinical threshold for initiating treatment may vary from one class of medications to another based on their efficacy and side effects. For example, the dopamine blocking agents, most notably haloperidol, have significant adverse effects that limit their long-term use in patients. The recent reports of tardive dyskinesia in TS patients treated with neuroleptics (Golden, 1985) are of special concern. Consequently, the clinical threshold for using these agents should be fairly high. Clonidine, in contrast, with its minimal side effect profile and ease of use, has become the initial treatment for TS in many centers and may be appropriately used in patients with moderate to severe symptoms.

There is no known patient population that predictably responds to clonidine. Severe initial symptomatology (Leckman, Detlor, Harcherik, Ort, & Shaywitz, 1985) and previous positive response to haloperidol (Borison et al., 1983) have been associated with a positive response. Clonidine's slow onset of action limits its usefulness in patients with acute, severe symptom exacerbations. Neuroleptics are better suited for this purpose. The recent report on the efficacy of clonidine in attention deficit disorder (Hunt, Minderra, & Cohen, 1985) may lead one to consider clonidine in those 40 to 50 percent of TS patients who in addition to tics complain of attentional problems, restlessness, anxiety, or irritability.

Evaluation of Treatment

The evaluation of treatment response is complicated by many of the factors that complicate the assessment of the severity of TS symptoms in general. The complexity of the symptoms, their waxing and waning course, and the need to rely on nonexpert informants for evaluation of the range of symptoms outside of the office make accurate assessment difficult. In addition, the general tendency for TS symptoms to decrease over the life of the patient, and the presence of what many feel are associated problems, attention deficit disorder with and without hyperactivity, obsessive–compulsive traits, and nonspecific problems of mood, behavior, and functioning, further complicate the evaluation of symptoms, their severity, and response to medication. Because of these difficulties, reliable assessment procedures that are comprehensive and address the complexity and variability of TS symptoms over time are essential. Significant advances in this area have occurred. Several good instruments are presently available that address both the tics and the associated behavioral problems (Leckman, Towbin, Ort, & Cohen, Chapter 4, this volume).

Assessing drug efficacy in TS is complicated by a variety of factors. Specific problems include placebo effects, the attribution of drug action to the natural waxing and waning of symptoms, the natural decreases in symptoms over time, or the effects of other environmental events. With clonidine specific problems arise. The long latency period (8 to 12 weeks) between the initiation of clonidine and the potential response and the incomplete and nonuniform nature of that response may enhance the possibility that attributional errors of drug response or other nonpharmacologic treatment effects may occur.

Treatment Regimen

Baseline evaluation prior to the initiation of a clonidine trial consists of a detailed medical and psychiatric history with an assessment of present and past TS symptoms and current life circumstances, and a physical exam with an EKG and fasting blood glucose. The latency and pattern of response, side effects, and the problem of abrupt withdrawal are especially important components of the discussion prior to beginning the clonidine trial.

The beginning dosage of clonidine is 0.05 mg per day. It is slowly increased by 0.05 mg per day over several weeks until dosages in the range of 0.15 to 0.30 mg per day ($3\mu g/kg$ per day) are achieved. The total daily dose is divided into three or four doses given every 4 to 6 hours depending upon the individual patient's response and needs. Doses in excess of 0.3 mg per day (or $7.5\mu g/kg$ per day) can be efficacious but tend to lead to an increasing incidence of side effects.

The greater efficacy of low doses appears to be related to a shift in clonidine's site of action from presynaptic $alpha_2$ activity (adrenergic inhibition) at low doses to a relative increase in postsynaptic $alpha_1$

activity (adrenergic stimulation) at higher doses. This is supported by those accounts of individual cases in which low doses have moderated symptoms, but with increasing doses, beneficial effects have been lost, and symptom exacerbations have occurred.

Combined Treatment with Neuroleptics

Clinically, the combined administration of clonidine and low-dose neuroleptics in drug-naive or treatment-resistant patients has been reported. Although a few clinicians have anecdotally reported successful treatment outcomes with this regimen, few systematic data are available that empirically address this question (Bruun, 1984; Regeur, Pakkenberg, Fog, & Pakkenberg, 1986).

Pattern of Response

Clonidine has a relatively slow onset of action. Initial effects, which occur weeks to months after beginning the medication, may be described as an increased sense of calm or a decrease in tension. This is often followed by decreases in attentional and behavioral symptoms and complex tics. Simple tics seem less responsive.

At best, there is a gradual reduction but not elimination of symptoms over the subsequent 3 to 4 months with the possibility of continued symptom reduction for up to a year. In our experience, although there were a few dramatic early responses, the general pattern was one of ≥ 30 percent decrease in symptoms during the first 8 to 12 weeks and > 50 percent decrease over 12 months. The intensity of symptoms is less severe. However, this pattern is not always apparent. The effects on motor and phonic tics and behavioral symptoms need not coincide. There may be isolated reductions in one symptom or type of symptom with little or no effect on other symptoms.

Side Effects

The most commonly reported unwanted effect of clonidine is sedation. It occurs in 10 to 20 percent of cases, is dose related, and, with time, tolerance usually develops. Other less frequent side effects (< 5 percent) include orthostatic hypotension and dry mouth, both of which are dose related. Headache, irritability, labile mood, and sleep difficulties (particularly early morning awakening in the absence of depression) can occur. Rare but potentially important unwanted effects include the exacerbation of preexisting cardiac arrythmias and decreased glucose tolerance. Baseline and follow-up EKGs and fasting glucose levels are recommended. Clonidine-related increases in growth hormone have not appeared to accelerate somatic growth in pubertal subjects. Tolerance or undesirable "tardive" signs and symptoms have not been observed even in very long-term treatments (>5 years).

Withdrawal

Tolerance to the beneficial effects of clonidine does not develop in hypertensive patients. There have been reports, however, of rebound increases in blood pressure and heart rate occurring after abrupt discontinuation of clonidine. Leckman and coworkers (1986) studied abrupt withdrawal in seven patients with TS. We observed acute (<72 hours) increases in motor restlessness and activity, increased talkativeness, increased anxiety, and difficulty sleeping. These symptoms were responsive to clonidine reinitiation. There also were increases in motor and phonic tics that occurred shortly after discontinuing, but this also was seen in patients after a more gradual tapering of medication. In five of seven patients, the marked worsening of tics after abrupt withdrawal persisted for 2 weeks to 4 months after reinitiation of clonidine. Increasing symptoms after abrupt withdrawal did not appear to be related to plasma-elimination half-life, which ranged from 6.4 to 18.6 hours.

SUMMARY

There are conflicting data concerning the efficacy of clonidine in TS. Overall, clonidine appears to be a safe and effective agent to suppress tic symptoms in 40 to 60 percent of TS patients over an interval of 8 to 12 weeks. Treatment parameters of dose (<7.5 μg/kg per day) and duration (8 to 12 weeks minimum), a history of a positive response to haloperidol, and severe initial TS symptomatology have been associated with a positive outcome. The controversy arises from concerns about clonidine's modest ability (compared to haloperidol) to inhibit rapidly motor and phonic tics. The long duration of treatment required to observe beneficial effects (12 to 52 weeks) also increases the possibility of other nonspecific factors having an effect on symptoms. The frequent presence of non-tic behavior problems such as ADD complicates the matter further. The exact nature of these problems and their relationship to TS, their impact on TS symptoms, and their specific response to clonidine are all questions that remain unanswered. The results from a completed double-blind trial (Goetz et al., 1987) challenge the role of clonidine in the treatment of TS. A second ongoing double-blind trial should help resolve the questions concerning clonidine's efficacy compared to placebo in TS.

REFERENCES

Abuzzahab, F.S. (1981). Clonidine HCI in Gilles de la Tourette syndrome. *First International Gilles de la Tourette Syndrome Symposium, 17.* (Abstract)

Ang, L., Borison, R., Dysken, M., & Davis, J.M. (1982). Reduced excretion of MHPG in Tourette syndrome. In A.J. Friedhoff, T.N. Chase (Eds.), *Gilles de la Tourette Syndrome.* New York: Raven.

Antelman, S.M., & Caggiula, A.R. (1977). Norepinephrine-dopamine interactions and behavior. *Science, 195,* 646–653.

Borison, R.L., Ang, L., Hamilton, W.J., Diamond, B.I., & David, J.M. (1983). Treatment approaches in Gilles de la Tourette syndrome. *Brain Research Bulletin, 11*(2), 205–208.

Bruun, R.D. (1984). Gilles de la Tourette syndrome. An overview of clinical experience. *Journal of the American Academy of Child Psychiatry, 23*(2), 126–133.

Bunney, B.S., & DeRiemer, S.A. (1982). Effects of clonidine on nigral dopamine cell activity: Possible mediation by noradrenergic regulation of serotonergic raphe system. In A.J. Friedhoff, & T.N. Chase (Eds.), *Gilles de la Tourette Syndrome.* New York: Raven.

Caine, E.D. (1985). Gilles de la Tourette's syndrome. A review of clinical and research studies and consideration of future directions for investigation. *Archives of Neurology, 42,* 393–397.

Cohen, D.J., Young, J.G., Nathanson, J.A., & Shaywitz, B.A. (1979). Clonidine in Tourette's syndrome. *Lancet, ii,* 551–553.

Cohen, D.J., Detlor, J., Young, J.G., & Shaywitz, B.A. (1980). Clonidine ameliorates Gilles de la Tourette syndrome. *Archives of General Psychiatry, 37,* 1350–1357.

Deutch, A.Y., Goldstein, M., & Roth, R.H. (1986). Activation of the locus coeruleus induced by selective stimulation of the ventral tegmental area. *Brain Research, 363,* 307–314.

Dorsey, R. (1981). Clonidine and Gilles de la Tourette syndrome. *Archives of General Psychiatry, 38,* 1185.

Dysken, M.W., Berecz, J.M., Samarza, A., & Davis, J.M. (1980). Clonidine in Tourette syndrome. *Lancet, ii,* 926–927.

Goetz, C.G., Tanner, C.M., Wilson, R.S., Carroll, V.S., Como, P.G., & Shannon, K.M. (1987). Clonidine and Gilles de la Tourette syndrome: Double-blind study using objective rating methods. *Annals of Neurology, 21,* 307–310.

Gold, M.S., Redmond, D.E., & Kleber H.D. (1978). Clonidine blocks acute opiate-withdrawal symptoms. *Lancet, ii,* 599–602.

Golden, G.S. (1985). Tardive dyskinesia in Tourette syndrome. *Pediatric Neurology, 1*(3), 192–194.

Hunt, R.D., Minderra, R., & Cohen, D.J. (1985). Clonidine benefits children with attention deficit disorder and hyperactivity: Report of a double-blind placebo-crossover therapeutic trial. *Journal of the American Academy of Child Psychiatry, 24,* 617–629.

Leckman, J.F., Detlor, J., Harcherik, D.F., Young, J.G., Anderson, G.M., Shaywitz, B., & Cohen, D.J. (1983). Acute and chronic clonidine treatment in Tourette's syndrome: A preliminary report on clinical response and effect on plasma and urinary catecholamine metabolites, growth hormone and blood pressure. *Journal of the American Academy of Child Psychiatry, 22,* 433–440.

Leckman, J.F., Cohen, D.J., Gertner, J.M., Ort. S.I., & Harcherik, D. (1984). Growth hormone response to clonidine in children ages 4–17: Tourette syndrome vs. children with short stature. *Journal of the American Academy of Child Psychiatry, 23,* 174–181.

Leckman, J.F., Detlor, J., Harcherik, D.F., Ort, S., Shaywitz, B.A., & Cohen, D.J. (1985). Short and long term treatment of Tourette's syndrome with clonidine: A clinical perspective. *Neurology, 5,* 343–351.

Leckman, J.F., Ort, S., Caruso, K.A., Anderson, G.M., Riddle, M.A., & Cohen, D.J. (1986). Rebound phenomena in Tourette's syndrome after abrupt withdrawal of clonidine: Behavioral, cardiovascular and neurochemical effects. *Archives of General Psychiatry, 43,* 1168–1176.

Martin, P.R., Ebert, M.H., Gordon, E.K., Linnoila, M., & Kopin, I.J. (1984). Effects of clonidine on central and peripheral catecholamine metabolism. *Clinical Pharmacology & Therapeutics, 35*(3), 322–327.

McKeith, I.G., Williams, A., & Nicol, A.R. (1981). Clonidine in Tourette syndrome. *Lancet i,* 270–271.

Regeur, L., Pakkenberg, B., Fogg, R., & Pakkenberg, H. (1986). Clinical Features and long term treatment with pimozide in 65 patients with Gilles de la Tourette syndrome. *Journal of Neurology, Neurosurgery, & Psychiatry, 49,* 791–795.

Shapiro, A.K., Shapiro, E., & Eisenkraft, G.J. (1983). Treatment of Gilles de la Tourette's syndrome with clonidine and neuroleptics. *Archives of General Psychiatry, 40*(11), 1235–1240.

Singer, H.S., Gammon, K., & Quaskey, S. (1986). Haloperidol, fluphenazine, and clonidine in Tourette syndrome: Controversies in treatment. *Pediatric Neurologic Science, 12*(2), 71–74.

Stefl, M.E. (1983). *The Ohio Tourette study.* Cincinnati: School of Planning, University of Cincinnati.

CHAPTER TWENTY-ONE

The Role of "Other" Neuroleptic Drugs in the Treatment of Tourette's Syndrome

Harvey S. Singer
Richard Trifiletti
Karen Gammon

OVERVIEW

Pharmacologic agents that act to decrease central dopaminergic activity by blocking dopamine receptors have been shown to improve the symptomatology of Tourette's syndrome (TS). The two most widely utilized agents, the butyrophenone, haloperidol, and the diphenylbutylpiperidine, pimozide, are discussed in separate chapters. These two drugs, however, may either be ineffective or have adverse effects that restrict use or lead to noncompliance. It is therefore important to consider published reports that have suggested that other chemical classes of neuroleptics may be effective in this syndrome. Hence in this chapter we will review reported data as well as our personal experiences with several other neuroleptic medications. It is our recommendation, based on available information, that the piperazine phenothiazine, fluphenazine, should be considered as a therapeutic alternative to both haloperidol and pimozide.

CLINICAL PHARMACOLOGY

Tourette's Syndrome and Dopamine Receptors

Hypotheses of the pathophysiologic mechanism of Tourette's syndrome have generally included a component of neurotransmitter system "imbalance." Dopaminergic, cholinergic, serotoninergic, noradrenergic, and peptidergic neurotransmitters have all been proposed as components of this imbalance. As autopsy material from TS patient is scarce, the above abnormalities have been suspected largely from studies of transmitter metabolites in the CSF and from reduction of symptoms in patients in response to pharmacologic agents designed to interact with a given neurotransmitter system.

Of the aforementioned putative neurochemical abnormalities in Tourette's syndrome, the dopaminergic system has received the most attention. The dopaminergic hyperfunction hypothesis is based on responsiveness of patients to medications that block dopaminergic receptor sites, aggravation of tics by CNS stimulants, altered levels of biogenic amine metabolites in CSF, and the existence of a tardive Tourette's syndrome. A more specific proposal is that Tourette's syndrome is related to hypersensitive dopamine receptors: either an increased number of receptors are present or existing receptors have an increased affinity for dopamine.

Which dopamine receptors are likely to be involved in TS? In the current scheme, dopamine receptors are broadly divisible into two distinct classes: D_1 and D_2 receptors. D_1 receptors are positively coupled to adenylate cyclase (i.e., D_1 agonists, like dopamine, stimulate adenylate cyclase), but their function is otherwise unknown. By contrast, the D_2 dopamine receptors are considered the pharmacologically relevant dopamine receptors in the sense that the affinities of neuroleptics for these sites are closely correlated with amelioration of psychotic symptoms and movement disorders. Recent studies, however, using D_1-selective antagonists, have suggested a complex interaction of D_1 and D_2 receptors in behaviors formerly thought to be solely mediated by D_2 receptors (Mailman et al., 1984; Meller, Kuga, Friedhoff, & Goldstein, 1985). It has also been proposed that D_1 receptors influence D_2 receptors via a mechanism that is dependent upon functionally intact catecholaminergic neurons (Breese & Mueller, 1985).

The efficacy of drugs for suppression of TS symptoms is positively correlated with potency of their competition for [^{3}H]haloperidol binding to D_2-dopamine receptors, but is not correlated with potency at inhibiting dopamine-sensitive adenylate cyclase (D_1) receptors (Stahl and Berger, 1982). This suggests the possibility that selective D_2 dopamine receptor supersensitivity is part of the pathophysiology of TS. If correct, this finding is of potential significance since a number of D_2 antagonists, which are more D_2 selective than haloperidol, are currently available (e.g., domperidone, molindone, metoclopramide, and sulpiride) and may be worthy of further evaluation in TS.

(Editors' Note: Additional pharmacological evidence concerning the pathobiology of TS is discussed in Chapter 7 of this volume.)

General Receptor Effect of Neuroleptics

Neuroleptics exert their antipsychotic effects by D_2 dopamine receptor blockade, but neuroleptics (to varying degrees, depending on the particular drug) also block other receptors (see Fig. 21.1). As mentioned earlier, the potency of a given neuroleptic at dopamine D_2 receptors correlates positively with its antipsychotic and "anti-tic" efficacy. However, the affinity for D_2 receptor blockade also tends to correlate positively with a drug's potential to produce extrapyramidal symptoms (EPS), including bradykinesia, akathisia, and dystonia. Neuroleptics may also block alpha-adrenergic receptors, resulting in sedation (Peroutka, U' Prichard, Greenberg, & Snyder, 1977).

In addition to effects on monoaminergic receptors, neuroleptics inhibit muscarinic cholinergic receptors (Fig. 21.1). This blockade, in contrast to prior actions, has a negative correlation for the production of extrapyramidal symptoms (EPS) (Snyder, Greenberg, & Yamamura, 1974). Hence, muscarinic cholinergic blockade has a beneficial effect in counteracting EPS produced by D_2 dopamine receptor blockade. On the other hand, Stahl and Berger (1982) have suggested that the more

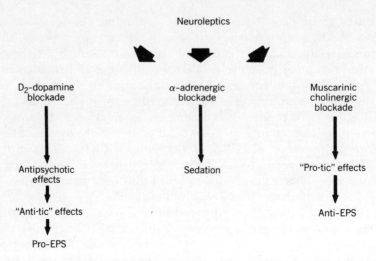

Figure 21.1.   A simplified correlation between synaptic and clinical effects of neuroleptic drugs (EPS = extrapyramidal symptoms).

efficiently a neuroleptic inhibits cholinergic receptors the less effective it is in controlling tic symptoms. Thus in theory, the "ideal" neuroleptic therapy for TS should have an appropriate balance of D_2 dopamine and muscarinic cholinergic receptor blockade so that tics are relieved and EPS is avoided. Such a neuroleptic should also have minimal alpha-adrenergic inhibition in order to minimize sedative side effects.

DOPAMINERGIC-RELATED NEUROLEPTICS

Phenothiazines

Phenothiazines, classified on the basis of their chemical structure into aliphatic, piperidine, or piperazine compounds (Fig. 21.2), are most widely known for their antipsychotic activity. In general, phenothiazine neuroleptics appear to be less consistently effective in the treatment of Tourette's syndrome compared with butyrophenones (Shapiro, Shapiro, Bruun, & Sweet, 1978). Definitive comparison studies, however, have not been performed for this class of drugs. At present, scattered case reports in the literature suggest that several classes of phenothiazines may occasionally be effective (Abuzzahab & Anderson, 1973; Bockner, 1959; Eisenberg, Ascher, & Kanner, 1959; Goetz, Tanner, & Klawans, 1984; Levy & Ascher, 1968; Lucas, 1964; Mesnikoff, 1959; Polites, Kruger & Stevenson, 1965; Shapiro, Shapiro, Bruun & Sweet, 1978; Walsh, 1962). For example, fluphenazine, a potent phenothiazine with a piper-

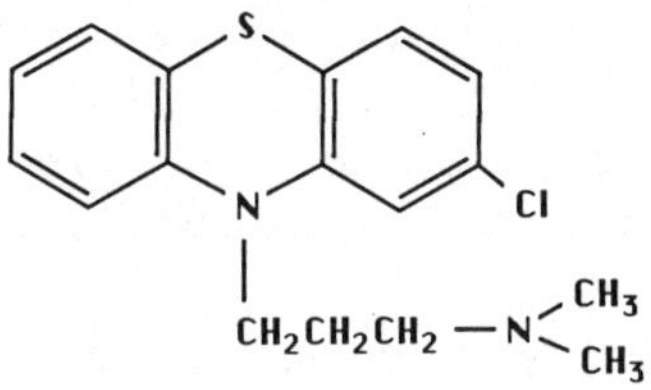

Chlorpromazine

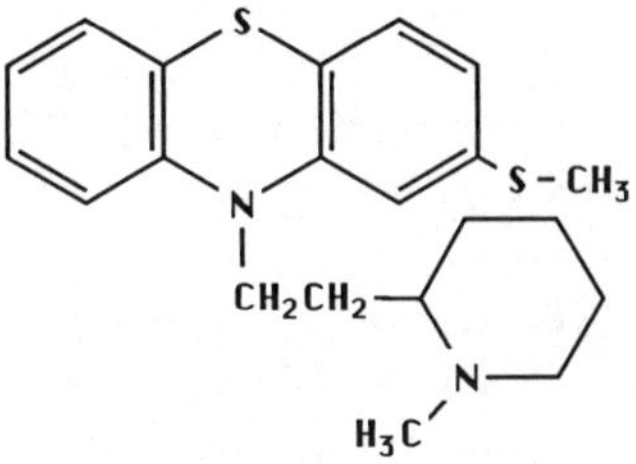

Thioridazine

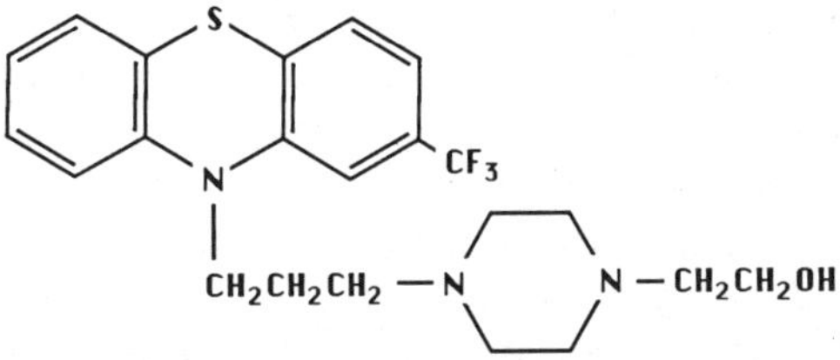

Fluphenazine

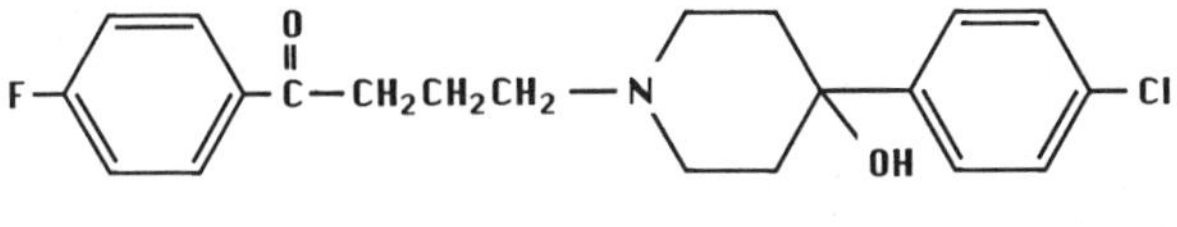

Haloperidol

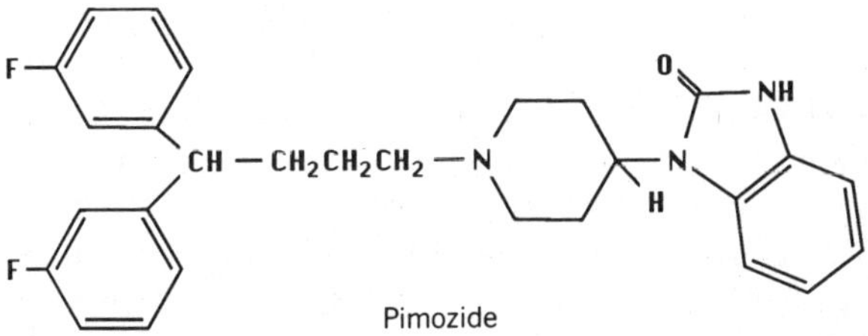

Pimozide

Figure 21.2. Structures of some representative neuroleptic drugs.

azine side-chain, is thought by several investigators to be useful in the treatment of Tourette's syndrome. In contrast, phenothiazines with aliphatic side-chains (chlorpromazine) or those with piperidine side-chains (thioridazine) tend to be less effective (Stahl & Berger, 1982).

Fluphenazine. Fluphenazine has been recommended as an alternative therapy for patients with multiple tics who cannot tolerate the butyrophenone haloperidol. In a study of 21 such patients who received fluphenazine as part of an open-label study, 11 reported improved drug efficacy and fewer side effects (Goetz et al., 1984). Overall, 16 patients were reported to have a level of tic control equal to or greater than with haloperidol. Similarly, in a double-blind, placebo-controlled study in 10 patients receiving a flexible dosage schedule, the relative efficacies of haloperidol and fluphenazine were compared (Borison et al., 1982). The drugs produced statistically significant therapeutic effects, which appeared to be equivalent. In terms of drug potency, 1 mg of fluphenazine was deemed to be equivalent to 0.75 mg of haloperidol. Haloperidol, however, produced a significantly increased incidence of sedative and extrapyramidal side effects.

To evaluate our experience with fluphenazine and haloperidol, a retrospective review of 120 patients (97 males and 23 females) enrolled in the Tourette Syndrome Clinic at the Johns Hopkins Hospital was undertaken (Singer, Gammon, & Quaskey, 1986). The average age of onset in this group was 7.1 years and the mean follow-up of patients was 2.4 years.

In this population, 60 patients had received haloperidol; for 55 it was the initial drug. In contrast, 31 patients were treated with fluphenazine; for 6 it was the initial drug, for 18 the second, and for 7 the third drug. A good or fair improvement in tic symptoms, based upon parental, physician, and linear analogue ranking scales, was found in 83 percent of patients on haloperidol and 81 percent of those on fluphenazine. Patients on fluphenazine (mean maximal dose 5.1 mg per day) received higher doses of medication compared with those on haloperidol (mean maximum dose 3.8 mg per day) and had fewer overall side effects, 17 of 31 versus 50 of 60, respectively. The major side effects encountered with fluphenazine administration were sedation (13 of 31), lethargy (1 of 31), irritability (2 of 31), dysphoria (2 of 31), personality change (4 of 31), appetite change (2 of 31), dystonia (1 of 31), and akathisia (1 of 31). For comparison, the major side effects associated with haloperidol use were sedation (41 of 60), lethargy (17 of 60), irritability (4 of 60), dysphoria (22 of 60), personality change (14 of 60), appetite change (15 of 60), dystonia (2 of 60), and akathisia (7 of 60). Side effects accounted for withdrawal of medication in 19 percent of the fluphenazine group and 33 percent of the patients receiving haloperidol.

Further evaluation of our data showed that 23 patients had received fluphenazine following a therapeutic trial with haloperidol (Table 21.1); 17 took fluphenazine as the second drug (number 1 to 17), and 6 as the third drug (numbers 18 to 23). The dosage, length of treatment, therapeutic response, and side effects in this group are summarized in Table 21.1. Dosages listed are the largest amounts received by the patient. Tic response signifies the maximum control of motor and vocal symptoms based upon clinical ratings of improvement. No significant differences were apparent between the ability of haloperidol and that of fluphenazine to control the symptoms of Tourette's syndrome: 9 patients had similar responses, 6 were better with fluphenazine, and 8 were worse. In contrast, side effects occurred significantly less often and were less severe when the patient was receiving fluphenazine. The results of this retrospective uncontrolled study confirm those of Goetz and colleagues (1984) and Borison and colleagues (1982) and suggest that fluphenazine is a valuable alternative to haloperidol for the pharmacotherapy of TS. A controlled, double-blind, long-term, prospective study should be performed to clarify further the role of this drug.

Diphenylbutylpiperidines

Penfluridol. Similar to the drug pimozide (Moldofsky & Sander, Chapter 19, This volume), penfluridol is a diphenylbutylpiperidine derivative. This compound, although reported by Shapiro, Shapiro, and Eisenkraft (1983) and the Norway Tourette Association (Melbye, H.C.A., personal communication, 1987) to have a beneficial effect in patients with TS, has been withdrawn from clinical use in the U.S.A. The rationale for a clinical trial with penfluridol was based on animal studies that showed the drug to be a specific blocker of dopamine without significant noradrenergic or serotonergic blocking effects (Nose & Takemoto, 1975). Furthermore, it was known to have a long half-life and to cause less severe extrapyramidal side effects. However, because of its potential to induce mammary and pancreatic tumors in adult rodents, the drug has been withdrawn by the Food and Drug Administration from even investigational status.

Other Dopaminergic-Related Neuroleptics

RO22-1319. A water-soluble dopamine receptor antagonist, RO22-1319 has a chemical structure that differs from that of other antipsychotic agents. Mechanistically, the drug preferentially blocks dopamine receptors in the mesolimbic system and those not linked to adenylate cyclase (Davidson, Boff, MacNeil, Wenger, & Cook, 1983). Uhr, Berger,

Table 21.1. *Comparison of Haloperidol and Fluphenazine Treatment*

		Haloperidol			Fluphenazine		
Number	Age of Onset/ Sex	Dose/ Duration	Tic Response[a]	Side Effects[b]	Dose/ Duration	Tic Response	Side Effects
1	5/F	4.0/1 years, 4 months	G	SED, LETH, DYS, APP, AKA	2.0/6 months	E	None
2	11/M	3.5/2 years	F	SED, LETH, DYS, PER, APP, BRA	6.0/6 months	G	None
3	4/M	1.0/3 years	G	SED, LETH, PER, APP	2.0/9 months	G	None
4	5/M	5.0/1 year, 4 months	G	SED, PER, APP, BRA	4.0/2 years, 8 months	G	None
5	8/M	2.0/7 months	G	SED, LETH, DYS, HA	15.0/2 years, 2 months	G	SED, APP, HEP
6	8/M	1.0/2 months	F	SED, IRRIT, AKA, RASH	1.0/1 month	F	IRRIT, DYS, PER, AKA
7	3/F	8.0/9 years	G	SED, IRRIT	1.0/1 month	P	None
8	4/M	1.5/3 years	G	SED, APP	4.0/3 months	P	SED, LETH
9	6/M	6.0/2 years, 6 months	G	SED, LETH, PER, BRA, TREM	4.5/6 months	F	SED, DIZ
10	5/F	2.0/4 months	G	SED, DYS, PER	5.0/6 months	G	PER, AKA
11	5/M	3.0/6 months	P	SED, DYS, PER, TREM	10.0/1 year, 6 months	P	None
12	4/M	3.0/1 year, 6 months	G	SED	4.0/2 years, 6 months	P	SED, PER
13	7/M	9.0/1 year, 6 months	F	SED, ABD	3.0/1 month	P	None
14	8/F	5.0/2 years, 6 months	F	SED, APP, AKA, SP	3.0/3 months	F	None
15	7/M	1.5/7 months	P	SED, LETH, DYS, PER	4.0/2 years, 3 months	G	SED
16	5/M	3.5/6 years	F	SED, LETH, APP	3.0/2 years	G	SED
17	7/F	7.5/5 years, 8 months	G	LETH, PER, APP, DYS, ABD	5.0/2 years, 9 months	G	SED, DIZ
18	6/M	8.0/9 months	F	SED, LETH, DYS, APP	4.0/1 month	P	None
19	6/M	3.0/7 months	G	SED, LETH, DYS	3.0/11 months	F	SED, DYS
20	3/M	6.0/4 years	F	SED, BRA, VIS	16.0/2 years, 6 months	F	None
21	5/M	6.0/2 years, 6 months	F	SED, LETH, DYS, BRA	6.0/1 month	P	SED
22	9/M	2.5/5 months	G	SED, LETH, DYS	6.0/1 month	G	SED
23	6/F	5.0/1 year	F	SED, APP	3.0/1 year, 4 months	G	SED, APP

[a]Tic response: E = excellent, G = good, F = fair, P = poor.
[b]Side effects: SED (sedation); LETH (lethargy), DYS (dysphoria); APP (appetite change); BRA (bradykinesia); AKA (akathisia); IRR (irritable); HEP (hepatic abnormality); DYST (dystonic reaction); VIS (visual alteration); TREM (tremulous); DIZ (dizzy); SP (slurred speech); ABD (abdominal pain); RASH (rash); HA (headache).
Source: From Singer, Gammon, & Quaskey, 1986.

Pruitt, and Stahl (1985) have reported on three patients with Tourette's syndrome who received the investigational drug RO22-1319 in an open trial. All had clinically detectable decreases in tics, with sedation being the only adverse effect. Additional evaluations are in progress.

Clozapine. The dibenzodiazepine clozapine, which has few extrapyramidal reactions, has not been shown to be efficacious in Tourette's syndrome (Caine, Polinsky, Kartzinel & Obert, 1979).

NONDOPAMINERGIC-RELATED NEUROLEPTICS

Tricyclic Antidepressants

Therapeutic trials have been reported with two tricyclic antidepressant drugs, chlorimipramine and desipramine. Chlorimipramine acts by inhibiting the uptake of serotonin at the presynaptic neuron, thereby increasing neurotransmitter availability. This pharmacologic action, however, is not specific for serotoninergic neurons, since prolonged administration of chlorimipramine has also been shown to increase the concentration of a norepinephrine metabolite in the CSF (Asberg et al., 1977). Desipramine, a metabolite of imipramine, primarily blocks the reuptake of norepinephrine, but has little effect on serotonin (Carlsson, Corrodi, Fuxe, & Hokfelt, 1969). In a double-blind crossover study comparing the effects of chlorimipramine and desipramine with that of a placebo, no statistically significant clinical improvements occurred in six Tourette's syndrome patients (Caine, Polinsky, Obent, Rapaport, & Mikkelsen, 1979). Side effects were observed in all patients receiving chlorimipramine and the majority taking desipramine. Indeed, one patient receiving chlorimipramine experienced a marked exacerbation of both motor and vocal tics. In contrast, there are reports that chlorimipramine produces a therapeutic effect in TS with only mild side effects (Yaryura-Tobias & Neziroglu, 1977).

Desipramine has also been suggested as a useful treatment for patients with Tourette's syndrome who have symptoms of attention deficit disorder (ADD) and hyperactivity (H) (Hoge & Biederman, 1986). Since the pharmacologic treatment of ADDH includes stimulants that frequently exacerbate tics, substitute therapies are often required. Desipramine was effective in treating some adolescents with ADD (Gastfriend, Biederman, & Jellinek, 1984) and a single 10-year-old with TS (Hoge & Biederman, 1986). A double-blind crossover study comparing desipramine with other drugs used to control ADDH in Tourette's syndrome such as stimulants and clonidine should be performed.

Trazodone

Trazodone, an antidepressant, is a phenylpiperazinylpropyl derivative of triazolopyridine and as such is chemically unrelated to the more common tricyclic or tetracyclic drugs. The low incidence of anticholinergic and cardiac side effects from trazodone is considered an advantage over tricyclic medications. Pharmacologically, its proposed mechanism of action is selective inhibition of serotonin reuptake into presynaptic axon terminals. Prolonged exposure results in a decrease of serotoninergic postsynaptic receptors and presynaptic adrenergic alpha-2 receptors. Trazodone was reported to have been successful in treating a small number of patients with Tourette's syndrome (Borison, Hamilton, Nichols & Diamond, 1983).

Lithium

Lithium is a well-established effective agent in the prophylaxis and treatment of bipolar affective disorders. Its mechanism of action is not fully understood but may involve depletion of membrane polyphosphatidylinositides (Sherman, Leavitt, Honcher, Hallcher, & Phillips, 1981). The rationale for the use of lithium in patients with Tourette's syndrome is based on its ability to ameliorate some dyskinesias and its effect on dopamine excretion in manic states (Messiha, Erickson, & Goggin, 1976). Clinical reports, however, show conflicting effects on tic symptoms. Erickson, Goggin, & Messiha (1976) reported a beneficial effect in controlling major tics and vocalizations in 3 patients, and Hamra and coworkers (1983) in a single case. In contrast, lithium administered in a single-blind, placebo-controlled fashion to 10 patients, with increasing doses to a maximum serum concentration of 1.0 meq/L, showed no significant beneficial effects; 4 patients actually had a worsening of their tics (Borison, Ang, Hamilton, Diamond & Davis, 1983).

Benzodiazepines

Benzodiazepines are frequently used when an antianxiety, sedative, or hypnotic action is desired. The mechanism of action appears to be facilitation of GABA-mediated neurotransmission via allosteric alteration of the GABA receptor. The benzodiazepine clonazepam has been reported as a possible agent for treatment of tics associated with Tourette's syndrome. In a small pilot study, clonazepam was used as the sole agent or in conjunction with haloperidol (Gonce & Barbeau, 1977). In five patients who received only clonazepam, clinical improvement occurred in three, albeit transient or associated with ataxia or drowsiness. When the drug was added to an existing regimen of haloperidol, in two patients there was further diminution of tic activity. We have initiated clonazepam as adjunctive medication in five patients who were simultaneously receiving either haloperidol (4/5) or clonidine (1/5). In our experience, in only one instance was there persistent improvement of motor tics.

CONCLUSIONS

Clinical studies investigating the effects of various therapeutic agents in Tourette's syndrome are difficult to evaluate. Frequently the reports are limited by small sample sizes, absence of double-blind and crossover procedures, nonrandom allocation of drugs, and a lack of reliable, valid methods to measure change. Furthermore, evaluation of therapeutic response in Tourette's syndrome is compounded by the spontaneous variation in symptoms typical of the disorder. Thus a precise comparison of different neuroleptic drugs remains an elusive goal.

Haloperidol has long been regarded as the primary therapy for Tourette's syndrome, with reports of benefit in up to 80 percent of patients (Shapiro et al., 1978). Because of the large incidence of side effects, however, physicians continue to seek alternative forms of therapy. Based in part upon pathophysiologic theories implicating abnormalities of the dopaminergic system, a variety of dopaminergic-related neuroleptic drugs have been evaluated as potential therapeutic agents. In this chapter, we have analyzed published reports on the efficacy of several dopaminergic-related neuroleptic agents, excluding haloperidol and pimozide, in the treatment of Tourette's syndrome. Available data show that phenothiazines with a piperizine side-chain are more effective than those with aliphatic or piperidine side-chains. In our clinical experience fluphenazine is effective for treatment of Tourette's syndrome, inducing an equivalent control of motor and phonic tic symptoms, but fewer side effects than haloperidol. Further studies are clearly indicated to clarify the ultimate role of this drug. The value of newer dopamine receptor antagonists remains to be determined.

Neuroleptic drugs that act on neurotransmitter systems other than dopamine have also been screened to evaluate their clinical effectiveness in Tourette's syndrome. Support for such an approach stems from hypotheses of neurotransmitter abnormalities involving changes in serotoninergic, adrenergic, and cholinergic systems. Unfortunately drugs such as tricyclic antidepressants, lithium, or trazodone are less effective than is haloperidol. Similarly, initial enthusiasm for the proposed use of clonazepam as an adjunctive therapy has not been substantiated. It is to be hoped that, as the biochemical pathophysiology of this syndrome becomes more clearly defined, newer therapeutic approaches will be developed.

REFERENCES

Abuzzahab, F.S., & Anderson, F.O. (1973). Gilles de la Tourette's syndrome: International registry. *Minnesota Medicine, 56,* 492–496.

Asberg, M., Ringberger, V., Sjoqvist, F., Thoren, P., Traskman, L. & Tuck, J.R. (1977). Monoamine metabolites in cerebrospinal fluid and serotonin uptake inhibition during treatment with chlorimipramine. *Clinical Pharmacology and Therapeutics, 21,* 201–207.

Bockner, S. (1959). Gilles de la Tourette's disease. *J Mental Sci, 105,* 1078–1081.

Borison, R.L., Ang, L., Chang, S., Dysken, M., Comaty, J.E., & Davis, J.M. (1982). New pharmacological approaches in the treatment of Tourette syndrome. In A.J. Friedhoff & T.N. Chase (Eds.), *Gilles de la Tourette's syndrome.* New York: Raven.

Borison, R.L., Ang, L., Hamilton, W.J., Diamond, B.I., & Davis J.M. (1983). Treatment approaches in Gilles de la Tourette syndrome. *Brain Research Bulletin, 11,* 205–208.

Borison, R.L., Hamilton, W.J. Nichols, F.T., & Diamond, B.I. (1983). Trazodone and Tourette's syndrome. *Neurology, 33* (Suppl. 2), 199.

Breese, G.R., & Mueller, R.A. (1985). SCH-23390 antagonism of a D-2 dopamine agonist depends upon catecholaminergic neurons. *European Journal of Pharmacology, 113,* 109–114.

Caine, E.D., Polinsky, R.J., Ebert, M.H., Rapaport, J.L., & Mikkelsen, E.J. (1979). Trial of chlorimipramine and desipramine for Gilles de la Tourette syndrome. *Annals of Neurology, 5,* 305–306.

Caine, E.D., Polinsky, R.J., Kartzinel, R., & Ebert, M.H. (1979). The trial use of clozapine for abnormal involuntary movements. *American Journal of Psychiatry, 136,* 317–320.

Carlsson, A., Corrodi, H., Fuxe, K., & Hokfelt, T. (1969). Effect of antidepressant drugs on the depletion of intraneuronal brain 5-hydroxytryptamine stores caused by 4-methyl-gamma-ethyl-meta-tyramine. *European Journal of Pharmacology, 5,* 357–366.

Carlsson, A., Corrodi, H., Fuxe, K., & Hokfelt, T. (1969). Effects of some antidepressant drugs on the depletion of intraneuronal brain catecholamine stores caused by 4-gamma-dimethyl-meta-tyramine. *European Journal of Pharmacology, 5,* 367–373.

Davidson, A.B., Boff, I., MacNeil, D.A., Wenger, J., & Cook, L. (1983). Pharmacological effect of RO22-1319: A new antipsychotic agent. *Psychopharmacology, 79,* 32–39.

Eisenberg, L., Ascher, E., & Kanner, L. (1959). A clinical study of Gilles de la Tourette's disease (maladie des tics) in children. *American Journal of Psychiatry, 115,* 715–723.

Erickson, H.M., Goggin, J.E., & Messiha, F.S. (1976). Comparison of lithium and haloperidol therapy in Gilles de la Tourette syndrome. In F.S. Messiha & A.D. Kenney (Eds.), *Parkinson's Disease: Neurophysiological, Clinical and Related Aspects,* New York: Plenum.

Gastfriend, D., Biederman, J., & Jellinek, M.S. (1984). Desipramine in the treatment of adolescents with attention deficit disorder. *American Journal of Psychiatry, 141,* 906–908.

Goetz, C.G., Tanner, C.M., & Klawans, H.L. (1984). Fluphenazine and multifocal tic disorders. *Archives of Neurology, 41,* 271–272.

Gonce, M., & Barbeau, A. (1977). Seven cases of Gilles de la Tourette's syndrome: Partial relief with clonazepam, a pilot study. *Canadian Journal of Neurolgical Sciences, 4,* 279–283.

Hamra, B.J., Dunner, F.H., & Larson, C. (1983). The remission of tics with lithium therapy: Case report. *Journal of Clinical Psychiatry, 44,* 73–74.

Hoge, S.K., & Biederman, J. (1986). A case of Tourette's syndrome with symptoms of attention deficit disorder treated with desipramine. *Journal of Clinical Psychiatry, 47,* 478–479.

Kaim, B. (1983). A case of Gilles de la Tourette syndrome treated with clonazepam. *Brain Research Bulletin, 11, 213*–214.

Levy, B.S., & Ascher, E. (1968). Phenothiazines in the treatment of Gilles de la Tourette's disease. *Journal of Nervous and Mental Disease, 46,* 36–40.

Lucas, A.R. (1964). Gilles de la Tourette's disease in children: Treatment with phenothiazine drugs. *American Journal of Psychiatry, 121,* 606–608.

Mailman, R.B., Schulz, D.W., Lewis, M.H., Staples, L., Rollema, H., & DeHaven, D.L. (1984). SCH-23390: A selective D_1 dopamine antagonist with potent D_2 behavioral actions. *European Journal of Pharmacology, 101,* 159–160.

Meller, E., Kuga, S., Friedhoff, A.J., & Goldstein, M. (1985). Selective D_2 dopamine receptor agonists prevent catalepsy induced by SCH 23390, a selective D_1 antagonist. *Life Science, 36,* 1857–1864.

Mesnikoff, A.M. (1959). Three cases of Gilles de la Tourette's syndrome treated with psychotherapy and chlorpromazine. *Archives of Neurology and Psychiatry, 81,* 710.

Messiha, E.F., Erickson, H.M., & Goggin, J.E. (1976). Lithium carbonate in Gilles de la Tourette's disease. *Res Commun Chem Path Pharmacol, 15,* 609–611.

Nose, T., & Takemoto, H. (1975). The effect of penfluridol and some psychotropic drugs on monoamine metabolism in central nervous system. *European Journal of Pharmacology, 31,* 351–359.

Peroutka, S.J., U'Prichard, D.C., Greenberg, D.A., & Snyder, S.H. (1977). Neuroleptic drug interactions with norepinephrine alpha receptor binding sites in rat brain. *Neuropharmacology, 16,* 549–556.

Polites, D.J., Kruger, D., & Stevenson, I. (1965). Sequential treatments in a case of Gilles de la Tourette's syndrome. *British Journal of Medical Psychology, 38,* 43–52.

Shapiro, A.K., & Shapiro, E. (1982). Clinical efficacy of haloperidol, pimozide, penfluridol and clonidine in the treatment of Tourette's syndrome. In A.J. Friedhoff & T.N. Chase (Eds.), *Gilles de la Tourette Syndrome.* New York: Raven.

Shapiro, A.K., Shapiro, E.S., Bruun, R.D., & Sweet, R.D. (1978). *Gilles de la Tourette Syndrome.* New York: Raven.

Shapiro, A.K., Shapiro, E., & Eisenkraft, G.J. (1983). Treatment of Tourette disorder with penfluridol. *Comprehensive Psychiatry, 24,* 327–331.

Sherman, W.R., Leavitt, A.L., Honchar, M.P., Hallcher, L.M., & Phillips, B.E., (1981). Evidence that lithium alters phosphoinositide metabolism; chronic administration elevates primarily myo-inositol-1-phosphate in cerebral cortex of rat. *Journal of Neurochemistry, 36,* 1947–1951.

Singer, H.S., Gammon, K., & Quaskey, S. (1986). Haloperidol, fluphenazine and clonidine in Tourette syndrome: Controversies in treatment. *Pediatric Neuroscience, 12,* 71–74.

Snyder, S.H., Greenberg, D., & Yamamura, H.I. (1974). Antischizophrenic drugs and brain cholinergic receptors: affinity for muscarinic sites predicts extrapyramidal effects. *Archives of General Psychiatry, 31,* 58–61.

Stahl, S.M., & Berger, P.A. (1982). Cholinergic and dopaminergic mechanisms in Tourette syndrome. In A.J. Friedhoff & T.N. Chase (Eds.), *Gilles de la Tourette syndrome.* New York: Raven.

Uhr, S.B., Berger, P.A., Pruitt, B., & Stahl, S.M. (1985). Treatment of Tourette's syndrome with RO22-1319, D-2 receptor antagnoist. *New England Journal of Medicine, 311,* 989.

Walsh, P.J.F. (1962). Compulsive shouting and Gilles de la Tourette's disease. *British Journal of Clinical Practice, 16,* 651–655.

Yaryura-Tobias, J.A., & Neziroglu, F.A. (1977). Gilles de la Tourette syndrome: A new clinico-therapeutic approach. *Progress in Neuro-Psychopharmacology and Biological Psychiatry, 1,* 335–338.

CHAPTER TWENTY-TWO

The Use of Stimulants in the Treatment of Tourette's Syndrome

Gerald S. Golden

INTRODUCTION

The clinical use of stimulant drugs in patients with Tourette's syndrome (TS) is part of a broader controversy concerning the potential of these agents to exacerbate the symptoms of tic disorders. The issues will not be resolved until the underlying neurochemical mechanisms are fully understood, and recommendations must be based on theoretical constructs and an analysis of the published clinical experience.

ADD AND TS

It has become clear that children with TS also frequently have symptoms that meet the clinical criteria of attention deficit disorder (ADD). These conditions coexist in between 21 (Erenberg, Cruse, & Rothner, 1985) and 54 percent (Comings & Comings, 1984) of cases. Males are more likely to be hyperactive than females, and the symptoms are most pronounced in the patients with more severe manifestations of TS.

In some children, the problems associated with the ADD are more of a handicap than is caused by the tics. Although behavioral approaches to therapy are sometimes effective, stimulants are the only predictably effective pharmacologic agents. This is the most common indication for the use of these drugs.

Use of Stimulants to Counteract Side Effects of Neuroleptics

Approximately one-half of patients being treated with haloperidol have side effects they find troublesome. The most frequent are lethargy, lack of motivation, cognitive blunting, and depression. The concurrent use of stimulants has been recommended by some workers to counteract these problems (Shapiro & Shapiro, 1981). This indication for treatment seems to be less commonly used in clinical practice than in the treatment of ADD.

NEUROCHEMICAL AND PHARMACOLOGIC CONSIDERATIONS

Neurochemical Basis of TS

Neurochemical hypotheses of the pathophysiology of TS have been built on the basis of clinical observations and research studies. The finding that haloperidol, a potent and highly selective dopamine receptor blocker, was effective in treating many patients with this condition suggested that hyperactivity of dopaminergic systems was involved.

Studies of cerebrospinal fluid metabolites of neurotransmitters have shown low levels of homovanillic acid (HVA), the major metabolite of dopamine, and decreased accumulation of this compound following the administration of probenecid (Butler, Koslow, Seifert, Caprioli, & Singer, 1979). Haloperidol administration produces an increase in cerebrospinal fluid HVA levels, suggesting that the underlying problem is hypersensitivity of dopamine receptors (Singer, Butler, Tune, Seifert, & Coyle, 1982). The increased HVA levels result from release of negative feedback to the dopaminergic neurons of the substantia nigra when the receptors are blocked.

Serotonergic systems are probably also involved. There are low resting levels of 5-hydroxyindoleacetic acid (5-HIAA), the major metabolite of this compound. In addition, the increase in 5-HIAA following administration of probenecid is reduced compared to controls (Butler et al., 1979; Cohen, Shaywitz, Caparulo, Young, & Bowers, 1978).

(*Editors' Note:* A more extended discussion of the pathobiology of TS and related disorders appears in Chapter 7 of this volume.)

Pharmacologic Effects of Stimulant Drugs

The stimulant drugs have complex effects upon the central nervous system, and all of their mechanisms of action are not completely understood. Methylphenidate and amphetamine appear to inhibit the uptake of dopamine and norepinephrine into synaptosomal preparations in vitro. These drugs also stimulate release of the same neurotransmitters (Ferris, Tang, & Maxwell, 1972). The net effect is increased activity of both norepinephrinergic and dopaminergic systems.

The mechanism of action of pemoline is less clearly understood. It appears to have a predominant effect on dopaminergic systems.

From a theoretical perspective, assuming that there are hypersensitive dopamine receptors in patients with tic disorders, stimulant drugs could be expected to have an adverse effect on the movement disorder. Any potential benefit on mental status might be a result of their action on norepinephrinergic systems.

CLINICAL CONSIDERATIONS

Evidence for a Deleterious Effect of Stimulant Drugs

A report of a 9-year-old boy with the rapid onset of TS following the administration of methylphenidate for the treatment of hyperactivity suggested that tic disorders could be triggered by the administration of a stimulant drug (Golden, 1974). There have been a number of similar reports, in which tic disorders have their onset soon after the initiation of therapy with stimulant drugs, or these agents appear to worsen the condition (Bremness & Sverd, 1979; Denckla, Bemporad, & Mackay, 1976; Fras & Karlavage, 1977; Feinberg & Carroll, 1979; Meyerhoff & Snyder, 1973; Pollack, Cohen, & Friedhoff, 1977; Rapoport, Nee, Mitchell, Polinsky, & Ebert, 1982; Shapiro & Shapiro, 1981; Sleator, 1980).

A survey of patients with TS found 32 who, at some point in time, also had taken stimulant drugs (Golden, 1977). Twenty-five of these patients had used stimulants after the onset of their symptoms, and clinically obvious worsening occurred in 53 percent of cases. When the drug was discontinued, symptoms returned to the baseline level. Seven patients had taken stimulants before their tics appeared. In 4 cases the drug had been discontinued for a period of time, but in 3 others the symptoms of TS began while the stimulant was still being administered. The major critique of this study was the possible ascertainment bias inherent in a questionnaire; this also does not allow the frequency of this phenomenon to be determined.

The precipitation of TS in 15 patients by administration of stimulant medications was reported by Lowe, Cohen, Detlor, Kremenitzer, and Shaywitz (1982). Nine of these children had a preexisting history of tics; 8, a family history of a tic disorder. Their recommendations were conservative, and the authors felt that stimulant drugs were contraindicated in the face of a tic disorder and that they should be used with caution in the presence of a family history of tics.

An attempt to determine the frequency with which this phenomenon occurs was carried out by analysis of a series of 200 patients with TS (Erenberg et al., 1985). Nine patients had been exposed to stimulants before their tics began, but only 4 were still receiving them at the onset of the TS. There were 39 patients who had tics at the time the stimulant drug was introduced, usually to treat ADD. Tics were unchanged in 26, exacerbated in 11, and appeared to be improved in 2. The symptoms of ADD were improved in 22 patients, and the authors stated that a cautious trial of stimulant therapy might be appropriate in some patients with both a tic disorder and ADD.

Provocative testing with both d- and l-amphetamine was carried out by Caine, Ludlow, Polinsky, and Ebert (1984). In a preliminary open trial with three patients with TS, two had an exacerbation of symptoms only with d-amphetamine, and the other with both isomers. Symptoms returned to the baseline level within 36 hours. A double-blind study of six patients produced significant changes in motor tics in three, one after administration of l-amphetamine, one after d-amphetamine, and one after taking either compound. Vocal tics were exacerbated by l-amphetamine only.

Price, Leckman, Pauls, Cohen, and Kidd (1986) surveyed 170 patients with TS and found that 34 had been treated with stimulant drugs. In 24 percent of the treated group, there was persistent exacerbation of the tics, while an additional 3 percent had transient difficulties. Another 24 percent had tics that did not appear to be related to treatment. A possible genetic vulnerability to stimulant-induced tics was suggested by the finding that in six pairs of identical twins discordant for treatment, both twins developed tics.

Although there are fewer published case reports, pemoline appears to be capable of producing the same effects (Bachman, 1981; Bonthala & West, 1983; Erenberg et al., 1985; Lowe et al., 1982; Mitchell & Matthews, 1980; Sleator, 1980).

Imipramine is sometimes used to treat ADD. Dillon, Salzman, and Schulsinger (1985) reported that it did not cause an increase in tics in a patient with TS. Cocaine may cause a severe exacerbation (Mesulam, 1986).

Dissenting Viewpoints

An alternate approach to analyzing the possible interactions between tic disorders and stimulant drugs is to evaluate patients who only have ADD and who were treated with stimulants (Denckla et al., 1976). Three percent of these children had preexisting tics, and 0.9 percent developed tics after stimulant therapy was instituted. In the group with preexisting tics, methylphenidate caused exacerbation in 13.3 percent. These data do not obviate the hypothesis that stimulant drugs can have a deleterious effect, but they do indicate that the problem is not one of great magnitude. It should be realized, however, that it may be extremely important to an individual patient.

In a series of 134 new patients with TS, 21 had been treated with stimulants (Shapiro & Shapiro, 1981). Two had been treated before the onset of TS, 1 developing symptoms after 6 months of therapy; the other patient had been treated for 3 years, and became symptomatic after the drug had been discontinued for 1 year. Four of the 18 patients who took stimulants following the onset of the tic disorder reported increased symptoms.

The authors also report on their experience in treating 62 patients with both TS and ADD with a combination of haloperidol and methylphenidate. They state that, although there may be a transient increase in tics at the initiation of therapy with the stimulant, this was not of major significance, and was outweighed by the beneficial effects on the haloperidol-induced affective and cognitive problems.

The timing of the diagnosis of TS and ADD and the relationship of the onset of symptoms to the administration of stimulant-medication were investigated by Comings and Comings (1984). They stated that patients treated with stimulants before the onset of tics developed symptoms an average of 5.3 years after the onset of the ADD. In the patient group in which stimulant drugs were first prescribed after the onset of the tic disorder, the delay between the appearance of the ADD and that of the tics was 1.6 years. If the patients with simultaneous onset of both syndromes were eliminated from the analysis, the time interval in the second group was 4.0 years. A positive family history for TS was present in approximately three-quarters of each group.

On the basis of these data, the authors concluded that patients with hyperactivity who develop tics after treatment with stimulants carry the gene for TS and would probably have developed the syndrome even if stimulant drugs had not been administered. The major criticism of this study is the attempt to define the exact time of onset of the ADD. Hyperactivity is frequently present from very early in life, and the symptoms evolve over time and vary in different social situations. In addition, some patients were as old as 71 years, and the diagnosis in many was made retrospectively. It is not appropriate to assume that the biases of this methodology were the same for the two groups.

RECOMMENDATIONS

Summary of Clinical Studies

It is clear that there is still a need for more extensive controlled studies using large groups of patients from many centers, so as to eliminate as many sources of ascertainment and observer bias as possible. With the data available, however, several conclusions can be tentatively reached. These have clinical implications, and so will be phrased conservatively.

1. Tic disorders may begin after initiation of stimulant drug therapy in a patient with ADD. Whether or not these patients carry a gene for TS and whether or not they would have developed tics if stimulants had not been used are not clear.

2. As many as one-half of patients with tic disorders will have an exacerbation of symptoms when stimulant drugs are added to the treatment regimen. In general, symptoms revert to the baseline level when the drug is discontinued.

3. The commonly used stimulants (methylphenidate, dextroamphetamine, and pemoline) have identical effects. There are fewer data about the effects of antidepressants and other psychoactive drugs.

4. There are theoretical concerns about using drugs that increase activity at dopaminergic synapses in a disorder that might be associated with hypersensitivity of dopaminergic receptors.

Clinical Recommendations

Patients with ADD

1. If there are no tics, and no family history of a tic disorder, the parents should be told to report promptly the occurrence of tics after stimulant drugs are begun. If tics are precipitated, the stimulant should be discontinued and the situation reassessed. Stimulants should only be reintroduced if attempts at behavioral management are ineffective, and the hyperactivity is a major social and educational problem. If tics are again precipitated, it may be necessary to introduce clonidine or haloperidol.

2. If there are no tics, but there is a family history of a tic disorder, the use of stimulant drugs should be even more conservative. If a trial of stimulants is initiated, the patient should be monitored very closely, and the same guidelines followed as in the earlier recommendation.

3. If tics are already present, an intensive behavioral approach to the treatment of ADD should be embarked upon before the use of stimulant drugs is considered. Clonidine should then be used if pharmacologic treatment seems to be appropriate. If this is ineffective, and the hyperactivity is a more significant problem than the tic disorder, a cautious trial of stimulants in the lowest effective dose possible is appropriate. If there is a major and sustained increase in tics that does not respond to small increases in the level of haloperidol, stimulants should be discontinued.

Patients Without ADD

The issues as to whether or not it is appropriate to use stimulant drugs to counteract the side effects of haloperidol are both theoretical and clinical. The theoretical concerns have already been stated. There is little published clinical experience, and that which is available is largely limited to one group (Shapiro & Shapiro, 1981). Until further studies can be done, a conservative approach is recommended. The need for stimulants should be clearly documented, they should be the only alternative treatment strategy, and minimum doses should be used for the shortest time possible.

(*Editors' Note:* See Shapiro & Shapiro, Chapter 18, and Comings & Comings, Chapter 8, this volume, for additional discussion concerning the controversial role of CNS stimulants in the management of TS.)

REFERENCES

Bachman, D.S. (1983). Pemoline-induced Tourette's disorder: A case report. *American Journal of Psychiatry, 138,* 1116–1117.

Bonthala, C.M., & West, A. (1983). Pemoline-induced chorea and Gilles de la Tourette's syndrome. *British Journal of Psychiatry, 143,* 300–302.

Bremness, A.B., & Sverd, J. (1979). Methylphenidate-induced Tourette syndrome. *American Journal of Psychiatry, 136,* 1334–1335.

Butler, I.J., Koslow, S.H., Seifert, W.E., Caprioli, R.M., & Singer, H.S. (1979). Biogenic amine metabolism in Tourette syndrome. *Annals of Neurology, 6,* 37–39.

Caine, E.D., Ludlow, C.L., Polinsky, R.J., & Ebert, M.H. (1984). Provocative drug testing in Tourette's syndrome: d- and l-amphetamine and haloperidol. *Journal of American Academy of Child Psychiatry, 23,* 147–152.

Cohen, D.J., Shaywitz, B.A., Caparulo, B., Young, J.G., & Bowers, M.B. (1978). Chronic, multiple tics of Gilles de la Tourette's disease: CSF acid monoamine metabolites after probenecid administration. *Archives of General Psychiatry, 35,* 245–250.

Comings, D.E., & Comings, B.G. (1984). Tourette's syndrome and attention deficit disorder with hyperactivity: Are they genetically related? *Journal of American Academy of Child Psychiatry, 23,* 138–146.

Denckla, M., Bemporad, J., & Mackay, M. (1976). Tics following methylpenidate administration: A report of 20 cases. *Journal of the American Medical Association, 235,* 1349–1351.

Dillon, D.C., Salzman, I.J., & Schulsinger, D.A. (1985). The use of imipramine in Tourette's syndrome and attention deficit disorder: Case report. *Journal of Clinical Psychiatry, 46,* 348–349.

Erenberg, G., Cruse, R.P., & Rothner, A.D. (1985). Gilles de la Tourette's syndrome: Effects of stimulant drugs. *Neurology, 35,* 1346–1348.

Feinberg, M., & Carroll, B.J. (1979). Effects of dopamine agonists and antagonists in Tourette's disease. *Archives of General Psychiatry, 36,* 979–985.

Ferris, R.M., Tang, F.L.M., & Maxwell, R.A. (1972). A comparison of the capacities of isomers of amphetamine, deoxypiprodol or methylphenidate to inhibit the uptake of tritiated catecholamines into rat cerebral cortex slices, synaptosomal preparations of rat cerebral cortex, hypothalamus and striatum and into adrenergic nerves of rabbit aorta. *Journal of Pharmacology & Experimental Therapeutics, 181,* 407–416.

Fras, I., & Karlavage. (1977). The use of methylphenidate and imipramine in Gilles de la Tourette's disease in children. *American Journal of Psychiatry, 134,* 195–197.

Golden, G.S. (1974). Gilles de la Tourette's syndrome following methylphenidate administration. *Developmental Medicine & Child Neurology, 16,* 76–78.

Golden, G.S. (1977). The effect of central nervous system stimulants on Tourette syndrome. *Annals of Neurology, 2,* 69–70.

Leckman, J.F., Detlor, J., Harcherik, D.F., Ort, S., Shaywitz, B.A., & Cohen, D.J.

(1985). Short- and long-term treatment of Tourette's syndrome with clonidine: A clinical perspective. *Neurology, 35,* 343–351.

Lowe, T.L., Cohen, D.J., Detlor, J., Kremenitzer, M.W., & Shaywitz, B.A. (1982).
Stimulant medications precipitate Tourette's syndrome. *Journal of the American
Medical Association, 247,* 1729–1731.

Mesulam, M.M. (1986). Cocaine and Tourette's syndrome. *New England Journal of
Medicine, 315,* 398.

Meyerhoff, J.H., & Snyder, S.H. (1973). Gilles de la Tourette's disease and minimal brain dysfunction: Amphetamine isomers reveal catecholamine correlates in an affected patient. *Psychopharmacology, 29,* 211–220.

Mitchell, E., & Matthews, K.L. (1980). Gilles de la Tourette's disorder associated
with pemoline. *American Journal of Psychiatry, 137,* 1618–1619.

Pollack, M., Cohen, N., & Friedhoff, A.J. (1977). Gilles de la Tourette's syndrome:
Familial occurrence and precipitation by methylphenidate therapy. *Archives
of Neurology, 34,* 630–632.

Price, A.R., Leckman, J.F., Pauls, D.L., Cohen, D.J., & Kidd, K.K. (1986). Gilles de
la Tourette's syndrome: Tics and central nervous system stimulants in twins
and nontwins. *Neurology, 36,* 232–237.

Rapoport, J.L., Nee, L., Mitchell, S., Polinsky, R., & Ebert, M. (1982). Hyperkinetic syndrome and Tourette syndrome. In A.J. Friedhoff & T.N. Chase (Eds.),
Gilles de la Tourette syndrome. New York: Raven.

Shapiro, A.K., & Shapiro, E. (1981). Do stimulants provoke, cause, or exacerbate
tics and Tourette syndrome? *Comprehensive Psychiatry, 22,* 265–273.

Singer, H.S., Butler, I.J., Tune, L.E., Seifert, W.E., & Coyle, J.T. (1982). Dopaminergic dysfunction in Tourette syndrome. *Annals of Neurology, 12,* 361–366.

Sleator, E.K. (1980). Deleterious effects of drugs used for hyperactivity on patients with Gilles de la Tourette syndrome. *Clinical Pediatrics, 19,* 453–454.

Part V

Clinical Care

CHAPTER TWENTY-THREE

The Clinical Care
of Individuals
with Tourette's Syndrome

Kenneth E. Towbin
Mark A. Riddle
James F. Leckman
Ruth D. Bruun
Donald J. Cohen

The chapters contributing to this volume cover the diverse ways in which Tourette's syndrome must be seen for a complete understanding of the disorder. Such a multidisciplinary approach to TS has only recently been appreciated. Different eras in medicine are characterized by different approaches to the patient; the care of patients with TS has reflected the changing fashions in neuropsychiatry. Since the time of Gilles de la Tourette the tendency has been to impose monadic models onto TS, such as the purely psychological theories before the 1960s, or the purely neurological perspectives of the 1960s and 1970s. Treatment, similarly, tended to have a narrow focus, leaving aside the patient as a whole person, an individual suffering from a variety of chronic problems.

Yet, after reading this book, it should be apparent that TS is best understood with a model in which genetic determinants, environmental stressors, and psychological factors combine to produce neurophysiologic changes. This model—containing biological, psychological, and social components—gains support from studies in neurochemistry, neuropharmacology, and neurophysiology, as elucidated by responses to pharmacologic probes and treatment agents (Ang, Borison, Dysken, & Davis, 1982; Leckman, Cohen, Gertner, Ort, & Harcherik, 1984; Leckman, Detlor, Harcherik, Young, & Anderson, 1983; Riddle et al., 1986), and human genetics as suggested by results from twin and family studies (Pauls & Leckman, 1986). It integrates the observations of patients and physicians on certain psychological components, such as the meaning of symptoms to patients and their families; the effects of chronic illness and socially and personally distressing symptoms on psychological development; and the emotional cost of "interventions" employed to treat, inhibit, or camouflage symptoms.

Clinical experience suggests that the patient's response, typology of symptoms, and severity of impairment are shaped and modified by psychological distress, defensive and coping mechanisms, and other psychological events. However, the way in which mental upset interacts with the constitutional vulnerability to TS to produce an exacerbation or persistent level of severity has yet to be learned.

The purpose of this chapter is to offer an overview that brings together the educational, family, psychotherapeutic, and pharmacologic perspectives on the treatment of TS described in the specific chapters. This composite intervention strategy follows from the premise that considering both patients' internal psychological experience of the disorder and the reaction of their environment to their movements and sounds provides TS sufferers and their families with optimal care and reflects what we have learned about the disorder. Such an orientation also opens the way to a wide array of useful treatment alternatives.

SCHOOL AND OCCUPATIONAL INTERVENTION

In children, any chronic disorder is likely to affect educational motivation and achievement. TS can have a significant impact on a child's education stemming both from the primary disorder (such as the outright physical impairment caused by movements, or obsessions interfering with concentration) and secondary consequences of the disorder (such as social isolation, being regarded as an object of contempt, impairment of self-esteem, etc.). When a child's educational capacity is not being fulfilled as a result of TS, offering assistance by providing the school with an understanding of the disorder and the pupil's educational needs can be a critical, far-reaching intervention.

The findings from research focusing on cognitive or learning impairments in TS suggest that specific learning deficits may be a frequent concomitant of clinically recognized illness. Work reported by Incagnoli and Kane (1982), Golden (1984), and Hagin (Chapter 15, this volume) suggests that TS patients may suffer from a particular weakness on the Coding subtest of the Wechsler Intelligence Scales for Children or impairment in motor control that would affect performance on the Coding subtest. Additional data from Hagin and others (Dykens, 1987) have suggested that TS patients may also exhibit a specific weakness in mathematics. As discussed in the chapters on phenomenology, the question of whether attention deficit disorder with hyperactivity (ADDH) is an intrinsic feature of TS remains open. The presence of ADDH has implications for the interpretation of weaknesses on the Mathematics and Coding subtests. Since many of the studies have not been stratified according to the presence of ADDH in TS patients, it becomes difficult to determine whether or not the identified neuropsychologic weaknesses may be attributed to the presence of ADDH as a comorbid condition. Some evidence from our work suggests that the weakness may be specific and not solely attributable to ADDH.

A further influence on education or work for those with TS may be adverse effects on learning from pharmacologic treatment. Some, but not all, investigators believe there are drug side effects that impair learning. Experienced clinicians have observed impairments in memory, concentration, and motivation in patients treated with haloperidol and pimozide. Sedation, when severe, can affect learning and may occur with these agents and clonidine. More subtle emotional effects on academic functioning such as the appearance of dysphoria (Bruun, 1982; Caine & Polinsky, 1979; Linet, 1985; Mikkelson, Detlor, & Cohen, 1981) also occur in children treated with haloperidol and pimozide.

The secondary consequences of TS on school performance are far more varied. The interplay between internal and social experiences can result in feedback loops in which frightening or frustrating social experiences (e.g., isolation from or being teased by peers, being held up to public ridicule by adults, or being viewed as willfully oppositional by persons in authority) fuel inner vulnerabilities toward low self-esteem, poor frustration tolerance, lack of motivation, hopelessness, and anxiety. The feedback loop is completed when these internal feelings lead to behaviors that increase the negative social experiences. Since school is the major social environment for most children, most of these negative social experiences occur in this setting. Without strong allies, the result often is that the school setting and the particular individuals become combined objects of fear and anger. Anxiety, avoidance, and opposition are common behavioral consequences.

Interventions at school can improve a child's social and educational adjustment. Hagin's survey of school modifications that worked successfully for TS patients (as reported in Chapter 15, this volume) suggests that a compassionate, positive, supportive attitude from teachers and efforts to reduce classroom stress can often be useful. These efforts to reduce stress included classroom structure, one-to-one assistance, setting reasonable goals divided into small segments, sensitivity to and flexibility with time pressures, and offering specific assistance with instructions. Many children with TS benefit from being freed from any time constraints on their examinations. Also, typewriters can be an immense relief when writing is impossible because of specific symptoms (such as jabbing at the paper or scribbling over and over) or penmanship is hindered by severe symptoms. Hagin stresses that many children benefit from time and a place away from class where they can be alone when their symptoms are frequent. A moderate amount of structure is most appropriate for students with TS, although some students benefit from programs that are at one or the other extreme. Not every child will need all of these aids, but most will need some of them. Complementing the perspective of the clinician, it is most helpful when teachers view the child as a whole person, develop a broad view of a pupil's overall academic and social functioning at school, and avoid the temptation to fix upon target symptoms.

For adults in the workplace similar modifications can be useful. Many adult patients with TS are capable of working in any environment and require no modifications of tasks or expectations. However, more severely affected individuals do benefit from the availability of structured tasks that can be broken into discrete pieces, flexibility with regard to time deadlines, specific assistance with instructions, and the ability to structure time so that they may take time away from clients and coworkers to be alone. Some have specifically requested and benefited from working in noisy locations. Experienced clinicians also have observed a high degree of variability in symptoms on the job. Although logically an employer might assume that certain tasks, such as detailed drawings, high-pressure sales positions, technical presentations, or public performances, would be beyond an employee with TS, especially one who is severely affected, paradoxically, many are able to complete these assignments with skill. Such work may be beyond some persons with TS, or may be impossible for some at certain times, but the characteristic waxing and waning of symptoms make an ultimate determination almost impossible. The complexity of this problem can be reduced by obtaining the assistance of the person with TS in making decisions about assignments. In addition, an expert's explanation and recommendations to employers, occupational medical staff, and job supervisors can also be of significant benefit in broadening their understanding of TS in general and their employee specifically. As a result of appropriate intervention, flexibility, and compassion, productivity can be increased for symptomatic patients in their workplace.

FAMILY INTERVENTION

As stressed in the chapter on evaluation, the patient lives in the context of his or her family and peer group. Although TS is not "caused" by pathological family or social relationships, the dynamics that develop among family members in response to symptoms form an integral part of a patient's experience of his or her disorder. For many patients troubled relationships within the family may be the most serious consequence of their disorder and can be the most impaired portion of their lives. This may be as true for the adult with TS who lives with spouse and children as for the child with TS who lives with family of origin. Cohen and coworkers (Chapter 12, this volume) have described how the assessment of these relationships develops from an understanding of individual and family functioning. From the patient's side there are the relationships to the family, the patient's internal understanding of the role he or she plays in the family, and family members' responses to him or her. From the parents' and spouse's perspective, there is their view of the child or spouse as a person, the meaning of their child or spouse to them, their expectations of and fantasies about him or her, and their understanding of the causes and consequences of the symptoms. When there are siblings at home, their view(s) of their family member and his or her symptoms and their responses to the potential encroachments by their impaired family member on the siblings' view of themselves, the family's life together, and social relationships comprise the third component. Relating the history and arriving at an understanding of the balance of forces—the family assessment—cannot occur in a single clinical visit or even within a brief series of meetings.

Usually it is derived in the context of a therapeutic relationship, from information reported and observations made of the process over an extended time, with a patient and his or her family. During this time a sensitive, trained clinician can come to know many features of the family, such as communication and alliances between family members, the family's management of privacy and revelation, the mechanisms by which members satisfy others' and achieve satisfaction of their own needs, their capacity for shielding from and permitting exploration of the "outside world," the balance of hatred and love, and the accessibility to and protection from the wider family network. Throughout this process, the clinician is required to appreciate and form an understanding from his or her own experience of being "part of the family" and must consider the meaning and impact of his or her interest on the family.

Family assessment may become "family treatment" as a result of the duration and intensity of the process set in motion by the clinician's inquiry and the family's interest, ability, and willingness to engage in the exploration. Results of the evaluation may suggest a need for family therapy; referral specifically for family treatment can be a useful intervention. In and of itself, the opportunity to discuss the disappointments, painful secrets, fears, and frustrations of living with TS in the presence of an informed, warm, accepting professional can have an immensely calming, salutary effect. It is easier to describe the goals than the techniques of family intervention for most families presenting with a member with TS. These goals are consonant with the ones described in previous chapters. In children these include the promotion of developmental progress with respect to feelings of self-esteem and competency, the capacity to explore and draw from one's peer group, to be challenged by and persevere in work or school, to tolerate frustration, disappointments, and losses, and to develop satisfying, intimate attachments. In adults, the goals are similar, including a kind of flexibility in which family members do not assume guilt for exacerbations of symptoms but recognize when special assistance is needed. Many of the same conflicts about work, peer relationships and intimate attachments, and intolerance of frustration, disappointments, and losses continue throughout life, presenting special challenges to persons with TS.

The elucidation of the genetic basis of TS has added special importance to the assessment and treatment of families. (Pauls & Leckman, Chapter 6, this volume). Briefly, it is now widely believed that TS is not only familial, but genetic, and that there is a range of expression of the underlying gene(s) that includes not only TS and chronic motor tics, but also obsessions and compulsions. Therefore, it is likely that in the family of a TS patient there are other individuals who have the same problems or problems related to these. It might be anticipated that an individual with similar problems will be more sensitive and empathic with others who have the same or similar difficulties. Within families this may be especially true; a parent with tics may provide understanding and strength, convey optimism, and offer a sense of support to the child with TS. But familial transmission can also influence family dynamics in ways that do not facilitate a good adaptation to the disorder (as reviewed in Chapter 12). A parent with tics may feel guilt for having transmitted the disorder; another with obsessions and compulsions may be completely unable to contend with the lack of control and impulsivity of the child with hyperactivity. During adolescence, when whatever problems faced by children are ordinarily blamed on their parents, teenagers may feel especially rageful at parents in whom they identify problems like their own. Older patients may be concerned about genetic counseling and family planning. It is surprisingly frequent that a parent with tics may not acknowledge them until coming for an evaluation with the child; even then, an affected parent may suppress the recognition of having symptoms that may be obvious to the spouse. Parents may not "remember" they had tics until reminded by their own parents. In situations such as these, the family assessment takes on very broad and sensitive tasks. The clinician needs to be sure of his or her alliance with a family, their motivation and preparation, before burdening them with this exploration and the awareness that results.

PSYCHODYNAMIC PSYCHOTHERAPY WITH TS PATIENTS

Whatever the etiology of TS, clinical experience suggests that some individuals with TS benefit from psychotherapy. The primary goal of psychotherapy is not the elimination of tics or TS symptoms, but treatment for the psychological conflicts that may result from this illness and in turn contribute to it, and any other psychological problems that may not be associated with TS. Patients may be helped to recognize circumstances that are associated with exacerbation, to understand how such circumstances arise, and to work toward ways to diffuse or avoid them.

The nature of this therapeutic work may include the interpretation of unconscious intrapsychic conflict. There is a difference, however, between, on the one hand, employing psychodynamic perspectives and methods and, on the other, presuming a primary psychodynamic etiology. A model encompassing biological and psychological contributions does not result in any contradiction between a psychodynamic perspective and a variety of etiologic explanations. Thus whatever the underlying etiologic assumptions of the dynamically oriented authors of the 1930s and 1940s, their observations of behavior and detailed perceptions of the inner lives of their patients offer a useful perspective. When their observations are added to the current understanding obtained from childen with other chronic illnesses, such as diabetes, asthma, or colitis, the role of psychotherapeutic intervention can be placed in some perspective. Clinicians have appreciated the immediate and enduring therapeutic value of assisting in the management of anxiety, sustaining a patient's progress on his or her optimal developmental path, assessing and reducing impediments to self-esteem, improving the patient's relationship to health care providers, and promoting the capacity to observe, understand, and respond to internal, familial, and social pressures that derive from and contribute to chronic illness.

Although they cannot be considered characteristic of TS, several psychological reactions are commonly reported in response to the symptoms. The losses of impulse control, in thought as well as in body, yield psychological reactions well described by Mahler and Rangall (1943), Ascher (1948), and Silver (Chapter 13, this volume). Accompanying the experience of feeling overwhelmed by thoughts and/or urges, patients frequently describe anxiety, anger, and the cognitive features, frequently seen in depression, of guilt, hopelessness, helplessness, and worthlessness. Along these lines, when faced with obsessive and compulsive symptoms clinicians may find assessment even more confusing. A great deal remains to be learned about the psychological defensive function obsessional phenomena play in TS sufferers and also the degree to which these phenomena actually represent an alternative expression of the underlying etiology that relentlessly gives rise to tics (Pauls, Towbin, Leckman, Zahner, & Cohen, 1986).

Another reaction to the loss of control in a person with TS may be to relinquish any efforts to modulate impulses, resulting in more generalized, overt, physical and verbal aggression and heightened impulsivity. When this happens the aggression may become syntonic with the person's character. Patients with TS who behave aggressively often leave others with the task of trying to answer an impossible question: Is the behavior voluntary or involuntary? Faced with the kind of impulsivity described by TS patients, queries offering this sort of dichotomous solution are unlikely to be fruitful. A more constructive line of inquiry focuses on the extent and circumstances under which these behaviors are controllable. If the behaviors are not completely syntonic, several legitimate foci of psychodynamic exploration may arise, such as their meaning to the patient, identification of the affects preceding and generated by this disinhibition, and the defenses employed to contain them. An appreciation of these dynamics may assist in increasing compliance with educational and medical resources and favorably affect the outcome of whichever treatments are applied.

The decision to employ psychodynamic treatment in TS rests on the presence of impairment in function with these findings: dysfunctional defenses employed against the experience of the disorder, lagging psychological development for a period following the appearance of TS, impairment in self-esteem arising from the reaction of family and social contacts to the symptoms of the disorder, and impairment in occupational or school role performance over and above physical disruption caused by symptoms. The complete evaluation of the TS patient demands an account of these features. In addition, the adjunctive value of psychodynamic treatment may be more strongly considered in patients who have had only marginal responses to pharmacotherapy, and in patients whose families develop pathological dynamics related to the disorder.

Persons with TS have at least an equal likelihood of experiencing a coexisting psychiatric disorder as the general population, and, given the demands of their chronic illness, are probably at greater risk for depression and anxiety disorders. Psychodynamic treatment may be especially considered in those with prominent neurotic dysfunction such as the anxiety disorders, dysthymic disturbances, depression, and when psychological defensive functions operate in an exaggerated and subsequently maladaptive manner.

BEHAVIORAL TREATMENTS

In an effort to control their movements or sounds, even before seeking professional consultation, TS patients frequently experiment, sometimes successfully, with behavioral techniques they develop for themselves. This may stem from the essential quality of suppressibility previously described about tics and suggests that control of symptoms can be favorably influenced by behavioral intervention. It is therefore useful to elicit information about these efforts in the initial evaluation of a TS patient.

Several techniques for controlling tics that capitalize on behavioral principles have been applied with success by behaviorally oriented clinicians (as reviewed in Chapter 16 of this volume, by Azrin & Peterson). These include massed negative practice, contingency management, relaxation training, self-monitoring, and habit reversal. Massed negative practice refers to the technique of self-imposed, forceful, repeated execution of a tic for a specified period, perhaps half an hour, with regular brief rest periods of minutes. Over time the subject becomes fatigued and, in theory, the frequency may decrease. Results from studies of observational cohorts are equivocal in the demonstration of efficacy, although some patients appear to respond.

Contingency management applies, in combination or alone, the familiar principles of positive and/or negative reinforcement to tic behaviors. Rewards can include parental praise, special gifts, money, or other desired items, while negative consequences (punishments) run the gamut from noise to social isolation to the controversial extreme of physical pain. Virtually all treatment paradigms contain some of these principles since, whatever kind of treatment is applied, when symptoms decrease, praise from clinicians, parents, teachers, and peers is a nearly universal response. Systematic study of these methods is hindered by the difficulty of adequately and ethically applying control maneuvers, such as praising a child when he or she displays symptoms.

Self-monitoring may be a corollary maneuver to reinforcement. Essentially, it formalizes and records the results of an activity that occurs spontaneously in many TS patients. Self-observation of tics and recording of tic counts during specified periods of the day promote an increased awareness of movements and may promote efforts to extinguish movements. Efforts to understand the mechanisms underlying the success of this method are underway.

Habit reversal is described by its proponents as the behavioral techniques just listed with the addition of isometric muscle tensing to oppose motor tics (Azrin & Nunn, 1973). It is conceived as the application of massed negative practice to the degree that opposing action is required for every tic movement, self-monitoring is required to oppose movements, and punishers are brought into play when subjects interrupt their activity and exert themselves forcefully. Investigations to date have employed only a few patients but suggest some success (Azrin & Peterson, Chapter 16, this volume).

Patients frequently report the spontaneous discovery of relaxation training employing tensing followed by relaxation, imagery, or deep breathing. For some these methods can be temporarily helpful. However, for prolonged control these maneuvers usually lose effectiveness and are often abandoned. Future studies will employ systematic investigations with rigorous methodology (Azrin & Peterson, Chapter 16, this volume; Rosen & Wesner, 1979).

As with other interventions, the successful application of behavioral treatment appears to require a familiarity with the techniques, adequate methods of assessment, persistence, and a committed client. Further study of these techniques by expert clinicians may provide new and useful alternatives.

SOCIAL ISSUES

The social policy issues facing TS patients at the local and national level and resources available to assist them cannot be emphasized sufficiently. Clinicians corresponding with local and federal agencies on behalf of TS patients need assistance in order to maximize the help offered to their patients. Meyers (Chapter 17, this volume) has underscored that many of these agencies have not had much experience with cases involving TS and that clinicians can be immensely helpful by offering more than diagnostic labels when asked to explain a patient's needs. There is an ambiguity about TS since it is viewed as a "mental illness" by some agencies and not by others. TS patients are frequently subjected to discrimination in education or vocational rehabilitation, employment, life and health insurance, housing, and disability reimbursement. Findings from the Ohio TS study of 114 adults in that state (Stefl, 1983) suggest that among TS sufferers unemployment is four times the state average, and that unemployment is not necessarily correlated with the degree of disability. Bruun's cohort yields (Chapter 2, this volume) similar statistics. Forty percent reported suffering job discrimination. Similarly, finding and keeping adequate housing for patients with prominent vocal tics can be impossible. As a result of the ambiguity about TS, patients may be denied access to certain supervised care facilities. Since each case is so specific, it is recommended that clinicians develop a relationship with their local or the national Tourette Syndrome Association (TSA) from whom information, instructions for corresponding with local and federal agencies for insurance and disability benefits, and programs and insurance companies with more experience with TS are available. For clinicians treating the most severely affected TS patients, this level of intervention, regarding shelter, public assistance, and vocational rehabilitation, is the most basic, complex, and difficult of all. Assistance from the TSA fills an especially important need for these patients.

PHARMACOLOGIC TREATMENT

Pharmacologic interventions probably are the most widely used treatments for TS. In a recent survey of TS subjects by the Ohio Tourette Syndrome Association, 70 percent reported a history of medication treatment (Stefl, 1983). For the patient and his or her clinician the most pertinent questions have to do with whether any relief is available from a medication and what side effects he or she may be required to endure; in addition, effects of pharmacologic agents are heuristically important and have led to hypotheses about the pathophysiologic mechanisms of TS. There is general agreement among those treating TS about the efficacy and limitations of many currently available agents.

The Context for Pharmacotherapy

The aim of treatment, whatever the modality, is to help place the patient back on his or her optimal developmental path. This will encompass dimensions of self-esteem, family and peer relationships, and academic or occupational functioning. Decisions about intervention must address the benefits and impingements in each of these arenas.

Subsequent to the decision to intervene, a consistent method of monitoring a patient's course is critical to the treatment process. For patients with mild symptoms, supportive counseling and observation may be the only interventions necessary. As reviewed in the chapter on assessment (Chapter 4, this volume), standardized instruments may be useful, objective tools for following the course and severity of symptoms, particularly when deciding to institute or change medication. Videotape records can be extremely useful, but are not always available in clinical practice. Even when video equipment is readily available, the natural variations of symptoms during a day or in different situations make a generalized interpretation of short records unreliable.

Most cases that come for treatment will be mild. In these cases the conservative interventions described earlier, including appropriate involvement of social agencies and education and counseling of the patient, family, and school or employer, should be applied first. During this time the patient should be followed carefully. If over the course of weeks to months there is a trend toward deterioration or if symptoms become much more severe and impairing, pharmacologic intervention becomes a logical choice.

Basic Principles of Pharmacotherapy in TS

The basic principles governing pharmacotherapy of any psychiatric disorder are equally applicable to the treatment of TS. These principles are:

Start patients on the smallest doses of medication possible.
Increase doses gradually.
Ensure an adequate duration of a drug trial.
Use sufficient doses.
Maintain the lowest effective dose.
Avoid polypharmacy.
Make changes in regimens as sequences of single steps.

In general, it is useful to start patients on the smallest doses of medication possible and increase gradually. This practice usually results in fewer and milder side effects, especially with the dopaminergic blocking agents or clonidine. It also appears to improve subsequent compliance.

Ensuring an adequate duration of a drug trial using sufficient doses increases the clinician's chances of learning whether a patient is responsive to a particular agent. Physicians not accustomed to TS may terminate drug trials prematurely, either because the patient fails to improve or because side effects are observed; consequently, it becomes difficult to determine whether another agent should be tried. When the patient, the patient's family, or the school feels an urgent need for rapid relief of symptoms, it can be especially difficult to permit a sufficient time to elapse for an agent to demonstrate its potential and to find the optimal dose.

Maintaining the lowest effective doses is a prudent course. This is especially imperative with the dopaminergic blocking agents, since the clinician is obligated to consider the risks of subsequent tardive dyskinesia. Often this may mean finding an effective dose and then, when the time is appropriate, gradually tapering downward. For patients who have been locked into a cycle of continually escalating doses and symptoms, this sometimes means enduring a considerable increase in symptoms during a rebound period before striking the new equilibrium where a lower dose is equally effective. This can be especially difficult in patients who have developed tardive dyskinesia subsequent to treatment for TS.

The concurrent use of two or more medications is usually considered when single agents have only partially ameliorated symptoms, or when complex combinations of symptoms are observed, such as TS with attention deficit disorder or obsessive–compulsive disorder. A risk with the use of multiple medications—polypharmacy—is that as the regimen grows the untoward effects that result from drug–drug interactions, toxicity, and side effects can become impossible to decipher. As described in chapters on pharmacologic treatment, it is unknown whether combinations of agents are more effective than single-drug schedules. As a result, clinicians are often uncertain about which agents they should use, when to use them, and what doses are most helpful in combination regimens.

A corollary of this principle about polypharmacy is that changes in regimens are usually most instructively made as sequences of single steps. For example, confusion may result if one reduces the dose of one medication while adding another, whatever course the patient's illness takes. It is not possible to discern whether improvement or exacerbation results from the new drug, a synergy of both agents, or the reduction of the old one. This also implies a need for washout periods. When a patient is switched from a drug with properties that include a long serum half-life and the potential, as levels decrease, to cause a rebound of symptoms, to a different drug, adequate washout periods are crucial for appreciating the efficacy of the second agent.

Pharmacotherapy in the Treatment of TS

At this point in the United States there are only four established pharmacologic interventions based upon evidence from large trials: haloperidol, clonidine, pimozide, and fluphenazine.

Haloperidol. The most widely investigated agent for the treatment of TS is the butryophenone haloperidol, a potent dopaminergic receptor blocking agent, with affinity for inducing blockade at the D_2 receptor site. Roughly 70 percent of patients with TS will improve moderately or more when treated with haloperidol. Its efficacy in decreasing tics is cited as the strongest evidence favoring a dopaminergic mechanism in the pathophysiology of TS. Haloperidol also has the desirable properties of being less sedating and less anticholinergic than many other dopaminergic blocking agents.

In the 1970s, clinicians would prescribe doses as high as 150 mg per day. Today it is recognized that much lower doses are effective, safer, and desirable. Ordinarily the lowest possible doses of haloperidol should be given when beginning pharmacotherapy. In general 0.5 mg is given before sleep or upon arising. Increments in 0.5-mg steps at weekly intervals are given if symptoms remain severe. Maximum doses vary among clinicians and situations. In children without other serious difficulties 4 mg per day is a typical maximum dose. In adults or children with very serious tics and/or behavioral difficulties as much as 15 mg per day may be used. Usually medication is given in a single dose, although some clinicians prefer twice-daily dosing.

Side effects are a major problem in maintaining patients on haloperidol. Roughly 40 to 60 percent of patients treated with haloperidol will discontinue it because of side effects. In general these include parkinsonian side effects, sedation, weight gain, decreased concentration, social or school phobias, decreased memory, anergia, dysphoria, akathisia, personality changes, loss of libido, sexual dysfunction, and, especially after chronic use of high doses, tardive dyskinesia (TD). There is a diversity of opinion about how antiparkinsonian medication should be used with haloperidol. Some clinicians will use low doses of antiparkinsonian medication, such as 0.5 mg/per day of benztropine, beginning with the first dose of haloperidol. Others prefer to wait until haloperidol doses reach 2 to 3 mg per day before beginning antiparkinsonian treatments. A third group prefers to wait until parkinsonian side effects emerge before prescribing antiparkinsonian agents. Warning about TD and periodic or annual assessments for dyskinetic movements (sometimes using a scale such as the Abnormal Involuntary Movement Scale [AIMS]) are advisable. Given the severity of potential side effects associated with haloperidol and the other neuroleptics, many clinicians will reserve its use for individuals with moderate to severe symptoms and substantial impairment in daily living.

Pimozide. Pimozide was approved for the treatment of TS in 1984 and is now in relatively common use. Neither a butyrophenone nor phenothiazine, it is a diphenylbutylpiperidine with potent dopaminergic blocking properties and, putatively, relative D_2-receptor selectivity. As with haloperidol, roughly 70 to 80 percent of TS patients will respond to pimozide (Moldofsky & Sandor, Chapter 19, this volume; Shapiro & Shapiro, 1984), but somewhat more than half of these patients, perhaps 60 percent, will tolerate side effects well and remain on the medication.

The side effects that have been identified, especially akathisia, extrapyramidal effects, and sedation, are similar to, but perhaps less severe than, those found with haloperidol. This also includes the more unusual side effects such as phobias, depression, and galactorrhea (Linet, 1985; Shapiro & Shapiro, 1984). Studies suggest that, when compared with haloperidol, side effects from pimozide appear in fewer patients. This may also be true for the development of tardive dyskinesia (Chouinard & Steinberg, 1982). Reports of electrocardiographic (ECG) abnormalities, U waves and inverted T waves, in early studies led to concern about cardiotoxicity. Further investigations with larger numbers of patients have not justified these concerns (Moldofsky & Sandor, Chapter 19, this volume). Nevertheless, it is advisable to obtain a routine ECG study before initiating treatment and periodically, especially after larger increases in doses.

In general, doses begin at 0.5 mg and increase slowly to 3 mg per day; a majority of patients respond to this dose over a 6-week trial. Some patients may require as much as 8 mg per day maintenance. Maximum recommended doses for children are 10 mg per day and for adults, 20 mg per day. The half-life of the drug permits single daily dosing or, to diminish sedation, divided doses may be given twice each day.

Other Neuroleptics. Alternatives to haloperidol and pimozide are phenothiazine compounds. The most investigated and effective agent in this category is fluphenazine. Its side effect profile is roughly identical to that of haloperidol but some patients report fewer of them and tolerate them better. In general, the dose range is similar to the recommendations for haloperidol: up to 5 mg per day for the low-dose responders and up to 12 mg per day for the higher-dose responders. Beginning at lower doses such as 1.0 mg per day is advised.

Clonidine.   An alternative agent in the treatment of TS is clonidine, an imidazoline compound with alpha-adrenergic agonist activity. (Leckman, Walkup & Cohen, Chapter 20, this volume). While clonidine exerts both post- and presynaptic activity, it acts preferentially at the presynaptic site. In low doses clonidine "down-regulates" alpha-adrenergic neurons in the locus coeruleus, decreasing the release of central norepinephrine. As with all these agents, clonidine has several other direct central effects at other sites affecting other neurotransmitter and neuroendocrine systems.

Clonidine may be effective for perhaps 40 to 60 percent of TS patients (Cohen, Detlor, Young, & Shaywitz, 1980). However, in the opinion of some clinicians, although there may be a reduced response rate compared to haloperidol or pimozide, this is offset by fewer side effects. The balance between side effects and efficacy may favor clonidine as a first-line drug. Efforts to draw conclusions about the efficacy of clonidine have been hampered by problems in sample size and large placebo response rates for all medications and by making comparisons between studies where there are wide disparities with regard to comorbid conditions, baseline severity, average age, and assessments of symptom severity.

Variables to be considered in the administration of clonidine include the maximum doses, rate of increasing doses, and latency of action. Most clinicians have used low doses, less than 0.25 mg per day, while others have employed doses as high as 0.90 mg per day. Some clinicians suggest that the rate of increasing doses is irrelevant and that patients may be started and doses increased quickly. Others advocate a slow, gradual progression for maximum effect with a minimum of side effects. Lastly, there are reports suggesting that clonidine response may have a long latency time, as long as 12 weeks; other clinicians have suggested that 6-week trials are adequate.

Some clinicians begin with clonidine, despite a lower response rate, because no known indications or constellations of symptoms predict response. Low-dose treatment usually begins with 0.05 mg daily and increases by 0.05 mg in 3- to 7-day intervals. The medication is increased by increasing the dosing frequency (0.05 mg twice daily, three times daily, etc.) to a maximum of four times daily. In some patients doses as high as 0.60 mg per day may be needed. In general, if patients respond to clonidine their compliance is greater because they experience fewer, or less disturbing, side effects. The most commonly observed side effects are sedation and dry mouth (xerostomia), which are usually improved by lowering the dose by 0.05 mg per day. Rarely, increased symptoms and manic episodes have been reported. In higher doses hypotension becomes more likely.

Combinations of Medications. Some clinicians propose using combinations of medications when a single agent is only partially effective. There is clinical experience suggesting that haloperidol plus clonidine or pimozide plus clonidine may act synergistically. There is also evidence that clonidine may reduce akathisia caused by neuroleptics (Zubenko, Cohen, Lipinski, & Jonas, 1984). Careful steps to ensure adequate doses for a sufficient duration are vital prerequisites to the use of combination approaches. It should be noted that there have been no large-scale published trials of combination treatments.

The Dilemma of Stimulant Medication

It is clear that tic symptoms, usually dose related and transient, have developed in children with ADDH who were under treatment with stimulant medication (Denkla, Bemporad, & Mackay, 1976; Golden, 1977; Lowe, Cohen, Detlor, Kremenitzer, & Shaywitz, 1982). It is also true that as many as 50 percent of childen with TS will experience an increase in symptoms when treated with stimulant medication. A common problem arises when patients previously responsive to stimulant medication develop tics, when patients with attention deficit disorder with hyperactivity (ADDH) also have a strong family history for tic disorders, or when patients with moderate to severe impairment resulting from ADDH and TS present for pharmacologic treatment. As discussed by Comings and Comings (Chapter 8, this volume) recent evidence has been interpreted to suggest that stimulant medication may unleash TS in vulnerable individuals, exacerbate TS in patients who already have the disorder, or, some believe, cause TS in previously unsusceptible individuals. Currently available data are difficult to interpret. Although there may be important individual differences, more remains to be learned before the relationship between tics and stimulants will be understood.

At the present time there are no generally agreed-upon guidelines for the combined treatment of tic disorders and ADDH (Golden, Chapter 22, this volume). Some clinicians will use stimulants in any patient with ADDH and simply observe him or her closely. Others will optimize environmental interventions and then use clonidine or one of the tricyclic antidepressants, imipramine or desipramine, setting aside stimulants. The middle of the road has been to discontinue stimulants in ADDH patients who develop tics while on stimulant medication and, if educational and therapeutic interventions have been optimal, to start clonidine or anti-depressants. When patients without tics present with ADDH and have a positive family history for tic disorders, then a cautious trial of stimulant medication may be employed.

There is a diversity of opinion about the treatment of patients with

TS and ADDH. Some clinicians will begin with stimulants and, if they prove helpful, discontinue them only if tic symptoms increase. Others avoid stimulants altogether in this group and prefer starting with clonidine or antidepressants. Another approach to the problem is the combined administration of haloperidol and stimulants (Comings & Comings, 1984; Shapiro & Shapiro, Chapter 18, this volume). Prescribing the lowest possible effective dose of stimulants, clinicians using this regimen maintain that tics are not exacerbated by the combination, and that the complementary interactions may offer significant relief to seriously impaired children. This combination has also been applied to combat the side effect of akinesia that results from haloperidol administration (Shapiro & Shapiro, Chapter 18, this volume). Although transient increases in tics have been observed, they are reportedly short-lived and easily managed. Careful investigations on larger populations of patients with tics and ADDH are obviously necessary before a clear approach can be defined.

Obsessions and Compulsions in TS

Often TS patients present with the uncomplicated picture of multiple motor and phonic tics. But this is not universal. As many as 50 to 60 percent of all patients with TS also experience obsessions and/or compulsions that can be seriously disabling. Studies of older patients and those with a longer duration of illness have reported prevalences of these obsessions and/or compulsions as high as 90 percent. The relationship of these symptoms to TS has been conceptualized in various ways by different investigators; some view the experiences as completely separate from TS while others have explained them as mental tics without behavioral expression (obsessions) or highly complex tics (compulsions). One useful way to think about these phenomena is based upon their content or temporal relationship to tics. Examples of "tic-related" experiences reported to us include repetitive thoughts preceding or following tics, ritualized movements substituted to ward off tics, magical arrangements of items to control movements, and an involuntary, consuming, elaborate psychological scheme for balancing mental and physical intensity. Symptoms exhibited by TS patients that are apparently unrelated to tics have included the more "traditional" obsessive–compulsive symptoms of washing, cleaning, checking, and counting rituals, needs for symmetry, obsessions of violent acts or images, and obligatory, unnecessary, exacting routines that must be executed according to specific rules. Many of these symptoms are commonly described by persons who suffer from obsessive–compulsive disorder (OCD). Although it appears that in OCD the most common compulsions are washing, checking, and counting behaviors, a wide variety of behaviors and thoughts have been reported. Preliminary investigations of TS patients suggest that an equally diverse array of compulsions are reported but that other compulsions, such as needs for symmetry, or needing to carry out tasks until they are "just right," may be the most common.

As a result of descriptive studies in TS it is apparent that the prevalence of obsessions and compulsions (OC) is greater in TS probands then in the general population (Pauls & Leckman, 1986). Beyond this, the results of genetic-family studies also suggest that the prevalence rate of OC among first-degree relatives of TS probands is dramatically increased (Pauls et al., 1986). This has led to speculation of a genetic contribution to the etiology of some OC symptoms (Pauls & Leckman, 1986). A provocative clinical finding from these studies is the discovery of individuals with obsessions and/or compulsions but without tics who have first-degree relatives with tics or TS. A result of this work is that the distinction between TS and OCD is more ambiguous than previously described. At one extreme there are patients with TS and OC while at the other there are the traditional OCD patients with no tics or family history of tics. An intermediate population has now been discovered that displays OC symptoms without tics and has first-degree relatives with TS or tics. Future investigations will contrast these groups in the hopes of elucidating a genetic etiology for some OCD and offering an understanding of the pathophysiology and more specific treatment(s) for this disorder.

The natural history, pathophysiology, pharmacologic responses, and modifying influences on the expression of OC symptoms in TS patients are frontiers for further exploration. As discussed by Towbin (Chapter 9, this volume), the consideration of treatment for these symptoms in TS patients has proved to be a confusing endeavor. Results from drug trials in OCD suggest that tricyclic antidepressants, such as imipramine or chlorimipramine, monoamine oxidase inhibitors, or newer heterocyclic antidepressants, such as fluoxitine, may be useful in ameliorating symptoms in some patients. Yet these trials were designed for OCD patients and their findings cannot be generalized to TS patients without caution. In response to recent studies, TS patients are now routinely evaluated for OC and we anticipate the availability of more data on the response of these symptoms to standard agents for tics, such as haloperidol, pimozide, and clonidine. There are anecdotal reports of patients developing worsening tics when treated with tricyclics and monoamine oxidase inhibitors, although no systematic trials have been conducted in TS patients to treat OC.

Patients with serious impairments resulting from obsessions and/or compulsions warrant consideration of treatment with imipramine or investigational agents such as chlorimipramine or fluoxitine. Certainly the determination of safety and efficacy of these investigational agents in TS patients will have to await specific controlled trials, but the response to these agents in OCD patients offers some hope to the most seriously disabled patients with TS and OC. In addition, the benefits and hazards of drug combinations, such as tricyclic or heterocyclic antidepressants plus clonidine, pimozide, or haloperidol, deserve further study.

Maintenance and Discontinuation

One possible outcome of pharmacologic treatment is the return to development appropriate to the patient's phase and minimized symptoms. When development is proceeding smoothly, symptoms are in some control, and daily life is not seriously impaired, it is reasonable gradually to discontinue pharmacologic treatment. On the other hand, there is no formula for predicting the optimum duration of drug treatment. The majority of patients who respond to a medication may remain on it for several years or more. Rating scales and videotapes may help document the new baseline for future reference. It can be useful to remind patients that, should symptoms return, the same agents may be employed. It does not appear that responders convert to nonresponders, although experience is scanty.

Gradual reductions are recommended for discontinuation of any of these agents. When clonidine is rapidly discontinued rebound hypertension may follow, and exacerbation of tics lasting as long as 6 or 8 weeks has been reported (Leckman et al., 1986). When abrupt reductions in haloperidol are attempted, withdrawal dyskinesias may be observed over a duration of 2 to 3 months (and as long as 9 months) and can be confused with exacerbation of tics. Even when reductions in neuroleptics are carried out gradually, dyskinetic movements, perhaps previously masked by the neuroleptic, may be seen. These movements tend to be less intense and more variable in duration than those caused by abrupt discontinuation (Shapiro & Shapiro, Chapter 18, this volume).

Some patients will continue to have disturbed development with severe symptoms even while receiving medication. In persons who are minimally responsive or unresponsive to medication, it is even more important to review nonpharmacologic interventions. This can ensure that the patient's immediate and future living environment and academic or vocational development are as good as possible. Sometimes clinicians are tempted to prescribe larger and larger doses of medication with the hope that more medication will yield better control. However, especially where the dopaminergic blocking agents are concerned, it appears that greater benefits do not accrue and increasing side effects and risks of tardive dyskinesia may outweigh any additional amelioration of symptoms. In the case of clonidine, higher doses usually result in hypotension and sedation.

TREATMENT: INTEGRATION AND PROSPECTS

In the future, the treatment of individuals with TS may be greatly simplified by the discovery of fully effective methods. However, for the immediate future, it is very likely that the treatment of individuals with TS will call upon a broad range of clinical interventions, used concurrently or sequentially over many years. The experienced clinician will move from a careful diagnostic assessment of the individual patient and his or her family through the application of specifically focused interventions. The assessment process may in itself be therapeutic as the past and current experiences are clarified for the patient and his or her family; for many it will be the first time they can make sense out of their experiences. The availability of a concerned and knowledgeable expert can bring great relief to a distressed and confused patient and family. Following this phase, the clinician will offer various approaches geared to the specific needs of the patient, including reassurance, education, guidance, advocacy in the school or workplace, behavioral techniques, psychotherapy, and pharmacotherapy. The judicious, planned use of various therapeutic approaches can provide the majority of patients with amelioration of their difficulties, including improvement in daily living and specific reduction in tic severity. The clinician will remain available by following the course of symptoms over the patient's development, assisting the patient and his or her family as new questions arise, if symptoms should worsen, or at times of stress. The primary goals of treatment focus on the patient as a whole, developing person, as a member of a family, and as a social being. The tics become but one portion of the assessment, one aspect needing to be understood in the context of each of the others in the patient's life.

It now appears very probable that the great majority of individuals with TS have a genetic disorder or carry a single dominant gene. If so, this means that the vulnerability to TS is inborn and that it will express itself in different ways throughout a patient's development. It is important to have this developmental perspective on TS in mind when counseling patients and planning treatment. All interventions—such as the initiation of medication—must be seen in the context of their anticipated effect on the individual immediately and over many years. Whether the patient is a child or an adult, treatment plans must be based upon his or her current and projected development. Since there is as yet no cure for TS, the experienced clinician will always try to help patients in the tasks of living and protect them from potential dangers.

From this perspective, helping to keep the patient's development on track—supporting warm family relationships and peer socialization, facilitating school achievement or rewarding employment, and promoting self-esteem—appears of greater clinical value than mere suppression of tics at whatever cost.

While TS can be a devastating and lifelong condition, recent advances in understanding TS offer reason for optimism. First, the pace of understanding the disorder is accelerating. It is likely that the genetic risks, mechanisms of transmission, and biological pathways leading to expression will be clarified during the next decade. Second, increased understanding offers hope for more effective treatment. Third, clinical engagement with patients over decades and the discovery of a larger population of TS patients who do not come for treatment suggest that most persons with TS will achieve at least as much in life as those who do not have TS. The diagnosis of TS need not arouse panic in parents and patients. It is important to recognize that, dramatic portrayals notwithstanding, TS is most often a mild condition, perfectly compatible with a full, normal life. Fourth, TS has moved from an exotic disorder with which most clinicians were unfamiliar to a widely recognized clinical entity; with this increased recognition, individuals with TS are more likely to find knowledgeable physicians, educators, psychologists, and others to whom they can turn for information, understanding, and care.

REFERENCES

Ang, L., Borison, R., Dysken, M., & Davis J.M. (1982). Reduced excretion of MHPG in Tourette's syndrome. In A.J. Friedhoff & T.N. Chase (Eds.), *Gilles de la Tourette syndrome.* New York: Raven.

Ascher, E. (1948). Psychodynamic considerations in Gilles de la Tourette disease (maladie des tics). *American Journal of Psychiatry, 105,* 267–276.

Azrin, N.H., & Nunn, R.G. (1973). Habit reversal: A method of eliminating nervous habits and tics. *Behavior Research & Therapy, 11,* 619–628.

Bruun, R.D. (1982). Dysphoric phenomena associated with haloperidol treatment of Tourette syndrome. In A.J. Friedhoff & T.N. Chase (Eds.), *Gilles de la Tourette syndrome.* New York: Raven.

Caine, E.D., & Polinsky, R.J. (1979). Haloperidol induced dysphoria in patients with Tourette syndrome. *American Journal of Psychiatry, 136,* 1216–1217.

Dykens, E. (1987). Intellectual and Adaptive Functioning of Tourette's Syndrome children with and without ADDH, poster presented at the Annual Meeting of the American Academy of Child and Adolescent Psychiatry, 1987.

Chouinard, G., & Steinberg, S. (1982). Type I tardive dyskinesia induced by anticholinergic drugs, dopamine agonists and neuroleptics. *Progress in Neuropsychopharmacology and Biological Psychiatry, 6,* 571–578.

Cohen, D.J., Detlor, J., Young, J.G., & Shaywitz, B.A. (1980). Clonidine ameliorates Gilles de la Tourette syndrome. *Archives of General Psychiatry, 37,* 1350–1357.

Comings, D.E., & Comings, B.G. (1984). Tourette's syndrome and attention deficit disorder with hyperactivity: Are they related? *Journal of the American Academy of Child Psychiatry, 23,* 138–146.

Denkla, M., Bemporad, J., & Mackay, M. (1976). Tics following methylphenidate administration: A report of 20 cases. *Journal of the American Medical Association, 235,* 1349–1351.

Golden, G.S. (1977). The effect of central nervous system stimulants on Tourette syndrome. *Annals of Neurology, 2,* 69–70.

Golden, G.S. (1984). Psychologic and neuropsychologic aspects of Tourette's syndrome. *Neurologic Clinics of North America, 2,* 91–102.

Incagnoli, T., & Kane, R. (1982). Neuropsychological functioning in Tourette syndrome. In A.J. Friedhoff & T.N. Chase (Eds.), *Gilles de la Tourette syndrome.* New York: Raven.

Leckman, J.F., Detlor, J., Harcherik, D.F., Young, J.G., Anderson, G.M., Shaywitz, B., & Cohen, D.J. (1983). Acute and chronic clonidine treatment in Tourette's syndrome: A preliminary report on clinical response and effect on plasma and urinary catecholamine metabolites, growth hormone and blood pressure. *Journal of the American Academy of Child Psychiatry, 22,* 433–440.

Leckman, J.F., Cohen, D.J., Gertner, J.M., Ort, S.I., & Harcherik, D.F. (1984). Growth hormone response to clonidine in children ages 4–17: Tourette's syndrome vs. children with short stature. *Journal of the American Academy of Child Psychiatry, 23,* 174–181.

Leckman, J.F., Ort, S.I., Cohen, D.J., Caruso, K.A., Anderson, G.M., & Riddle, M.A. (1986). Rebound phenomena in Tourette's syndrome after abrupt withdrawal of clonidine: Behavioral, cardiovascular, and neurochemical effects. *Archives of General Psychiatry, 43,* 1168–1176.

Linet, L.S. (1985). Tourette syndrome, pimozide, and school phobia: The neuroleptic separation anxiety syndrome. *American Journal of Psychiatry, 142*(5), 613–615.

Lowe, T.L., Cohen, D.J., Detlor, J., Kremenitzer, M.W., & Shaywitz, B.A. (1982). Stimulant medications precipitate Tourette's syndrome. *Journal of the American Medical Association, 247,* 1729–1731.

Mahler, M.S., & Rangell, L. (1943). A psychosomatic study of maladie des tics (Gilles de la Tourette's disease). *Psychiatric Quarterly, 17,* 519–605.

Mikkelson, E.J., Detlor, J., & Cohen, D.J. (1981). School avoidance and social phobia triggered by haloperidol in patients with Tourette's disorder. *American Journal of Psychiatry, 138*(12), 1572–1576.

Pauls, D.L., & Leckman, J.F. (1986). The inheritance of Gilles de la Tourette's syndrome and associated behaviors: Evidence for autosomal dominant transmission. *New England Journal of Medicine, 315,* 993–997.

Pauls, D.L., Towbin, K.E., Leckman, J.F., Zahner, G.E.P., & Cohen, D.J. (1986).

Gilles de la Tourette's syndrome and obsessive–compulsive disorder. *Archives of General Psychiatry, 43*(12), 1180–1182.

Riddle, M.A., Shaywitz, B.A., Leckman, J.F., Anderson, G.M., Shaywitz, S.E., Hardin, M.T., Ort, S.I., & Cohen, D.J. (1986). Brief debrisoquin administration to assess central dopaminergic function in children. *Life Sciences, 38,* 1041–1048.

Rosen, M., & Wesner, C. (1979). A behavioral approach to Tourette's syndrome. *Journal of Canadian Clinical Psychology, 41,* 303–312.

Shapiro, A.K. & Shapiro, E. (1984). Controlled study of pimozide vs. placebo in Tourette's syndrome. *Journal of the American Academy of Child Psychiatry, 23*(2), 161–173.

Stefl, M.E. (1983). *The Ohio Tourette study.* Cincinnati: School of Planning, University of Cincinnati.

Zubenko, G.S., Cohen, B.M., Lipinski, J.F., & Jonas, J.M. (1984). Use of clonidine in the treatment of akathisia. *Psychiatry Research, 13,* 253–259.

Author Index

Subject Index

Note: Page numbers followed by *t* or *f* indicate tables or figures respectively.